Sleep Deprivation and Disease

Matt T. Bianchi
Editor

Sleep Deprivation and Disease

Effects on the Body, Brain and Behavior

Springer

Editor
Matt T. Bianchi, M.D., Ph.D., M.M.Sc.
Harvard Medical School
Massachusetts General Hospital
Boston, MA, USA

ISBN 978-1-4614-9086-9 ISBN 978-1-4614-9087-6 (eBook)
DOI 10.1007/978-1-4614-9087-6
Springer New York Heidelberg Dordrecht London

Library of Congress Control Number: 2013949480

Printed on acid-free paper

Springer is part of Springer Science+Business Media (www.springer.com)

Foreword

In the past and for the most part in the present, sleep deprivation has never received its due. While sleep is a necessary brain and body state for optimal health, it has remained the mostly forgotten youngest prince in the ancient biological hierarchy of important things—breathing, circulation, hunger, thirst, wakeful consciousness, and pain. The conscious perception of pain requires the brain, while the substance of the brain itself is devoid of pain sensations as we conventionally understand it. In fact, stimulation of the brain in wake patients is a standard mapping procedure for epilepsy surgery. Yet, to think that the brain cannot express distress when its core functions are compromised makes no biological sense. Perhaps we need to listen better.

Enter sleepiness and sleep deprivation. Sleep deprivation robs the brain of essential housekeeping and a host of other functions. Imagine a home with garbage that collects, electrical wiring that is frayed, drains clogged, and water pipes broken and leaking. Sleep deprivation also prevents the proper conduct of maintenance functions in other body systems, including metabolism. Sleep deprivation makes the brain and body sick. Sleepiness in the context of sleep deprivation is the brain in pain.

Yet, that pain is more often than not ignored or trivialized by individuals, society, regulators, and those who should certainly know better—health care professionals. A student falling asleep in class (or a committee member at a board meeting) is offered little sympathy or understanding, while if that same individual had a seizure, there would be a real risk of drowning under expressed concern and empathy.

In this era of "the book is dead," I say, "Long live the book!" Reading books will remain, in my opinion, the most time and effort-efficient method to obtain a large amount of filtered and curated knowledge in a given area of interest. Books on sleep science and sleep disorders abound, while that on sleep deprivation less so. Matt Bianchi and the contributors to this wonderful book have summarized a complex body of work that reflects the role "brain pain" plays in health and disease. There are very few stones left unturned, either as dedicated chapters or within individual chapters. If nothing else, a sense of seriousness should infuse the reader that sleepiness and sleep deprivation should move up the hierarchy and rub shoulders with respiration, circulation, consciousness, hunger, thirst, and pain. If this book accomplishes that, as I fully expect it will, the function of books in general and this book in particular will have been achieved.

Boston, MA, USA — Robert Joseph Thomas, M.D., M.M.Sc.

Preface

There is scarcely a segment of health or performance that has escaped linkage to sleep. Over recent decades, anecdote has given way to experiment, yielding an explosion of information demonstrating that the field of sleep deprivation is indeed fertile ground. Yet despite key advances in many areas, the field faces a diversity of challenges ranging from philosophical to practical. This state of affairs need not lead to pessimism; it should instead inspire future research. In this volume, experts review the links between sleep and a spectrum of medical specialties as well as operational settings. Each chapter builds on a rich evidence basis, while at the same time highlighting the uncertainties we face in the interpretation of the existing literature as well as the pathways that promise to move us forward. The intention is to provide readers from clinical and research backgrounds alike not only with a firm grounding in each subspecialty area covered but also with the tools to use a critical approach to understand and perhaps investigate key areas of need for future work. Sleep is a dynamic process, and its study requires interdisciplinary perspectives to build coherent and cohesive narratives.

The first part, "Sleep Physiology, Measurement, and Experimental Deprivation," provides a foundation for modern approaches to sleep and the impact of deprivation. The second part, "Sleep and the Brain," highlights clinically relevant implications of sleep loss in the fields of neurology and psychiatry, including a chapter devoted to the therapeutic use of sleep deprivation in psychiatry. The third part, "Sleep and Medical Topics," carries the bulk of the volume to emphasize the diversity of human physiology beyond the central nervous system that is impacted by sleep deprivation. The final part, "Performance, Economics, and Operational Topics," covers a broad societal perspective regarding the implications of sleep for health and performance. In each chapter, discovery is balanced against uncertainty—and it is precisely this interface that drives future progress. It is hoped that this volume inspires progress by arming the reader with a breadth of knowledge, a multidisciplinary perspective, and of course a healthy skepticism that forms the foundation of scientific progress.

Boston, MA, USA

Matt T. Bianchi, M.D., Ph.D.

Contents

Contributors

Vivien C. Abad, M.D., M.B.A. Division of Sleep Medicine, Department of Psychiatry and Behavioral Sciences, Stanford University School of Medicine, Redwood City, CA, USA

Yvonne Alameddine, B.A. Department of Neurology, Massachusetts General Hospital, Boston, MA, USA

Siobhan Banks, Ph.D. University of South Australia, Centre for Sleep Research, Adelaide, Australia

Mihaela H. Bazalakova, M.D., Ph.D. Division of Sleep Medicine, Department of Neurology, Massachusetts General Hospital, Harvard Medical School, Boston, MA, USA

Division of Sleep Medicine, Department of Medicine, Brigham and Women's Hospital, Harvard Medical School, Boston, MA, USA

Matt T. Bianchi, M.D., Ph.D., M.M.Sc. Division of Sleep Medicine, Department of Neurology, Massachusetts General Hospital, Boston, MA, USA

Gregory Belenky, M.D. Sleep and Performance Research Center, Washington State University, Spokane, WA, USA

Francesco Benedetti, M.D. Department of Clinical Neurosciences, Ospedale San Raffaele, Milan, Italy

Nishi Bhopal, M.D. Department of Sleep Medicine, Beth Israel Deaconess Medical Center, Boston, MA, USA

Andrew D. Calvin, M.D., M.P.H. Division of Cardiovascular Disease, Mayo Clinic, Rochester, MN, USA

Ivan Cundrle Jr., M.D. Division of Cardiovascular Diseases, Mayo Clinic, Rochester, MN, USA

Sara Dallaspezia, M.D. Department of Clinical Neurosciences, Ospedale San Raffaele, Milan, Italy

Thien Thanh Dang-Vu, M.D., Ph.D. Department of Exercise Science, Center for Studies in Behavioral Neurobiology, Concordia University, Montreal, QC, Canada

Jeffrey M. Ellenbogen, M.M.Sc., M.D. Department of Neurology, Johns Hopkins University, Baltimore, MD, USA

Christian Guilleminault, M.D., D.M., D.Biol. Division of Sleep Medicine, Department of Psychiatry and Behavioral Sciences, Stanford University School of Medicine, Redwood City, CA, USA

Erin C. Hanlon, Ph.D. Section of Endocrinology, Diabetes, and Metabolism,Department of Medicine, Sleep , Metabolism,and Health Center, University of Chicago, Chicago, Chicago, IL, USA

Bradford D. Hare, M.D., Ph.D. Pain Research Center, Pain Management Center, Department of Anesthesiology, University of Utah, Salt Lake City, UT, USA

Anna Hemp Sleep Research and Performance Center, Washington State University, Spokane, WA, USA

Umakanth Khatwa, M.D. Sleep Laboratory, Division of Respiratory, Department of Medicine, Boston Children's Hospital, Boston, MA, USA

William D.S. Killgore, Ph.D. Center for Depression, Anxiety, and Stress Research, McLean Hospital, Harvard Medical School, Belmont, MA, USA

Elizabeth B. Klerman, M.D., Ph.D. Division of Sleep Medicine, Department of Medicine,Brigham and Women's Hospital, Harvard Medical School, Boston, MA, USA

Kristen L. Knutson, Ph.D. Section of Pulmonary and Critical Care, Departmentof Medicine, Sleep, Metabolism, and Health Center, University of Chicago, Chicago, IL, USA

Amanda Lamp, B.S. Sleep and Performance Research Center, Washington State University, Spokane, WA, USA

Maren Nyer, Ph.D. Depression and Clinical Research Program, Department of Psychiatry, Massachusetts General Hospital, Boston, MA, USA

Akiko Okifuji, Ph.D. Pain Research Center, Pain Management Center, Department of Anesthesiology, University of Utah, Salt Lake City, UT, USA

Edward F. Pace-Schott, Ph.D. Department of Psychiatry, Harvard Medical School, Massachusetts General Hospital, Charlestown, MA, USA

Michelle A. Short, Ph.D. Centre for Sleep Research, University of South Australia, Adelaide, SA, Australia

Tracy L. Skaer Department of Pharmacotherapy, College of Pharmacy, Washington State University, Spokane, WA, USA

Virend K. Somers, M.D., Ph.D. Division of Cardiovascular Diseases, Mayo Clinic, Rochester, MN, USA

Rebecca M.C. Spencer, Ph.D. Department of Psychology and Neuroscience and Behavior Program, University of Massachusetts, Amherst, Amherst, MA, USA

Aleksandar K. Stanic, M.D., Ph.D. Division of Reproductive Endocrinology and Infertility, Gynecology and Reproductive Biology, Vincent Department of Obstetrics and Gynecology, Harvard Medical School; Hospital, Massachusetts General Hospital, Boston, MA, USA

Mareen Weber, Ph.D. McLean Hospital, Harvard Medical School, Belmont, MA, USA

Jennifer L. Zaslona, B.Sc. Sleep/Wake Research Centre, Massey University, Wellington, New Zealand

Part I

Introduction

Sleep Deprivation: Practical and Philosophical Considerations

1

Matt T. Bianchi

Introduction

Despite being a fairly young field, sleep medicine has made enormous progress from mechanistic to applied clinical sciences. In this volume, the literature linking sleep to a diversity of health and performance topics is explored. The growth and development of this field has been explored in several books, and the interested reader is directed to explore these general readership works that nevertheless capture the evolution of sleep science and its relation to medicine [1, 2]. As a complement to the numerous textbooks of sleep medicine, these accounts provide an important historical perspective. Such context is particularly interesting because sleep may be unique among medical subspecialties in that it has a nearly universal audience in the lay-community, and knowledge about sleep is claimed as much from personal or cultural experience as it is from careful experimentation. This is both a challenge and an opportunity at the intersection of academic research, clinical practice, and social behavior. It is telling that in the annual meeting of the Associated Professional Sleep Societies in 2013, there was a symposium dedicated to the history and science of segmented sleep and the (arguably mythical) assumption that sleep should be (or at least feel like it is) uninterrupted. Among the speakers was historian A. Roger Ekirch, author of "At Day's Close: Night in Times Past" [3], who provided intriguing context to the presentations by leaders in the field. Although the topics presented in this volume focus on the scientific and medical perspectives, the clear relevance for wellness and performance has broad relevance beyond these arenas.

The expanding knowledge base in this field may enjoy more rapid dissemination precisely because of the universality of sleep itself. The narratives emerging from new research, particularly in the area of sleep deprivation, carry immense personal valence and strong apparent face validity. This has positive and negative consequences: information dissemination may have fewer hurdles in the way of relevance and believeability, but the risk of bias in the narrative may be more difficult to mitigate. It is not hard to imagine lay-targeted headlines that would easily capture unchallenged attention, like "No one wants a sleepy surgeon," or "Everyone knows how badly it feels to be sleep deprived." Even such apparently "obvious" narratives have alternative or competing narratives that may also, in isolation, seem quite compelling. Consider the hypothetical headline, "Patients prefer professionally dressed physicians"—it may seem like an obvious finding, especially for patients forced to choose between professional versus casual attire. But what if the question asked if you prefer a professionally dressed physician or an empathetic one? Taking the query one step further: how

M.T. Bianchi, M.D., Ph.D., M.M.Sc. (✉)
Division of Sleep Medicine, Department of Neurology, Massachusetts General Hospital, Boston, MA, USA
e-mail: mtbianchi@partners.org

M.T. Bianchi (ed.), *Sleep Deprivation and Disease: Effects on the Body, Brain and Behavior*,
DOI 10.1007/978-1-4614-9087-6_1,

well-dressed would a physician have to be to make up for lack of empathy, or how empathetic would a physician have to be to make up for casual attire? Now reconsider the sleepy surgeon: what if the choice were between sleep deprived yet invested in your care and thoroughly familiar with your case, and a night shift "covering" physician who is neither invested nor familiar with your case. This issue has been raised regarding queries about sleep, by considering the difference between asking whether you would like more sleep, versus asking what waking activities would you give up for more sleep [4]. Placing sleep in a broader context through a trade-off approach revealed in a cleverly designed survey study that few people chose sleep over potentially attractive alternative activities, despite a high prevalence of apparent sleep complaints [5]. The exercise of considering a broader context, including risk-benefit trade-offs, strengthens the narratives and insulates against the insidious risk of over-committing to a particular narrative. Modern medicine has recognized that face validity and personal experience have a worthy competitor for our attention in the form of careful experimentation. The history of medicine is littered with examples of expert consensus later exposed as folly when carefully studied. Even the findings of well-intended clinical trials in the modern era are often not replicated [6], so from a Bayesian standpoint we might do well to collectively approach the biomedical literature with skepticism because the prior probability seems to favor refutation rather than confirmation.

With the goal of cautious optimism, this chapter outlines some key ideas to keep in mind as one explores the remaining contents. A series of recent debates and editorials capture the sobering reality that studying the role of sleep in health and disease is no simple undertaking. The interested reader is encouraged to sample these engaging discourses directly, concerning the importance of sleep in general [7, 8], the challenges in studying short sleep [9], the concept of sleep debt versus adaptive regulation [4], and the possibility of enhancing health by improving sleep [10].

What Is Normal Sleep?

Identifying what is normal sleep is not as simple as one might hope, yet it is the foundation of any discussion of sleep deprivation. What is considered normal may evolve over time as research findings help disentangle what is "common" from what may be associated with adverse health outcomes. Consider blood pressure, blood sugar, and cholesterol—these are examples of continuous variables with evolving thresholds partitioning health and disease. Likewise, the many facets of sleep physiology may be best understood as a distribution of values, the tails of which represent (perhaps blurry) transitions to disease status.

It has been suggested that presence of symptoms plays an important role in defining pathology, whether in the historical use of "syndrome" suffix for the metrics of obstructive sleep apnea (OSA) combined with sleepiness (which is no longer required [11]), or in more recent discussions about short sleep duration [10]. The symptom-focused approach seems sensible at first glance, but on closer consideration we face problems of inference. If sleepiness is that which occurs when we lack sleep and resolves when we get sleep, then if there is no sleepiness, there is no sleep problem. Yet if we don't accept that lack of sleep-related symptoms implies normal sleep in some settings (e.g., OSA), we should be cautious implying that short (or long) sleepers should be subdivided into normal versus abnormal based solely on symptoms. The commonly used Epworth Sleepiness Scale has minimal correlation with objective measures of sleep [12, 13]. Also, it has been shown that many patients with even severe OSA do not report sleepiness [14, 15], yet untreated OSA harbors adverse health risks regardless [16]. It may be that symptoms are by definition required for certain disorders (such as restless legs or insomnia), and they may also help phenotype individuals, perhaps based on vulnerability to challenges such as sleep restriction or OSA. However, some sleep disorders may be asymptomatic, and some symptoms (such as sleepiness or fatigue) are not specific to sleep problems. The medical canon is filled with examples of asymptomatic phases of chronic diseases, and certainly the field of sleep disorders is no exception.

If one could state what the normal quantity and quality of sleep was, the discourse would surely include a caveat that the answer might vary among individuals, not only in the sense that a distribution of values might be acceptable, but also in the sense that a given value might be normal for only some people or only in some settings. For some individuals, 6 h of sleep per night could be normal, while for others, restriction to 6 h per night would incur substantial symptoms; the former group might even feel worse with the extra 2 h of sleep. Does the body care about total sleep time, or the sleep stage content, or continuity? Does stage content only matter when TST is restricted? Are different organ systems, or different brain functions, differentially sensitive? Would the answers to these questions change between individuals, or even within an individual depending on health status, recent sleep history, or the consumption of caffeine or alcohol? The combinatorial possibilities are daunting. Thus, defining normal sleep, whether by total duration, stage content, arousals, breathing, or other metrics, is not a trivial question.

Assuming the "basic" question of what is normal sleep can be answered, one must then identify how much deviation from normal is relevant? The issue of defining relevance can also be considered as a spectrum, ranging from that which is noticeable but either tolerable or overcome with simple countermeasures, to that which impairs performance, and eventually that which tangibly compromises medical or psychiatric health. One would like to know whether deviations from normal are sensed by the body in an absolute manner (say, one less hour of sleep), or in a relative manner (say, 10 % less sleep)?

The Act of Measuring Disturbs the System Under Observation

The experimental literature on the performance impact of sleep deprivation may be influenced by the Hawthorne effect, in which subjects may behave or perform differently when under observation. There may also be factors that reduce performance in experimental settings, such as lack of interest, tedium of the task at hand, and so forth. The extent to which this may play a role in extrapolating experimental results to real-world situations, especially when effect sizes are small, remains open to debate.

However, there is an even more fundamental issue at stake when we record sleep using PSG, as outlined in a recent article analogizing this gold standard test with quantum uncertainty [17]. It is obvious to many patients experiencing the sleep laboratory, regardless of their background physics training, that observing the sleep-wake system perturbs it in proportion to the burden and invasiveness of the measurement tools. One well-known example is the so-called "first night effect," in which the laboratory environment tends to increase N1, decrease sleep efficiency, and decrease REM sleep. However, it is also worth noting that some patients with insomnia may exhibit a "reverse" form of this, in which their sleep is actually improved in the laboratory setting despite the unusual environment. This is presumed to occur because one or more factors contributing to insomnia in the home setting are not present in the laboratory [18]. The recurrent theme of trade-offs thus surfaces both clinically and experimentally in the very question of how we measure sleep.

Sleep Debt, Sleep Extension, and Sleep Restriction

The topic of sleep debt raises interesting questions about the experimental investigation of sleep loss. Observations of sleep duration extension when provided the opportunity of extra time in bed have been interpreted to imply baseline sleep debt. That narrative assumes that the body precisely regulates the amount of sleep it needs, without capacity to adapt. In other words, more sleep cannot occur, even if the circumstances allow, without sleep debt. This logic hardly holds in other domains, such as hunger and food intake compared to caloric needs, as elegantly argued by Horne in his recent discourses suggesting that sleep duration is adaptive and depends on context and waking needs [4, 19].

Sleep extension beyond the acute setting may be feasible in small amounts (perhaps 1–2 h), but when the total time in bed exceeds physiological sleep capacity, fragmentation and decreased sleep efficiency ensue [20]. This should come as no surprise, as the technique of sleep restriction therapy is aimed at reversing the self-reinforcing trend among some insomniacs who make the mistake of spending more time in bed than their sleep capacity, thus perpetuating the pattern of initiation and/or maintenance sleep difficulties.

Numerous studies have investigated the impact of multiple nights of sleep restriction on physiological and performance outcomes, many of which are described in the chapters of this volume. Although the studies differ in methodology, nearly all of them report impairments, with one of the most commonly cited studies suggesting that even minor (6 h per night) restriction results in accumulated sleep debt equivalent to total sleep deprivation [21]. That study is also commonly cited as evidence that subjective sleepiness ratings underestimate objective performance metrics. However, other literature suggests that sleep restriction via gradual reduction of sleep time, in naturalistic home environments, was not only well tolerated, but also participants actually maintained the schedule voluntarily for at least 1 year following the studies [4].

The Differential Diagnosis of Self-Reported Sleep Duration: Lumping Versus Splitting

Because self-reported sleep duration is so important clinically and epidemiologically, it is a useful exercise to consider the potential underlying phenotypes for individuals reporting short sleep duration. While lumping by sleep duration may be convenient and feasible, when one considers the differential diagnosis of sleep duration, the splitting counter-argument is compelling. The possible phenotypes lumped into a group called "short sleep" could include at least the following:

1. Accurate reporting of the average of consistent objective short sleep time
2. Accurate reporting of objective short nocturnal sleep time without taking into account naps
3. Accurate reporting of the average of highly fluctuating sleep times
4. Underestimation relative to a longer objective sleep duration due to misperception insomnia
5. Underestimation relative to a longer objective sleep duration due to errors in reporting

Any of these categories could be further split according to the presence or absence of comorbid sleep disorders such as sleep apnea. Additional splitting could incorporate comorbid medical or psychiatric pathology, medications, age, genetic variance in susceptibility to sleep deprivation, and so forth. Comorbidities could influence the impact of sleep duration on health or potentially even on the accuracy of subjective reporting of sleep duration. Many survey studies attempt to control for comorbidities, but underlying sleep disorders are difficult to assess by survey, especially the disease with arguably the most dramatic objective sleep disruption—sleep apnea. The downside to splitting is of course that the sample sizes needed to explore the combinatorial possibilities rise rapidly.

The lumping approach may alter epidemiological correlations with various outcomes. Indeed, recent data suggests that medical morbidity is mainly associated with objective short sleep duration [22]. However, even this finding requires further inquiry—given the night to night variability of sleep, and of insomnia, it could be that short sleep duration in the lab is as much a marker of sensitivity to environmental challenge (i.e., the vulnerability of sleep in general) rather than a direct link to pathology.

One can undertake a similar differential diagnosis exercise with self-reported long sleep durations. In epidemiological surveys of sleep, long durations also correlate with adverse health outcomes (although this does not often resonate with media accounts focusing on the narrative that we need more sleep as a society). There has been much speculation as to the underlying reasons for U-shaped associations [9, 23, 24]. In many cases the longer self-reported sleep durations show greater health risk than shorter durations [24], as is the case for all-cause mortality (1.1 vs. 1.23), cardiovascular mortality (1.06 vs. 1.38), and cancer mortality (0.99 vs. 1.21). Even if we assume that short and long sleep self-reports are accurate, and that sleep duration correlates with incident adverse health outcomes, one must resist the inferential temptation to conclude that altering sleep duration will reverse or reduce these risks, which remains untested [10].

Experimental Sleep Deprivation Versus Clinical Insomnia

Patients with insomnia represent a natural target population for extrapolating the findings from experimental sleep deprivation studies. Grandner et al. recently reviewed the literature of self-reported and laboratory-measured short sleep, including an excellent overview of the challenges in this domain [9]. One particular issue regarding clinical extrapolation is that experimental sleep disturbance in a healthy individual is not analogous to the lack of sleep and hyperarousal associated with insomnia [25]. Sleep restricting a health adult generally results in objective hypersomnia (e.g., by multiple sleep latency testing), but this is not commonly observed in patients with insomnia. It is noteworthy that demonstrating objective consequences of insomnia has not enjoyed the success of demonstrating the impact of experimental deprivation. In fact, a recent review captures this challenge in its title, "Searching for the daytime impairments of primary insomnia" [26]. This is perhaps not surprising, when one considers by comparison that the dramatic physiology of severe sleep apnea, with recurrent arousals and hypoxia, does not correlate well with daytime sleepiness.

Correlation and Causation

It should go without saying that correlation is not causation, yet even modern literature sometimes offers exceptions to this sacred dictum. On one hand, there is a vast literature of carefully controlled laboratory experiments, manipulating the sleep of highly selected individuals living in highly unusual environments. In this world, we are as close to causation as can be expected in human research. On the other hand, we have decades of epidemiological studies of self-reported sleep habits, such as napping or sleep duration. In this world, even with prospective studies, if there is no randomization then causation is nowhere to be found, no matter how large the study or how small the *p*-value. From either of these worlds, extrapolating the findings to the worlds of clinical practice and operational guidelines is arguably the most important challenge facing the field. The extent of control in an experimental paradigm can be taken as a good estimate of the extent to which the results will not generalize to other conditions. Consider a light pulse given during a dim light constant routine experiment, which might dramatically shift the circadian clock; the same light pulse might go completely unnoticed in the background of potentially wild light exposure fluctuations in a real-world day. A striking example of experimental-versus-naturalistic dissociation emerged from a study showing non-rhythmic activity in mice over natural outdoor light–dark cycles in which mice self-chose their light exposure [27]. This observation is in striking contrast to the imposed unnatural step-function light–dark cycles of the modern rodent lab. This does not mean that circadian rhythms are an artifact of lab conditions, but it does mean that the system is so flexible (or noisy) that the rhythms are not always robustly manifested. Of course the problem of external validity is not limited to experimental investigations—the patient undergoing clinical PSG may exhibit distinctly different physiology in the home setting, where caffeine, alcohol, or other factors may differ from that observed during clinical testing, yet clinical decisions are often based on the laboratory data.

Numerous heuristics and biases impact the subjective response to seemingly straightforward questions about sleep duration often employed in epidemiological studies of sleep, not to mention the myriad factors impacting the objective sleep duration and even whether the subjective report matches the objective duration. Sleep duration is commonly underestimated especially among insomniacs [28], and the underestimation can be exaggerated when the time frame over which the estimate is requested is increased [29, 30]. Even if one could assume accuracy of self-reported sleep duration, duration is only one dimension of sleep and does not take into account sleep quality, sleep pathology, or individual susceptibilities to sleep disturbance or restriction. Even if simple duration is important [22], it is an entirely different question as to whether increasing sleep duration would abrogate medical risk(s). Randomizing individuals to such sleep interventions for extended periods (months or years) would not be feasible (or blind-able). Naturalistic observational studies provide an alternative perspective, but still cannot prove causality. For example, tracking patients longitudinally could reveal subsets of patients who either shorten or lengthen their sleep duration over the observation period, and this could be linked to some outcomes of interest [31]. However, without randomization, one cannot establish whether a factor that prompted a patient to "naturally" assume a course of action was itself responsible for the outcome of interest, rather than the course of action itself.

Other Statistical and Methodological Considerations

An entire text could be devoted specifically to the statistical pitfalls commonly encountered in biomedical research (and indeed they exist [32, 33]). It is worth, however, mentioning certain topics of relevance that may not be commonly discussed. The first deals with a common currency of research findings: the effect size. The magnitude of an observed effect is central to clinical research. The mistake of equating statistical significance and clinical (or philosophical) significance is so common, and has prompted so much editorializing, it seems almost trite to write about it yet again here. Clinical and statistical "significance" can dissociate under conditions when small *p*-values accompany miniscule effect sizes, usually in large sample studies. It is arguably better to observe a nonsignificant *p*-value, with a 95 % confidence interval of the effect size that spans a clinically meaningful value, than to obtain a very small *p*-value for a marginal effect size with a narrow confidence interval that does not include a clinically significant value. The former leaves open the possibility of an important effect, perhaps in a future study, while the latter convincingly suggests the effect can be ignored. In 1994, Cohen himself lamented that despite decades of severe criticism, the null-hypothesis testing (*p*-value) strategy has not yet been eradicated [34]. We have recently added to the lamenting literature, in the context of the Frequentist versus Bayesian debate [35].

Another flavor of effect size found in the literature is the Cohen's d statistic, which was intended to allow one to compare and combine experiments in a similar field but using different outcomes measurements. The essential idea is to standardize the magnitude of the effect through normalizing by some measure of variance. However, within a single experiment (where it never makes sense to use Cohen's d), and in clinical reasoning, the phrase effect size refers to the absolute magnitude of the observed effect. Importantly, when the variances are proportional, it can be that Cohen's d classifications are insensitive to the absolute versus relative effect problem. For example, a 10 % increase in mortality between groups with a pooled variance of 5 % has the same "effect size" as a 0.1 % increase with a pooled variance of 0.05 %. The qualitative gradation of effect size (small, medium, large) was devised by Cohen to apply to the social science context, not to biomedical research, where effect sizes can be larger, variances can be smaller, and there is a different philosophy behind the concept of effect size.

Another topic of importance to analysis of sleep physiology relates to reporting of sleep-wake stage architecture. Measurements of time spent in sleep and wake states are expected to anti-correlate simply because they are mutually exclusive, which can present interesting interpretation challenges. Similarly, REM and NREM are mutually exclusive and thus anti-correlated components of total sleep time. We recently explored the potential for embedded correlations, such that differentiating spurious versus meaningful correlations, for example related to a sleep stage, which itself correlates with total sleep time, is not straightforward [20]. Experimental sleep deprivation necessarily involves increasing time awake, which may be associated with different physiology, independent of the increased stress that often accompanies the intervention. Stage-specific deprivation protocols are often associated with "collateral damage," whether accomplished with pharmacology or with manual interruptions of sleep. For example, consider using an antidepressant to "suppress REM," which has been described in the literature—one would not want to trivialize the litany of other antidepressant effects on neurochemistry. Similarly, consider an acoustic protocol designed to provide arousing stimulation in real time whenever N3 sleep is observed to decrease its occurrence. This could easily be shown to decrease the time spent in N3, but the intervention also may increase N1 and N2, increase the arousal index, or cause episodic cardiac changes, among perhaps more subtle neurophysiologic changes. Even referring to such a protocol as "N3-deprivation" implies these numerous other correlated changes are not relevant. Being mindful of these inferential topics is critical whether perusing the growing literature or contributing to it.

Conclusion

Reviewing any field of medicine is as much about celebrating progress as scrutinizing potential points of vulnerability. The intention of this book is to capture the breadth and depth of research into the health and performance consequences of sleep deprivation, in hopes of reducing the portion of the literature at risk for being later exposed as folly.

References

1. Dement WC, Vaughan CC. The promise of sleep: a pioneer in sleep medicine explores the vital connection between health, happiness, and a good night's sleep. New York: Delacorte; 1999.
2. Kroker K. The sleep of others and the transformations of sleep research. Toronto: University of Toronto Press; 2007.
3. Ekirch AR. At day's close: night in times past. 1st ed. New York: Norton; 2005.
4. Horne J. The end of sleep: 'sleep debt' versus biological adaptation of human sleep to waking needs. Biol Psychol. 2011;87(1):1–14.
5. Anderson C, Horne JA. Do we really want more sleep? A population-based study evaluating the strength of desire for more sleep. Sleep Med. 2008; 9(2):184–7.
6. Ioannidis JP. Why most published research findings are false. PLoS Med. 2005;2(8):e124.
7. Rattenborg NC, Lesku JA, Martinez-Gonzalez D, Lima SL. The non-trivial functions of sleep. Sleep Med Rev. 2007;11(5):405–9; author reply 411–7.
8. Rial RV, Nicolau MC, Gamundi A, et al. The trivial function of sleep. Sleep Med Rev. 2007; 11(4):311–25.
9. Grandner MA, Patel NP, Gehrman PR, Perlis ML, Pack AI. Problems associated with short sleep: bridging the gap between laboratory and epidemiological studies. Sleep Med Rev. 2010;14(4):239–47.
10. Buysse DJ, Grunstein R, Horne J, Lavie P. Can an improvement in sleep positively impact on health? Sleep Med Rev. 2010;14(6):405–10.
11. Epstein LJ, Kristo D, Strollo Jr PJ, et al. Clinical guideline for the evaluation, management and long-term care of obstructive sleep apnea in adults. J Clin Sleep Med. 2009;5(3):263–76.
12. Benbadis SR, Mascha E, Perry MC, Wolgamuth BR, Smolley LA, Dinner DS. Association between the Epworth sleepiness scale and the multiple sleep latency test in a clinical population. Ann Intern Med. 1999;130(4 Pt 1):289–92.
13. Chervin RD, Aldrich MS. The Epworth Sleepiness Scale may not reflect objective measures of sleepiness or sleep apnea. Neurology. 1999;52(1):125–31.
14. Gottlieb DJ, Whitney CW, Bonekat WH, et al. Relation of sleepiness to respiratory disturbance index: the Sleep Heart Health Study. Am J Respir Crit Care Med. 1999;159(2):502–7.
15. Eiseman NA, Westover MB, Mietus JE, Thomas RJ, Bianchi MT. Classification algorithms for predicting sleepiness and sleep apnea severity. J Sleep Res. 2012;21(1):101–12.
16. Budhiraja R, Budhiraja P, Quan SF. Sleep-disordered breathing and cardiovascular disorders. Respir Care. 2010;55(10):1322–32. discussion 1330–1322.
17. Brown LK. Quantum physics and polysomnography: can we prevent the act of measuring sleep from changing sleep? J Clin Sleep Med. 2005;1(2):133–5.
18. McCall C, McCall WV. Objective vs. subjective measurements of sleep in depressed insomniacs: first night effect or reverse first night effect? J Clin Sleep Med. 2012;8(1):59–65.
19. Horne J. Sleep debt—Where is the answer—in or outside the laboratory? Biol Psychol. 2011;87(2):314–5; author reply 316.
20. Bianchi MT, Wang W, Klerman EB. Sleep misperception in healthy adults: implications for insomnia diagnosis. J Clin Sleep Med. 2012;8(5):547–54.

21. Van Dongen HP, Maislin G, Mullington JM, Dinges DF. The cumulative cost of additional wakefulness: dose–response effects on neurobehavioral functions and sleep physiology from chronic sleep restriction and total sleep deprivation. Sleep. 2003;26(2):117–26.
22. Vgontzas AN, Fernandez-Mendoza J, Liao D, Bixler EO. Insomnia with objective short sleep duration: the most biologically severe phenotype of the disorder. Sleep Med Rev. 2013;17(4):241–54.
23. Bliwise DL, Young TB. The parable of parabola: what the U-shaped curve can and cannot tell us about sleep. Sleep. 2007;30(12):1614–5.
24. Cappuccio FP, Cooper D, D'Elia L, Strazzullo P, Miller MA. Sleep duration predicts cardiovascular outcomes: a systematic review and meta-analysis of prospective studies. Eur Heart J. 2011;32(12): 1484–92.
25. Bonnet MH, Arand DL. Hyperarousal and insomnia: state of the science. Sleep Med Rev. 2010;14(1):9–15.
26. Shekleton JA, Rogers NL, Rajaratnam SM. Searching for the daytime impairments of primary insomnia. Sleep Med Rev. 2010;14(1):47–60.
27. Daan S, Spoelstra K, Albrecht U, et al. Lab mice in the field: unorthodox daily activity and effects of a dysfunctional circadian clock allele. J Biol Rhythms. 2011;26(2):118–29.
28. Harvey AG, Tang NK. (Mis)perception of sleep in insomnia: a puzzle and a resolution. Psychol Bull. 2012;138(1):77–101.
29. Fichten CS, Creti L, Amsel R, Bailes S, Libman E. Time estimation in good and poor sleepers. J Behav Med. 2005;28(6):537–53.
30. Bliwise DL, Friedman L, Yesavage JA. Depression as a confounding variable in the estimation of habitual sleep time. J Clin Psychol. 1993;49(4):471–7.
31. Chaput JP, Despres JP, Bouchard C, Tremblay A. Longer sleep duration associates with lower adiposity gain in adult short sleepers. Int J Obes (Lond). 2012; 36(5):752–6.
32. Huck S. Statistical misconceptions. New York: Routledge; 2008.
33. Huff D. How to lie with statistics. New York: W. W. Norton; 1993.
34. Cohen J. The earth is round (p<0.05). Am Psychol. 1994;49(12):997–1003.
35. Westover MB, Westover KD, Bianchi MT. Significance testing as perverse probabilistic reasoning. BMC Med. 2011;9:20.

Part II

Sleep Physiology, Measurement, and Experimental Deprivation

The Functional Impact of Sleep Deprivation, Sleep Restriction, and Sleep Fragmentation

2

Michelle A. Short and Siobhan Banks

Paradigms of sleep deprivation, sleep restriction, and sleep fragmentation have been utilized to answer fundamental questions about sleep, including how much sleep adults need and the deficits and recuperation associated with sleep loss. While definitive answers to many of these core questions remain, this work has highlighted how sleep is crucial for healthy functioning. Absent, insufficient, or fragmented sleep has widespread neurobehavioral and physiological consequences, and also broader social and economic ramifications. The present chapter will compare and contrast the functional impacts of sleep deprivation, sleep restriction, and sleep fragmentation in adults, then discuss the implications that this research has on our understanding and conceptualization of sleep need and sleep debt.

Sleep Deprivation

The first sleep deprivation study was published over 100 years ago [1] and since then many studies have examined the impact of sleep deprivation on healthy functioning. A meta-analysis by Pilcher and Huffcutt [2] highlighted the impact of sleep deprivation; with their data showing cognitive performance and self-rated mood of sleep-deprived individuals below the 9th percentile of non-sleep-deprived subjects. In a seminal study by Dawson and Reid [3], alcohol was used to illustrate the deleterious impact of sleep deprivation on performance. They found that cognitive ability following 17 h of sustained wakefulness was equivalent to that of a person with a blood alcohol concentration of 0.05 % (the legal driving limit in many countries), while performance following 24 h of wakefulness was equivalent to that with a blood alcohol concentration of 0.10 % [3]. Sleep deprivation is common in many occupations that demand 24 h operations, such as nursing, mining, trucking, and aviation and tragically sleep deprivation has been implicated in several catastrophic incidents and accidents [4, 5].

Sleep Deprivation, Cognition, and Neurobehavioral Functioning

Changes to sleepiness and alertness are among the most robust and frequently examined consequences of sleep deprivation [6–11]. During sleep deprivation, the drive for sleep builds [12], resulting in decreased subjective alertness and increased self-reported and objective sleepiness. There are numerous ways to measure sleepiness, ranging from subjective self-report, EEGs markers, such as the latency to slow wave sleep (SWS) (shorter latencies reflect greater sleep pressure) and objective sleepiness measures, such as the Multiple Sleep Latency Test (MSLT) and the Maintenance of Wakefulness Test (MWT). These tests measure the time taken to fall asleep, or

M.A. Short, Ph.D. (✉) • S. Banks, Ph.D.
Centre for Sleep Research, University of South Australia, Adelaide, SA, Australia
e-mail: michelle.short@unisa.edu.au

M.T. Bianchi (ed.), *Sleep Deprivation and Disease: Effects on the Body, Brain and Behavior*, DOI 10.1007/978-1-4614-9087-6_2, © Springer Science+Business Media New York 2014

sleep latency, using EEG to monitor brain activity. The MSLT objectively measures the time taken to fall asleep in a sleep-conducive environment, while the MWT measures sleep latency under conditions where an individual is trying to *resist* falling asleep. Both MSLT and MWT values decline during sleep deprivation, indicating that individuals fall asleep much more quickly when trying to sleep, and they also fall asleep faster even when they are attempting to stay awake [13, 14]. Just one night of sleep deprivation can reduce MSLT sleep latencies to well within a pathologically sleepy range of 5 min or less [15] and reduce the latency to deep sleep by 50 % [16]. Franzen and colleagues [7] compared a group of 15 healthy, young adults following 1 night of sleep deprivation with 14 who had normal sleep. Sleep deprivation led to a range of performance and mood deficits; however, it had the largest impact on subjective and objective sleepiness. Faster MWT sleep latencies highlighted the increased likelihood of unintended sleep onset following sleep deprivation, a problem with substantial ramifications to safety.

The ability to sustain attention and maintain vigilance is reduced following even 1 night without sleep, another factor which increases the risk for accidents. Reaction times slow, behavioral lapses (the failure to respond to a stimulus within a timely fashion) increase, and failure to inhibit an incorrect response increases with sleep deprivation [7, 17–22]. Lapsing of attention (failing to respond to a stimulus) is believed to occur when microsleeps intrude into the waking state [23]. A commonly used task of vigilant attention task that is very sensitive to sleep loss is the psychomotor vigilance test (PVT). In a sleep deprivation study involving 88 h of sleep deprivation (3 nights without sleep), Doran and colleagues [23] found that, after 18 h of wake, PVT performance progressively deteriorated in terms of both reaction time and response errors. Over time, they also witnessed greater between-subject variance in vigilant attention, with the magnitude of performance deficits varying significantly among subjects. Lim and Dinges [24] suggest that sleep deprivation leads to a general slowing in response times (responses >500 ms), an increase in incorrect responses, and an amplification of the time-on-task effect (whereby performance deteriorates during a test as a result of boredom, fatigue, or lack of novelty). While the PVT is a basic task, vigilance and attention are functions that are important to and subserve a multitude of higher-order cognitive tasks. They argue that sustained attention deficits, as a prerequisite for upstream cognitive processing, are responsible for many of the performance deficits in memory and executive functioning tasks following sleep deprivation [24].

Many simple and complex cognitive tasks and domains show deficits following sleep deprivation. These include working memory [6, 25], memory consolidation, mental arithmetic [22], reasoning [22, 26], tracking [26, 27], innovative thinking and strategic planning [28–31], creative thinking [32, 33], verbal fluency [28, 32, 34], temporal memory [35], planning [32], creative and flexible thinking, decision making, speech articulation, language, and judgement [28–30, 34, 36, 37]. These deficits can begin as early as the first night of sleep deprivation [38, 39] and continue to increase significantly with extended wakefulness [9, 40, 41].

While these neurobehavioral deficits are commonly found in response to sleep loss, there is substantial variance among people in terms of individual vulnerability to sleep loss [9]. In addition, there is also substantial variance within individuals in regard to which domains are most affected by sleep loss [42]. This pattern of response was illustrated by a study by Van Dongen and colleagues [43]. They exposed 21 healthy, young participants to 36 h of sleep deprivation on three separate occasions. Results revealed a remarkable consistency in their response to sleep loss across different occasions. Surprisingly, however, this consistency did not hold across different neurobehavioral domains. So participants who reported a high level of subjective sleepiness did not necessarily show cognitive processing deficits or poor sustained attention, and individuals particularly vulnerable to cognitive deficits following sleep loss were not necessarily sleepier or less behaviorally alert. This differing pattern of individual response is illustrated in Fig. 2.1. One of the important ramifications of

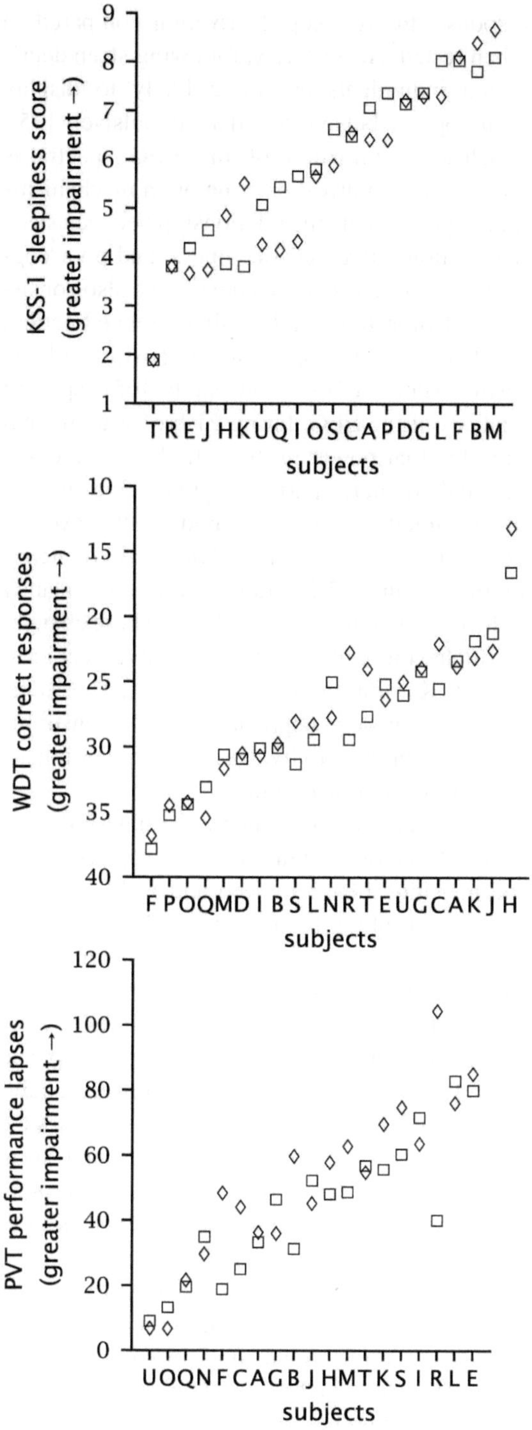

Fig. 2.1 Trait like neurobehavioral responses to total sleep deprivation. Data are shown for the Karolinska Sleepiness Scale (KSS-1), the word detection task (WDT), and the psychomotor vigilance task (PVT). The abscissa of each panel shows the 21 individual subjects, labeled

Fig. 2.1 (continued) A–U, in arbitrary order with the same label being used for the same subject across the three panels. Within each panel, the subjects are ordered by the magnitude of their impairment (averaged over 2, 36 h sleep deprivation periods), with the most resistant subjects on the left and the most vulnerable subjects on the right. Responses in the first exposure to sleep deprivation following 7 days of sleep extension are marked by boxes; responses in the second exposure to sleep deprivation following 7 days of sleep extension are marked by diamonds. The data show that subjects differed substantially in their responses to sleep deprivation, while the responses were relatively stable within subjects between the 2 exposures to sleep deprivation. (Reproduced with permission from Van Dongen et al. [43])

this work is that it highlights the shortcomings of relying upon an individual's subjective feelings of sleepiness and alertness to evaluate their cognitive or behavioral impairments. Indeed, the authors of this study argued that individuals are not well equipped to introspect their performance deficits following sleep deprivation.

Sleep Deprivation and Mood

Sleep deprivation has been associated with an increase in negative mood states [6, 44] and diminished positive mood [44]. These findings span discrete emotions including excitement, happiness, cheerfulness, activation, pride, and delight, as well as intensified symptoms of dissociation [45, 46]. Sleep deprivation has been linked to potentially serious changes to emotion, mood states, and their regulation [47, 48]. Changes with sleep deprivation to the brain's serotonergic system (low serotonin is associated with depression), in particular a desensitization of the serotonin (5-HT) 1A receptor system, could be a mechanism underlying this dysregulation of mood [49].

It has also been found that following 1 night of sleep deprivation, healthy young adults report increased negative mood and decreased positive affect [7]. In this study objective affect reactivity was measured using pupil dilation in response to emotional pictures [7]. Sleep deprivation led to elevated pupillary responses to negative pictures and the authors hypothesized that this reflected heightened emotional reactivity to negative emotional information. Another study by Minkel et al. [50] examined stress and mood response following 1 night of sleep deprivation in either a low stress or high stress environment. Stressor intensity was altered by increasing the difficulty of the cognitive task, providing negative feedback about performance, and increasing time pressure. Sleep deprivation increased subjective stress, anxiety, and anger ratings following exposure to the low-stressor condition, but not in response to the high-stressor condition. Sleep deprivation elevated negative mood and stress about equally for both sleep conditions. These data suggest that sleep deprivation lowers the psychological threshold for the perception of stress, but does not change the magnitude of negative affect in response to high-stress, cognitive demands.

Sleep Deprivation and the Brain

The impact of sleep deprivation on cognition, sustained attention, and mood is likely to reflect the effect that sleep deprivation has on the neural systems that subserve these functions. Numerous and diverse cortical and subcortical structures and systems have been shown to be sensitive to sleep loss [8, 43, 51, 52]. Positron emission tomography (PET) and functional magnetic resonance imaging (fMRI) studies have revealed significant decreases in global glucose metabolism throughout the brain during sleep deprivation [8, 53–57]. It has been argued that these reductions in brain glucose metabolism underlie functional deficits following sleep deprivation because of resource depletion [58–60]. While the relationship between attention, cognition, and neurophysiology following sleep deprivation is reasonably well explored, less is known about the neural mechanisms associated the changes in affect occurring after sleep deprivation [7]. Yoo and colleagues [61] found reduced functional connectivity between the medial frontal cortex (which exerts top-down control over limbic areas and has a role in emotional and behavioral regulation [62–64]) and the amygdala following sleep deprivation and a 60 % increased amygdala response during sleep deprivation compared to when rested. Accordingly, following sleep deprivation individuals are more likely to display inappropriate behaviors and act impulsively [35].

Close examination of the EEG spectra is another way to investigate the brain mechanisms that might mediate the relationship between sleep deprivation, increased sleepiness, and poor cognitive performance. Past studies have also consistently demonstrated a drowsiness-related pattern of changes in the spectral composition of the resting state EEG. In one study [65], spectral analysis of the EEG during 21 h of wakefulness revealed that power in the delta band increased (2 and 4 Hz) in the parietal region, while alpha in the occipital region (measured as the average power in a 1-Hz band around the peak frequency in the 8- and 12-Hz range) was significantly reduced by extended wakefulness. These changes paralleled those observed in subjective sleepiness ratings (Karolinska Sleepiness Scale). These data suggests that sleep deprivation has demonstrable effects on brain activity, with subsequent impact on feeling and functioning.

After a period of extended wakefulness, the stability of one of the brain regions responsible for the transition between sleep and wake becomes unstable, resulting in the uncontrollable intrusion of sleep into wakefulness [66]. The main region involved in this transition is the ventrolateral preoptic (VLPO) nucleus and it is sometimes referred to as the "flip-flop" switch between sleep and wake [66] The VLPO receives diminished inhibition following sleep loss [24], which increases the likelihood of both behavioral lapses and sleep onset. Research has shown that lapses are more likely to occur when the waking EEG shows signs of transition to sleep onset [67].

More recently, research has shown the importance of sleep to the generation and survival of new neurons [68]. In an adult rat model, 96 h of sleep deprivation led to a 50 % reduction in new cells in the hippocampal dentate gyrus, a brain region involved in the formation of new memories. Three weeks subsequent to the sleep deprivation period, the development of mature, functioning cells was reduced by 35 %. Taking into account both suppressed neurogenesis and failure to develop to functional maturity, the authors estimate that sleep deprivation reduced the new neurons in this region by 60 %, supporting the role of sleep in enabling the development of the structural substrates of brain plasticity. This suggests that recovery from sleep deprivation may not be quick and the effects of sleep deprivation on neurogenesis are not readily reversible.

Sleep Restriction

Typically it is recommended that adults obtain about 8 h sleep per night [69], however restricting sleep below this amount is common practice. Lifestyle and occupational factors such as long hours of work, commuting, shift work, family and social commitments, and the increased use of technology in the evening, all impact sleep duration and can cause chronic sleep restriction [70–72]. In a sample of more than 1.1 million American adults, 20 % reported obtaining less than 6.5 h sleep per night [73].

Early studies of sleep restriction reported few adverse effects [74, 75], but many of these studies were limited by methodological difficulties including lack of a non-sleep-restricted control group, lack of experimental control over key variables, such as sleep duration, use of caffeine or exposure to light, or use of tests that were insensitive to sleep loss, or the results of which were confounded by practice effects or circadian timing [76]. Now the deleterious effects of sleep restriction are better documented and well recognized.

Sleep Restriction and Neurobehavioral Function

A wide range of neurobehavioral functions have been shown to be sensitive to sleep loss. Sleep restriction to less than 6 h per night for a number of consecutive nights leads to increased objective sleepiness as measured on the MSLT, and faster night time sleep onset [77, 78]. The effects of sleep restricted to 5 h time in bed (TIB) for 7 nights on measures of subjective and objective sleepiness were measured in ten healthy, young adults [78]. On the second day of sleep restriction, the MSLT showed increases in sleepiness which continued to rise and a visual analogue scale showed an increase in sleepiness following sleep restriction, which leveled off after 4 days of sleep restriction. This discrepancy between subjective sleepiness, which tapers off, and objective sleepiness, which continues to rise, may indicate greater adaptation to sleep restriction in subjective sleepiness than objective sleepiness. This finding of dissociation between subjective and objective sleepiness and performance has been replicated in other studies [9, 79].

Van Dongen and colleagues [9] conducted a seminal study examining the impact of sleep deprivation and sleep restriction on sleep and performance in a strictly controlled laboratory environment. Sleep deprivation was examined across 3 days, together with sleep restricted to 4, 6, or 8 h TIB per night for 14 nights, in 48 healthy, young adults aged 21–38 years. Subjective sleepiness showed an initial increase, but then plateaued. While subjective responses showed a saturating exponential response, lapses in behavioral alertness (PVT) were near-linearly related to the length of accumulated wakefulness in excess of 16 h. The time course of these deficits is shown in Fig. 2.2. The dissociation between subjective and objective sleepiness and performance indicates that individuals are unaware of their level of cognitive and behavioral impairments, a finding that has significant ramifications for individuals' self-management of fatigue and safety under conditions of sleep restriction (Fig. 2.2).

This study also compared sleep restriction with sleep deprivation. While the 4 and 6 h TIB conditions showed significant, cumulative, dose-dependent impairments across all cognitive tasks, total sleep deprivation over 3 nights led to performance deficits and changes to EEG delta power relative to sleep lost that were disproportionately greater. This study supports the notion that individuals do not adjust to chronic sleep restriction, but that performance deficits continue to accrue with successive nights. Further, the estimated maximum length of continuous wakefulness per

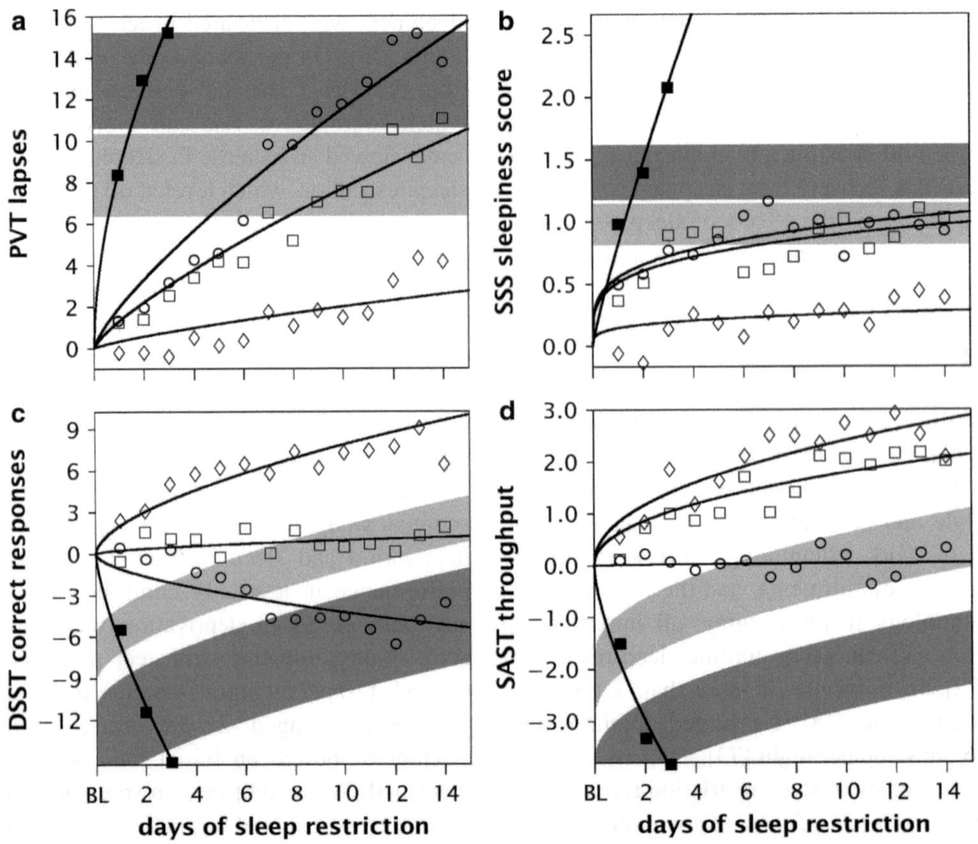

Fig. 2.2 Neurobehavioral responses to varying doses of nightly sleep. Four different neurobehavioral tests were used to measure cognitive performance and subjective sleepiness. *Panel A* shows psychomotor vigilance task (PVT) performance lapses; *panel B* shows Stanford Sleepiness Scale (SSS) self-ratings; *panel C* shows digit symbol substitution task (DSST) correct responses; and panel D shows serial addition/subtraction task (SAST) correct responses per min. Upward corresponds to worse performance on the PVT and greater sleepiness on the SSS, and to better performance on the DSST and the SAST. Each panel displays group averages for subjects in the 8 h (*open circles*), 6 h (*open squares*), and 4 h (*open diamonds*) chronic sleep period conditions across 14 days, and in the 0 h (*filled squares*) sleep condition across 3 days. The curves through the data points represent best-fitting profiles of the response to sleep deprivation. The mean ± SE ranges of neurobehavioral functions for 1 and 2 days of 0 h sleep (total sleep deprivation) are shown as *light* and *dark gray bands*, respectively, allowing comparison of the 3-day total sleep deprivation condition and the 14-day chronic sleep restriction conditions. (Reproduced with permission from Van Dongen et al. [9])

day to maintain optimal functioning and prevent the accumulation of neurobehavioral deficits was just under 16 h per day.

It has been suggested that neurobehavioral and cognitive functions show the least adaptation to chronic sleep restriction [80], with a number of studies reporting decreased PVT performance, in terms of both lapses and speed [77, 79, 81, 82]. Tasks including the digit symbol substitution task and serial addition and subtraction task, which measure working memory and cognitive throughput, also show declines in performance following sleep restriction [9].

Mood and sociability are also reduced with sleep restriction [47, 48, 76]. Dinges and colleagues [47] restricted 16 healthy, young adults to 7 nights of 4–5 h sleep per night. Sleep restriction resulted in cumulative deficits in subjective sleepiness, and an increase in fatigue, confusion, tension, mental exhaustion, and stress. While the effects of sleep restriction on attention, sleepiness, cognitive performance, and mood are clear, there are marked differences both within individuals and between individuals regarding the magnitude and time course of these deficits [9, 43, 83].

Sleep Restriction and the Brain and Body

Core features of sleep EEG change following sleep restriction. Reductions occur in sleep onset latency, Stage N2, wake after sleep onset, REM and latency to REM, while SWS remains unchanged [9, 76, 77, 79, 81, 84, 85]. The conservation of SWS has led some to speculate that SWS may be "protected" during sleep restriction, due to the crucial role of SWS in restoring brain function [86]. But data suggests that while sleep EEG changes occur rapidly in response to sleep restriction, they do not seem to accumulate with successive days of sleep restriction, unlike performance deficits [9]. Slow wave activity (power in the EEG delta band), the putative marker of sleep homeostasis, has however been found to increase with successive nights of sleep restriction [76], suggesting that there is some response in the brain during sleep to chronic shortening of sleep time.

Sleep restriction also has been found to impact upon a range of physiological functions. These changes include an increased stress response [49, 87], altered immune function [88] such as changes to killer cell activity [89], impaired glucose metabolism [90], increased blood pressure [91], heightened sympathetic nervous system activation [92], increased inflammatory markers [93] such as interleukin-6 [94, 95], altered appetite through reduced leptin and increased ghrelin [96, 97], neurogenesis [98], and poorer outcomes such as increased body mass index, and heightened risk of cardiovascular disease and diabetes [99, 100]. Vgontaz and coauthors [77] reduced the sleep of 25 healthy adults to 6 h per night for 7 days and found that this relatively mild dose of sleep restriction lowered morning peak cortisol secretion and significantly increased the daily secretion of the inflammatory cytokine, IL-6. These are markers of systemic inflammation and have been linked to the development of cardiovascular disease, osteoporosis, and insulin resistance [77]. In another study, 6 nights of sleep restricted to 4 h per night led to a significant decrease in glucose tolerance, most acutely in response to the initial meal following wake (breakfast) [87]. Even shorter periods of sleep restriction also have implications for metabolic regulation. Spiegel and colleagues [96] found that just 2 nights of short sleep (4 h TIB) led to higher glucose levels and lower insulin levels. They also examined ghrelin (a peptide that stimulates appetite) and leptin (an adipocyte-derived hormone that suppresses appetite) and found an increase of over 70 % in the ghrelin-to-leptin ratio and a 30 % increase in self-reported appetite for calorie-dense, high-carbohydrate foods. Thus, when these hormones are out of balance, appetite is increased which could lead to weight gain and possibly type 2 diabetes.

Population-based studies support these laboratory results (for review see Killick et al. [101]). For example in the Wisconsin Sleep Cohort sleep was measured in 1,024 adults using sleep diaries, surveys, and overnight PSG [99]. Fasting blood samples were taken subsequent to the PSG night. Among participants sleeping less than 8 h per night (nearly three quarters of the sample), there was a negative relationship between sleep duration and BMI. Short sleep was also associated with decreased leptin and increased ghrelin, although no significant association was found between sleep duration and insulin or glucose.

Sleep Fragmentation

Sleep fragmentation, like sleep restriction, is commonplace in the community. Sleep fragmentation frequently arises due to sleep disorders, such as obstructive sleep apnea (OSA), periodic limb movements in sleep (PLMS), and sleep maintenance insomnia, as well as other medical conditions involving chronic pain or urinary frequency. Studies have been conducted that experimentally fragment sleep to examine in a controlled way its impact on health functioning.

Experimental Sleep Fragmentation and Cognitive Function

Studies experimentally inducing sleep fragmentation have used a number of techniques, from waking individuals from sleep and requiring a behavioral response, to producing a brief EEG arousal by administering an auditory or vibration stimulus to elicit increased EEG frequency [102]. Irrespective of the paradigm used, studies frequently find that sleep fragmentation results in increased subjective and objective sleepiness [103–105], decrements in attention [103, 104, 106], slowed reaction time [103, 107], less cognitive flexibility [108], decreased working memory [107], and impaired mood [105, 106, 109, 110]. Sleep continuity therefore appears to be important for cognitive functions and memory consolidation [111]. Studies in which the frequency of arousals was experimentally manipulated found that performance deficits on a simple addition task, completed during a brief awakening, as well as longer latencies to respond, occurred sooner and increased more rapidly with more frequent arousal schedules, suggesting a dose–response relationship [104, 112]. The magnitude of stimulus required to elicit wake also increased with more frequent arousals [112], suggesting that individuals may habituate to the stimulus, or perhaps their pressure for sleep was such that they were more difficult to arouse. Participants who were woken every minute showed performance levels equivalent to individuals performance following 64 h of sleep deprivation [112]. Sleep appears to have a reduced recuperative value when significantly fragmented.

Challenges in interpreting studies that have completely woken participants, and particularly those that have measured performance during these arousals, include, (1) difficulty in teasing apart the impact of sleep fragmentation and that of sleep inertia, and (2) fully waking also introduces greater disruption to sleep parameters and sleep architecture. More recent studies of sleep fragmentation have used auditory tones to produce brief EEG arousal without requiring a full waking response [104, 109, 113]. These studies have been able to examine the effect of sleep fragmentation and non-fragmented sleep in conditions where total sleep time is the same [113], or at least very similar [104, 109]. These studies have found that sleep fragmentation causes greater sleepiness, even when sleep duration is near equivalent. Stepanski and colleagues [103] conducted a within-subjects experiment examining three sleep fragmentation conditions: 8–9 arousals per hour, 4–5 arousals per hour, or 8–9 arousal per hour for the first 4 h of sleep and then uninterrupted sleep for the remainder of the sleep period [103]. They used auditory tones to induce brief arousals and ran each condition for 2 nights. After 2 nights, individuals in all conditions showed significantly increased sleepiness on the MSLT the next day (fell asleep more quickly), but surprisingly, there were no significant differences between conditions, suggesting that perhaps the difference in the arousal frequency was not sufficient to result in significant differences in objective sleepiness [103]. However, even when total sleep is unaffected by sleep fragmentation, some studies have still found changes to sleep architecture, including increased Stage N1 sleep and decreased SWS and REM [106, 114, 115]. It appears, therefore, that changes in sleep stage dynamics and the constant disruption of the normal sleep process are major contributing factors to the cognitive deficits seen with sleep fragmentation.

Sleep Fragmentation and Health

Given the prevalence of sleep and medical conditions which can cause fragmented sleep, it is possible that sleep fragmentation may contribute to the morbidity associated with these conditions. In one study of healthy subjects, sleep fragmentation alone resulted in alterations to blood pressure, heart rate, glucose metabolism, and O_2/CO_2 metabolism [114, 116]. Stamatakis and Punjabi subjected 11 healthy, young volunteers to 2 nights of sleep fragmentation using auditory and mechanical stimuli at a rate of 30 or more EEG micro-arousals per hour, which is similar to mild to moderate sleep apnea [114]. Two nights of sleep fragmentation were associated with increased morning cortisol, decreased insulin sensitivity and glucose effectiveness, and a significant increase in sympathetic nervous system activation, but no changes in inflammatory markers.

Carrington and Trinder found that sleep fragmentation inhibited the normal dip in blood pressure that occurs during sleep onset [116]. The absence of normal blood pressure dipping at sleep onset, coupled with transient increases in blood pressure following arousals from sleep [117, 118], may translate into higher diurnal blood pressure. These experimental data are also supported by a population-based study of sleep fragmentation [119]. The association between blood pressure during wake and a PSG-derived sleep fragmentation index was examined in 1,021 healthy, middle aged adults, without sleep apnea from the Wisconsin Sleep Cohort. It was found that, after controlling for demographic variables, BMI, and use of blood pressure medication, individuals with a higher sleep fragmentation index were found to have higher levels of systolic blood pressure [119]. Taken together these data suggest that sleep fragmentation could lead to the development of hypertension and increase the risk for cardiovascular disease.

Sleep Deprivation, Restriction, and Fragmentation: Comparison and Implications for our Theoretical Understanding of Sleep

Many of the waking effects of sleep deprivation, sleep restriction, and sleep fragmentation on neurobehavioral response and physiology are similar, hinting at common underlying mechanisms. Deficits common to all three include increased subjective and objective sleepiness, deficits of vigilance, attention and cognition, mood degradation, and changes to glucose metabolism and heart rate. Despite many qualitative similarities between these conditions, the magnitude and time course of these deficits varies substantially. It is these differences, as well as the similarities, that have the potential to add to our understanding of human sleep need, its purpose for function, what accounts for the pattern and time course of neurobehavioral and physiological changes observed, and the recuperative value of sleep.

Early sleep restriction experiments tended to reveal few waking deficits associated with sleep restriction, but more significant effects following sleep deprivation. This observation led to the core sleep hypothesis [120]. This hypothesis posits that only a core sleep of 4–5 h per night is physiologically required to maintain healthy functioning and that additional sleep is optional, often used purely to fill the quiet hours until morning. However more recent, controlled sleep restriction experiments have shown significant functional deficits after sleep is reduced to 7 h or less TIB per night [9, 79]. In addition, sleep fragmentation experiments in which total sleep time has been minimally reduced have shown substantial waking deficits, sometimes comparable to that seen following partial or total sleep deprivation. Therefore, the core sleep hypothesis does not adequately account for these cognitive impairments.

Given the conservation of SWS during sleep restriction, it has been argued that SWS or deep sleep must have a primary recuperative value. This would help to explain why sleep deprivation has a much greater and more immediate impact on human functioning than sleep restriction, because individuals are deprived of the recuperative value of SWS. This could also account for some of the findings from sleep fragmentation experiments in which SWS was reduced and functioning was diminished. However, in sleep restriction paradigms, while SWS is preferentially preserved across different total sleep conditions, performance deficits still vary according to these conditions, with less sleep, but not always less SWS associated with greater and faster accumulating deficits [9, 79]. Additionally, sleep fragmentation studies, while reducing SWS, do not eliminate it entirely, yet they have shown deficits akin to that of total sleep deprivation, which is inconsistent with the hypothesis that SWS is the only recuperative component of sleep.

Sleep restriction studies, showing dose-dependent responses to sleep restriction, have led to the concept of sleep debt. Sleep debt is the accumulated deficit of sleep time relative to individual sleep need and has intuitive appeal relative to a basic understanding of sleep restoration: that the deficits in waking function will be relative to the quantity of sleep lost. However, studies that have compared sleep restriction with sleep deprivation do not support this notion [9]. Participants who obtained 4 h of sleep per night for 14 nights sustained a cumulative sleep debt (totally amount of sleep lost) much greater than participants who were deprived of sleep for 88 h; however, those in the sleep deprivation condition showed much greater deficits of waking performance [9]. This suggests that it is not sleep loss, per se, that accounted for these patterns of waking deficits, but rather that there are neurobehavioral costs associated with extended wakefulness [9].

More recently, a theory positing the importance of bottom-up processes as an explanation for patterns of deficits following sleep loss has been suggested [121]. This theory emphasizes the importance of use-dependent sleep occurring in localized neuronal groups to explain performance deficits. Thus, localized areas develop a heightened homeostatic sleep drive in response to *both* sleep loss and also to sustained use. Beyond a certain point, these local areas "fall asleep," and thus brain area-specific performance is impaired. The sustained use of a localized area may occur when a cognitive task is performed that loads heavily on that brain area. While generalized homeostatic sleep pressure builds across the whole brain as a function of sleep loss, localized homeostatic sleep drive is use-dependant. Thus, this theory offers a potential mechanism to explain the differences within individuals in terms of their performance deficits across different cognitive domains. It also has the potential to explain why performance across sleep deprivations studies is more degraded than during an equivalent accumulated sleep loss during sleep restriction. Presumably this is because sleep deprivation involves both accumulated wakefulness and greater local use of neuronal networks with repeated task performance. However, while this bottom-up theory provides a reasonable account of performance deficits witnessed in sleep deprivation and sleep restriction studies, as well as accounting for within-subjects variability in response to sleep loss, it is less clear how it can accommodate findings from sleep fragmentation research. In particular, the findings showing deficits following sleep fragmentation without substantial reductions in total sleep or extensions in total wake. It follows then that perhaps sleep fragmentation may cause cognitive performance deficits and physiological derangement through a different mechanistic pathway than total sleep deprivation or sleep restriction. The important component of this type of sleep loss may therefore be the fragmentation itself and the lack of sleep continuity, rather than reductions in sleep time per se.

It seems likely that there are aspects of both the waking period (in particular the length of prior wake and local use of neuronal networks) and the sleep period (especially sleep length and sleep continuity) that explain performance deficits and the restoration of function. However, more theoretical understanding of these different forms of sleep loss would be gained by comparing them together, in a single experiment.

Conclusion

This chapter has reviewed results from studies examining the impact of sleep deprivation, sleep restriction, and sleep fragmentation on healthy functioning. Limiting or disrupting sleep opportunities in adults has significant negative effects on cognitive performance, sleepiness, and neurophysiologic functioning. These findings are highly relevant in modern society, with sleep loss increasingly common in the general population, and where the ramifications of poor sleep extend into general safety, health, and well-being.

References

1. Patrick GT, Gilbert JA. On the effects of loss of sleep. Psychol Rev. 1896;3:469–83.
2. Pilcher JJ, Huffcutt AI. Effects of sleep deprivation on performance: a meta-analysis. Sleep. 1996; 19:318–26.
3. Dawson D, Reid K. Fatigue, alcohol and performance impairment. Nature. 1997;388:235.

4. Mitler M, Carskadon M, Czeisler C, Dement W, Dinges DF, Graeber RC. Catastrophes, sleep and public policy: consensus report. Sleep. 1988;11:100–9.
5. Horne JA, Reyner LA. Sleep related vehicle accidents. BMJ. 1995;310:565–7.
6. Durmer JS, Dinges DF. Neurocognitive consequences of sleep deprivation. Semin Neurol. 2005;25:117–29.
7. Franzen PL, Siegle GJ, Buysse DJ. Relationships between affect, vigilance, and sleepiness following sleep deprivation. J Sleep Res. 2008;17:34–41.
8. Thomas ML, Sing H, Belenky G, et al. Neural basis of alertness and cognitive performance impairments during sleepiness. I. Effects of 24 h of sleep deprivation on waking human brain activity. J Sleep Res. 2000;9:335–52.
9. Van Dongen HPA, Maislin G, Mullington JM, Dinges DF. The cumulative cost of additional wakefulness: dose–response effects on neurobehavioral functions and sleep physiology from chronic sleep restriction and total sleep deprivation. Sleep. 2003;26:117–26.
10. Duffy JF, Willson HJ, Wang W, Czeisler CA. Healthy older adults better tolerate sleep deprivation than young adults. J Am Geriatr Soc. 2009;57:1245–51.
11. Drake CL, Roehrs TA, Burduvali E, Bonahoom A, Rosekind M, Roth T. Effects of rapid versus slow accumulation of eight hours of sleep loss. Psychophysiology. 2001;38:979–87.
12. Borbély AA, Achermann P. Concepts and models of sleep regulation: an overview. J Sleep Res. 1992;1:63–79.
13. Carskadon M, Dement WC. Daytime sleepiness: quantification of a behavioral state. Neurosci Biobehav Rev. 1987;11:307–17.
14. Mitler M, Gujavarty KS, Browman CP. Maintenance of wakefulness test: a polysomnographic technique for evaluating treatment efficacy in patients with excessive somnolence. Electroencephalogr Clin Neurophysiol. 1982;53:658–61.
15. Carskadon MA, Dement WC. Effects of total sleep loss on sleep tendency. Percept Mot Skills. 1979;48:495–506.
16. Dinges DF. Differential effects of prior wakefulness and circadian phase on nap sleep. Electroencephalogr Clin Neurophysiol. 1986;64:224–7.
17. Akerstedt T. Sleep/wake disturbances in working life. Electroencephalogr Clin Neurophysiol Suppl. 1987;39:360–3.
18. Torsvall L, Akerstedt T. Sleepiness on the job: continuously measured EEG changes in Train drivers. Electroencephalogr Clin Neurophysiol. 1987;66:502–11.
19. Kribbs NB, Dinges DF. Vigilance decrements and sleepiness. In: Harsh JR, Ogilvie RD, editors. Sleep onset mechanisms. Washington, DC: American Psychological Association; 1994. p. 113–25.
20. Jugovac D, Cavallero C. Twenty-four hours of total sleep deprivation selectively impairs attentional networks. Exp Psychol. 2012;59:115–23.
21. Martella D, Casagrande M, Lupianex J. Alerting, orienting and executive control: the effects of sleep deprivation on attentional networks. Exp Brain Res. 2011;210:81–9.
22. Babkoff H, Caspy T, Mikulincer M. Subjective sleepiness ratings: the effects of sleep deprivation, circadian rhythmicity and cognitive performance. Sleep. 1991;14:534–9.
23. Doran SM, Van Dongen HPA, Dinges DF. Sustained attention performance during sleep deprivation: evidence of state instability. Arch Ital Biol. 2001;139:253–67.
24. Lim J, Dinges DF. Sleep deprivation and vigilant attention. Ann N Y Acad Sci. 2008;1129:305–22.
25. Turner TH, Drummond SPA, Salamat JS, Brown GG. Effects of 42 hr of total sleep deprivation on component processes of verbal working memory. Neuropsychology. 2007;21:787–95.
26. Lamond N, Dawson D. Quantifying the performance impairment associated with fatigue. J Sleep Res. 1999;8:255–62.
27. Mullaney DJ, Kripke DF, Fleck PA, Johnson LC. Sleep loss and nap effects on sustained continuous performance. Psychophysiology. 1983;20:643–51.
28. Harrison Y, Horne JA. Sleep loss impairs short and novel language tasks having a prefrontal focus. J Sleep Res. 1998;7:95–100.
29. Harrison Y, Horne JA. One night of sleep loss impairs innovative thinking and flexible decision making. Organ Behav Hum Decis Process. 1999;78:128–45.
30. Horne JA. Sleep loss and `divergent' thinking ability. Sleep. 1988;11:528–36.
31. McKenna BS, Dickinson DL, Orff HJ, Drummond SP. The effects of one night of sleep deprivation on known-risk and ambiguous-risk decisions. J Sleep Res. 2007;16:245–52.
32. Horne JA. Sleep loss and divergent thinking ability. Sleep. 1998;11:528–36.
33. Wimmer F, Hoffman RF, Bonato RA, Moffitt AR. The effects of sleep deprivation on divergent thinking and attention processes. J Sleep Res. 1992;1:223–30.
34. Harrison Y, Horne JA. Sleep deprivation affects speech. Sleep. 1997;20:871–7.
35. Harrison Y, Horne JA. Sleep loss and temporal memory. Q J Exp Psychol. 2000;53a:271–9.
36. Banderet LE, Stokes JW, Francesconi R, Kowal DM, Naitoh P. Artillery teams in simulated sustained combat: performance and other measures. In: Johnson LC, Tepas DJ, Colguhon WP, Colligan MJ, editors. Biological rhythms, sleep and shift work. New York: Spectrum; 1981. p. 459–77.
37. Newhouse P, Belenky G, Thomas M, Thorne D, Sing H, Fertig J. The effects of d-amphetamine on arousal, cognition, and mood after prolonged total sleep deprivation. Neuropsychopharmacology. 1989;2:153–64.

38. Angus RG, Heslegrave RJ. Effects of sleep loss on sustained cognitive performance during a command and control simulation. Behav Res Methods Instrum Comput. 1985;17:55–67.
39. Monk TH, Carrier J. Speed of mental processing in the middle of the night. Sleep. 1997;20:399–401.
40. Horne JA, Pettitt AN. High incentive effects on vigilance performance during 72 hours total sleep deprivation. Acta Psychol (Amst). 1985;58:123–39.
41. Koslowsky M, Babkoff H. Meta-analysis of the relationship between total sleep deprivation and performance. Chronobiol Int. 1992;9:132–6.
42. Dorrian J, Rogers NL, Dinges DF. Psychomotor vigilance performance: a neurocognitive assay sensitive to sleep loss. In: Kushida CA, editor. Sleep deprivation. New York: Marcel Dekker; 2005.
43. Van Dongen HPA, Baynard MD, Maislin G, Dinges DF. Systematic interindividual differences in neurobehavioral impairment to sleep loss: evidence of a trait-like differential vulnerability. Sleep. 2004; 27:423–33.
44. Zohar D, Tzischinsky O, Epstein R, Lavie P. The effects of sleep loss on medical residents' emotional reactions to work events: a cognitive energy model. Sleep. 2005;28:47–54.
45. Talbot LS, McGlinchey EL, Kaplan KA, Dahl RE, Harvey AG. Sleep deprivation in adolescents and adults: changes in affect. Emotion. 2010;10:831–41.
46. Giesbrecht T, Smeets T, Leppink J, Jelicic M, Merckelbach H. Acute dissociation after 1 night of sleep loss. J Abnorm Psychol. 2007;116:599–606.
47. Dinges DF, Pack F, Williams K, et al. Cumulative sleepiness, mood disturbance, and psychomotor vigilance performance decrements during a week of sleep restricted to 4–5 hours per night. Sleep. 1997;20:267–77.
48. Haack M, Mullington JM. Sustained sleep restriction reduces emotional and physical well-being. Pain. 2005;119:56–64.
49. Roman V, Walstra I, Luiten PG, et al. Too little sleep gradually desensitizes the serotonin 1A receptor system. Sleep. 2005;28(12):1505–10.
50. Minkel JD, Banks S, Htaik O, et al. Sleep deprivation and stressors: evidence for elevated negative affect in response to mild stressors when sleep deprived. Emotion. 2012;12:1015–20.
51. Chee MW, Choo WC. Functional imaging of working memory after 24 hr of total sleep deprivation. J Neurosci. 2004;24:4560–7.
52. Thomas ML, Sing H, Belenky G, et al. Neural basis of alertness and cognitive performance impairments during sleepiness. II. Effects of 48 and 72 h of sleep deprivation on waking human brain activity. Thalamus Related Systems. 2003;2:199–229.
53. Petiau C, Harrison Y, Delfiore G, et al. Modification of fronto-temporal connectivity during a verb generation task after 30 hour total sleep deprivation. A PET study. J Sleep Res. 1998;7:208.
54. Drummond SPA, Brown GG, Gillin JC, Stricker JL, Wong EC, Buxton RB. Altered brain response to verbal learning following sleep deprivation. Nature. 2000;403:655–7.
55. Cajochen C, Foy R, Dijk D-J. Frontal predominance of a relative increase in sleep delta and theta EEG activity after sleep loss in humans. Sleep Res Online. 2000;2:65–9.
56. Wu JC, Gillin JC, Buchsbaum MS, et al. The effect of sleep deprivation on cerebral glucose metabolic rate in normal humans assessed with positron emission tomography. Sleep. 1991;14:155–62.
57. Drummond SPA, Brown GG, Stricker JL, Buxton RB, Wong EC, Gillin JC. Sleep deprivation-induced reduction in cortical functional response to serial subtraction. Neuroreport. 1999;10:3745–8.
58. Dahl RE, Lewin DS. Pathways to adolescent sleep and behaviour. J Adolesc Health. 2002;31:175–84.
59. Gailliot MT, Baumeister RF, DeWall CN, et al. Self-control relies on glucose as a limited energy source: willpower is more than a metaphor. J Pers Soc Psychol. 2007;92:325–36.
60. Masicampo E, Baumeister R. Toward a physiology of dual-process reasoning and judgment: lemonade, willpower and expensive rule-based analysis. Psychol Sci. 2008;19:255–60.
61. Yoo SS, Gujar N, Hu P, Jolesz FA, Walker MP. The human emotional brain without sleep—a prefrontal amygdala disconnect. Curr Biol. 2007;17:877–8.
62. Davidson RJ. Anxiety and affective style: role of prefrontal cortex and amygdala. Biol Psychiatry. 2002;51:68–80.
63. Phelps EA, Delgado MR, Nearing KI, LeDoux JE. Extinction learning in humans: role of the amygdala and vmPFC. Neuron. 2004;43:897–905.
64. Miller EK. The prefrontal cortex and cognitive control. Nat Rev Neurosci. 2000;1:59–65.
65. Smith ME, McEvoy LK, Gevins A. The impact of moderate sleep loss on neurophysiologic signals during working memory task performance. Sleep. 2002;25:784–94.
66. Saper CB, Cano G, Scammell TE. Homeostatic, circadian, and emotional regulation of sleep. J Comp Neurol. 2005;493:92–8.
67. Williams HL, Lubin A, Goodnow JJ. Impaired performance with acute sleep loss. Psychol Monogr. 1959;73:1–26.
68. Guzman-Marin R, McGinty D. Sleep deprivation suppresses adult neurogenesis: clues to the role of sleep in brain plasticity. Sleep Biol Rhythms. 2006;4:27–34.
69. National Sleep Foundation. Sleep in America poll. Washington: National Sleep Foundation; 2002.
70. Colton HR, Altevogt BM. Sleep disorders and sleep deprivation: an unmet public health problem. Washington: National Academies Press; 2006.
71. Monk TH. Shift work: basic principles. In: Kryger MH, Roth T, Dement WC, editors. Principles and practice of sleep medicine. 4th ed. Philadelphia: Elsevier/Saunders; 2005.
72. National Sleep Foundation. Sleep in America poll. Washington: National Sleep Foundation; 2005.

73. Kripke DF, Garfinkel L, Wingard D, Klauber MR, Marler MR. Mortality associated with sleep duration and insomnia. Arch Gen Psychiatry. 2002;59:131–6.
74. Webb WB, Agnew HW. The effects of chronic limitation of sleep length. Psychophysiology. 1974;11:265–74.
75. Friedmann J, Globus G, Huntley A, Mullaney D, Naitoh P, Johnson L. Performance and mood during and after gradual sleep reduction. Psychophysiology. 1977;14:245–50.
76. Banks S, Dinges DF. Behavioral and physiological consequences of sleep restriction in humans. J Clin Sleep Med. 2010;3:519–28.
77. Vgontaz AN, Zoumakis E, Bixler EO, et al. Adverse effects of modest sleep restriction on sleepiness, performance and inflammatory cytokines. J Clin Endocrinol Metab. 2004;89:2119–26.
78. Carskadon MA, Dement WC. Cumulative effects of sleep restriction on daytime sleepiness. Psychophysiology. 1981;18:107–13.
79. Belenky G, Wesensten NJ, Thorne DR, et al. Patterns of performance degradation and restoration during sleep restriction and subsequent recovery: a sleep dose–response study. J Sleep Res. 2003;12:1–12.
80. Dinges DF, Rogers NL, Baynard MB. Chronic sleep deprivation. In: Kryger MH, Roth T, Dement WC, editors. Principles and practice of sleep medicine. 4th ed. PA: W.B. Saunders Company; 2004.
81. Mollicone DJ, Van Dongen HPA, Rogers NL, Banks S, Dinges DF. Time of day effects on neurobehavioral performance during chronic sleep restriction. Aviat Space Environ Med. 2010;81:735–44.
82. Dinges DF. Sleep debt and scientific evidence. Sleep. 2004;7:1–3.
83. Roehrs T, Timms V, Zwyghuizen-Doorenbos A, Roth T. Sleep extension in sleepy and alert normal. Sleep. 1989;12:449–57.
84. Guilleminault C, Powell NB, Martinez S, et al. Preliminary observations on the effects of sleep time in a sleep restriction paradigm. Sleep Med. 2003;4:177–84.
85. Brunner DP, Dijk DJ, Borbély AA. Repeated partial sleep deprivation progressively changes in EEG during sleep and wakefulness. Sleep. 1993;16:100–13.
86. Banks S, Dinges DF. Behavioral and physiological consequences of sleep restriction in humans. J Clin Sleep Med. 2007;3:519–28.
87. Spiegel K, Leproult R, Van Cauter E. Impact of sleep debt on metabolic and endocrine function. Lancet. 1999;354:1435–9.
88. Rogers NL, Szuba MP, Staab JP, Evans DL, Dinges DF. Neuroimmunologic aspects of sleep and sleep loss. Semin Clin Neuropsychiatry. 2001;6:295–307.
89. Irwin M, Mascovich A, Gillin JC, et al. Partial sleep deprivation reduces natural killer cell activity in humans. Psychosom Med. 1994;56:493–8.
90. Reynolds AC, Dorrian J, Liu PY, et al. Impact of five nights of sleep restriction on glucose metabolism, leptin and testosterone in young adult men. PLoS One. 2012;7:e41218.
91. Tockikubo O, Ikeda A, Miyajima E, Ishii M. Effects of insufficient sleep on blood pressure monitored by a new multibiomedical recorder. Hypertension. 1996;27:1318–24.
92. Kato M, Phillips BG, Sigurdsson G, Narkiewicz K, Pesek CA, Somers VK. Effects of sleep deprivation on neural circulatory control. Hypertension. 2000;35:1173–5.
93. Mullington JM, Haack M, Toth M, Serrador JM, Meier-Ewert HK. Cardiovascular, inflammatory, and metabolic consequences of sleep deprivation. Progr Cardiovasc Dis. 2009;51:294–302.
94. Redwine L, Hauger RL, Gillin JC, et al. Effects of sleep and sleep deprivation in interlukin-6, growth hormone, cortisol, and melatonin levels in humans. J Clin Endocrinol Metab. 2000;85:3579–603.
95. Shearer WT, Reuben JM, Mullington M, et al. Soluble TNF-alpha receptor 1 and IL-6 plasma levels in humans subjected to the sleep deprivation model of space flight. J Allergy Clin Immunol. 2001;107:165–70.
96. Spiegel K, Leproult R, L'Hermite-Baleriaux M, Copinschi G, Penev PD, Van Cauter E. Leptin levels are dependent on sleep duration: relationships with sympathovagal balance, carbohydrate regulation, cortisol and thyrotropin. J Clin Endocrinol Metab. 2004;89:5762–71.
97. Spiegel K, Knutson K, Leproult R, Tasali E, Van Cauter E. Sleep loss: a novel risk factor for insulin resistance and Type 2 diabetes. J Appl Physiol. 2005;99:2008–19.
98. Hairston IS, Little MT, Scanlon MD, et al. Sleep restriction suppresses neurogenesis induced by hippocampus-dependent learning. J Neurophysiol. 2005;94:4224–33.
99. Taheri S, Lin L, Austin D, Young T, Mignot E. Short sleep duration is associated with reduced leptin, elevated ghrelin, and increased body mass index. PLoS Med. 2004;1:e62.
100. Gangwisch JE, Malaspina D, Boden-Albala B, Heymsfield SB. Inadequate sleep as a risk factor for obesity: analyses of the NHANES I. Sleep. 2005;28:1289–96.
101. Killick BS, Lui P. Implications of sleep restriction and recovery on metabolic outcomes. J Clin Endocrinol Metab. 2012;97:3876–90.
102. Stepanski EJ. The effect of sleep fragmentation on daytime function. Sleep. 2002;25:268–76.
103. Stepanski EJ, Lamphere J, Roehrs T, Zorick F, Roth T. Experimental sleep fragmentation in normal subjects. Int J Neurosci. 1987;33:207–14.
104. Bonnet MH. Performance and sleepiness as a function of frequency and placement of sleep disruption. Psychophysiology. 1986;23:263–71.
105. Bonnet MH. Sleep restoration as a function of periodic awakening, movement, or electroencephalographic change. Sleep. 1987;10:364–73.
106. Bonnet MH, Berry RB, Arand DL. Metabolism during normal, fragmented, and recovery sleep. J Appl Physiol. 1991;71:1112–8.

107. Bonnet MH. Effect of sleep disruption on sleep, performance, and mood. Sleep. 1985;8:11–9.
108. Martin SE, Engleman HM, Deary IJ, Douglas NJ. The effect of sleep fragmentation on daytime function. Am J Respir Crit Care Med. 1996; 153:1328–32.
109. Martin SE, Brander PE, Deary IJ, Douglas NJ. The effect of clustered versus regular sleep fragmentation on daytime function. J Sleep Res. 1999; 8:305–11.
110. Kingshott RN, Cosway RJ, Deary IJ, Douglas NJ. The effect of sleep fragmentation on cognitive processing using computerized topographic brain mapping. J Sleep Res. 2000;9:353–7.
111. Djonlagic I, Saboisky J, Carusona A, Stickgold R, Malhotra A. Increased sleep fragmentation leads to impaired off-line consolidation of motor memories in humans. PLoS One. 2012;7:e34106.
112. Downey R, Bonnet MH. Performance during frequent sleep disruption. Sleep. 1987;10:354–63.
113. Roehrs T, Merlotti L, Petrucelli N, Stepanski E, Roth T. Experimental sleep fragmentation. Sleep. 1994;17:438–43.
114. Stamatakis KA, Punjabi NM. Effects of sleep fragmentation on glucose metabolism in normal subjects. Chest. 2010;137:95–101.
115. McCoy JG, Tartar JL, Bebis AC, et al. Experimental sleep fragmentation impairs attentional set-shifting in rats. Sleep. 2007;30:52–60.
116. Carrington MJ, Trinder J. Blood pressure and heart rate during continuous experimental sleep fragmentation in healthy adults. Sleep. 2008;31:1701–12.
117. Ringler J, Basner RC, Shannon R, et al. Hypoxemia alone does not explain blood pressure elevations after obstructive apneas. J Appl Physiol. 1990; 69:2143–8.
118. Davies RJO, Belt PJ, Roberts SJ, Ali NJ, Stradling JR. Arterial blood pressure responses to graded transient arousal from sleep in normal humans. J Appl Physiol. 1993;74:1123–30.
119. Morrell MJ, Finn L, Kim H, Peppard PE, Badr MS, Young T. Sleep fragmentation, awake blood pressure and sleep-disordered breathing in a population-based study. Am J Respir Crit Care Med. 2000;162:2091–6.
120. Horne A. Why we sleep: the functions of sleep in humans and other animals. Oxford: Oxford University Press; 1988.
121. Van Dongen HPA, Belenky G, Krueger JM. A local, bottom-up perspective on sleep deprivation and neurobehavioral performance. Curr Top Med Chem. 2011;11:2414–22.

Methods for Human Sleep Deprivation Experiments

3

Elizabeth B. Klerman and Matt T. Bianchi

Introduction

Experimentally imposed sleep loss is an important method used to determine the effects of sleep on multiple physiological processes. The two most common approaches, sleep deprivation and sleep restriction, both involve altering the amount of sleep obtained relative to the amount of wake. In sleep deprivation protocols, the goal is to maintain wakefulness continually throughout a period of time that would usually involve sleep. In sleep restriction protocols, sometimes termed partial sleep deprivation, a shortened sleep opportunity is imposed over multiple nights. Because the time course of sleep loss differs between the two approaches, their effects may differ on subjective and objective measures of performance and sleepiness and other physiological measures. Each technique has practical relevance in operational and clinical settings.

Since sleep exerts a strong influence on multiple physiological processes (e.g., endocrine, cardiovascular, immune) and since each of these processes is also affected by other factors, including circadian rhythms, pharmaceuticals, age, medical conditions, and general health, the experimental methods should consider those factors to allow appropriate interpretation of results. Here we review common techniques involved in human sleep loss experiments performed in the inpatient setting and considerations for interpreting their results.

E.B. Klerman, M.D., Ph.D.
Division of Sleep Medicine, Department of Medicine, Brigham and Women's Hospital, Harvard Medical School, Boston, MA, USA

M.T. Bianchi, M.D., Ph.D., M.M.Sc. (✉)
Division of Sleep Medicine, Department of Neurology, Massachusetts General Hospital, Boston, MA, USA
e-mail: mtbianchi@partners.org

Concept of Sleep Homeostasis

One purpose of sleep deprivation and sleep restriction protocols is to evaluate the effects of altered sleep homeostasis or increased sleep pressure on the variable(s) of interest. Therefore, a quantifiable measure of sleep homeostasis or pressure is required to document that the experimental manipulation has resulted in an altered state. The major assumption underlying the concept of sleep homeostasis is that the duration or stage composition of sleep is regulated by the duration of prior wakefulness: there is a positive relationship between amount of wake and the accumulation of sleep pressure or drive. This homeostatic mechanism reacts to both recent (e.g., length of prior wake immediately prior to the sleep episode) and longer term (e.g., amount of wake and sleep over preceding days or weeks) sleep-wake history relative to the individual's sleep "need" [1]. Any proposed marker of sleep homeostasis would be expected to increase with increasing wake duration and decrease during sleep. Markers of homeostasis have been proposed

M.T. Bianchi (ed.), *Sleep Deprivation and Disease: Effects on the Body, Brain and Behavior*, DOI 10.1007/978-1-4614-9087-6_3, with respect to sleep deprivation, but there are no accepted markers for chronic sleep restriction, which has different time course of effects on performance than sleep deprivation [1].

Current metrics that can be quantified after the individual is asleep relative to immediate prior wake duration (i.e., sleep deprivation) are: Slow Wave Sleep (NREM Sleep Stages 3 and 4 in the Rechtschaffen and Kales scoring system and N3 in the current American Academy of Sleep Medicine system), delta (~0.5–4.5 Hz) power in the EEG during NREM sleep and sleep latency. Note that in the literature, sleep onset latency may have multiple definitions (e.g., first epoch of any stage, first epoch of a block of three or more consecutive epochs of any stage, etc.). During wake, theta/low frequency alpha (TLFA, 5.5–9 Hz) power in the EEG during the Karolinska Drowsiness Test (KDT) and slow eye movemetns (SEMs) during wake have been proposed a marker of homeostasis [2, 3]. Markers of sleep homeostasis/drive that can be obtained when the individual is awake are particularly useful in circumstances when there are problems with sleep (such as insomnia) and/or under conditions in which measuring homeostatic sleep pressure is required during times when sleep should not be occurring (e.g., when the individual is at work).

Methods

Participant Selection and Preparation

One of the most important considerations in human protocols involves inclusion and exclusion criteria. The participant population should be uniform in certain important characteristics, especially with regard to factors known to influence sleep and/or performance, including caffeine and alcohol use. This is particularly important given the presence of inter-individual differences as well as variance in physiological measurements and performance outcomes. Special consideration should be made to whether the participants have undiagnosed sleep disorders or other conditions (e.g., pain) or medications that may interfere with sleep. Undiagnosed sleep disorders can be particularly challenging, since occult presence of sleep disordered breathing or periodic limb movements of sleep may not cause symptoms of which the participant is aware, but nevertheless may affect the experimental results. A thorough medical history and exam is important, including all medical conditions and prescription drug dosage and use. Objective testing for sleep disorders should be strongly considered; for example, even rigorously screened asymptomatic low-risk individuals may have sleep apnea on formal testing [4].

The history should include documentation of over-the-counter medications and supplements, illegal drugs, caffeine, tobacco, and alcohol use. All of these may affect sleep and wake obtained at home and may cause withdrawal symptoms if not used or allowed during inpatient study procedures. The history may be supplemented by objective serological and/or urine testing for substances.

The amount and timing of sleep obtained at home in the 1–2 weeks before the study starts is important to at least record and potentially regulate. For example, it is critical to know if participants have traveled across time zones in the past few months, recently stayed awake late or all night, worked rotating or night shifts, or had an irregular sleep-wake schedule. These issues have practical implications for experimental design and interpretation: if participants have not obtained enough sleep at home before the experimentally imposed sleep loss begins, they may already be sleep-deprived in a manner that might impact both baseline measurements in the study and their response to the intervention. In addition, if individual participants enter the experimental portion of the study with undocumented and uncontrolled prior sleep patterns, this could confound their responses in the experimental portion. Pre-study conditions of a regular ~ 8 h nightly sleep schedule with no use of substances that may affect sleep (unless required for health/medical reasons, allowed under exclusion criteria, and included in the experimental documentation) for at least 2 weeks are recommended to mitigate the above concerns. Verification measures are strongly encouraged in addition to sleep-wake diaries. Examples include wrist actigraphy and/or call-ins to a time-stamped recorder at the time of going to bed and awakening.

A psychological screening should be performed and individuals with a history of psychiatric disorders or with immediate family members affected by these disorders should be identified. Specifically, a personal history of adverse reaction to sleep deprivation (e.g., mania or psychiatric instability) should have additional consideration before admission to an inpatient sleep protocol involving deprivation. Finally, the potential occurrence of recent events (e.g., death of a family member or friend) that might affect the individual's physical and/or psychological state should be queried.

Of extreme importance is thorough discussion with the potential participant of the expected events and conditions. If possible, the potential participant should visit the facility. Thorough familiarity with the protocol is expected to reduce stress from unknown and unexpected (and potentially unnatural) situations of the study. For example, experimental settings that prohibit use of internet or phone, or live TV/radio, for multiple days may be challenging to those accustomed to daily media availability. As part of the enrollment and consent process, members of our research team ask potential participants during the screening process to describe to us, after the protocol is explained to them, what they believe is involved in the study; this is an additional opportunity to ensure that the participant understands the study requirements and conditions, which is a critical aspect of required informed consent regulations.

Experimental Conditions

The experimental conditions should include appropriate equipment for monitoring the desired physiology and allow the study procedure of sleep loss to occur without undesired interference such as uncontrolled noise or extraneous light. A diversity of monitoring resources is preferred, as measurements may span bio-sampling (blood, saliva, urine), moderately invasive (e.g., rectal thermistor) and noninvasive (e.g., EEG) sleep-wake physiology, and cognitive performance or other psychological testing.

Although individual experimental protocols may require different degrees of specialization, we describe as an example our inpatient facility at the Brigham and Women's Hospital. This center, supported as a NIH Clinical Translational Science Center (CTSC), enables study of multiple physiological functions concurrently. A highly skilled nursing and technical staff with documented standard operating procedures and ongoing training is present. Related facilities, including a clinical centrifuge, a cold room for special handling of blood following collection, ultrasound and other imaging resources, and metabolic kitchens for preparation of required measured diets for the study volunteers, are nearby. Each experimental room is private, sound-proof, light-proof, and has an ante-room and bathroom with shower. The ante-room lowers the risk of outside noise or light affecting the room in which the participant is living. Private rooms decrease inter-participant interaction that may affect measures of interest (e.g., performance testing, mood, sleep timing and content). Almost all studies are conducted under time-free conditions, such that the participant does not know the current time or day, since knowledge of time of day or time elapsed may influence the subjective measures under study. The staff is trained to not speak of anything time-related or the timing of events during the protocol, as well as not to discuss potentially emotional issues (e.g., politics, certain sports teams). Watches, mobile phones, computers, and visitors are not allowed. The control room includes, for each experimental suite, video monitoring equipment, intercom, one computer for polysomnographic (PSG) recordings, one for monitoring computerized performance testing, and one to study schedule event prompting and monitoring. For all protocols, an investigator can have the following information available online during the study and for analysis after each experiment is complete: precise actual timing of events and of specimen collection; core body and skin temperature data; room temperature data; light levels in suites minute by minute; data from computerized performance and alertness tests; and continuous recording of EEG, EOG, EMG, ECG, heart rate, O_2 saturation, and respiratory effort.

The hardware and software for this facility form a single-source data collection system: all experimental events (e.g., time of actual rather than scheduled time of blood samples, light levels, start/end of sleep episodes), temperature data, and results of performance tests are stored on a single computer system that meets data security and integrity guidelines. In addition, external equipment (e.g., PSG recorders) is synchronized with this system at the start of every recording, so that the timing of the recordings matches that of the system. Timing of events (e.g., specimen collection, meal presentation, other events) is entered by event marker equipment inside and outside each suite. For quality assurance, technicians must "sign off" with their personal identification on all procedures (e.g., blood sample, meal administration) that they have conducted. All data stored on this system are by de-identified study code, rather than participant name or other identifiers.

For neurocognitive testing, both simple and complex tasks that assess different functions are included and new neurobehavioral tasks can be programmed and added as needed. After every sleep episode, participants complete a questionnaire in which they indicate their estimates of time to fall asleep (sleep latency), number of awakenings during the sleep episode, total amount of wake before the end of each sleep episode, and total amount of sleep obtained in each sleep opportunity. These subjective estimates, which are frequently used in clinical PSG assessments as well as in outpatient research field studies, can be compared with objective measures of sleep obtained from scored PSG data. Note that numerous studies have documented mismatch between objective and subjective measurements of these sleep-wake variables [5, 6]. Self-assessment of performance questionnaires may also be useful for comparison with objective performance measures. Both subjective and objective measures are monitored because they assess different aspects of vulnerability to circadian and sleep homeostatic influences [7–9], including sleep inertia.

Sleep PSG recordings should be conducted and scored using standardized accepted measures, such as those approved by the American Academy of Sleep Medicine [10] by trained scorers blind to study interventions. Waking PSGs may also be useful; the waking EEG has been shown to have homeostatic sleep and circadian components [11]. For example, waking EEG activity can be assessed using the KDT. In the KDT, participants sit quietly and fix their gaze for 5 consecutive minutes (4 min eyes open followed by 1 min of eyes closed) allowing for the intermittent recording of short bouts of uncontaminated EEG at specified times within longer periods of sustained wakefulness during a study. Spectral analyses or other signal processing of the EEG can then be conducted. The waking PSG recordings are also used to monitor whether any unintentional sleep occurred during scheduled wake episodes. The EOG can be recorded for the assessment of slow eye movements (SEMs) [3], another measure of sleep homeostasis.

Actigraphy

Activity and light-measuring devices (i.e., "actigraphy") should be worn by all participants during at least the week before inpatient portion of the protocols begin to confirm compliance with outpatient protocol instructions. Actigraphy data should be downloaded and reviewed at least weekly with the participant during screening to improve compliance. Actigraphy can also be worn during the inpatient portion of the protocol for comparison of data under known activity and light conditions. Light data and either raw activity data or activity data scored into Sleep or Wake from validated algorithms [12–16] also can be used for further analyses.

Temperature Recordings, Blood Samples, Urine Samples, and Saliva Samples: For Circadian-based Analyses

Core body temperature (CBT) is commonly measured as a surrogate for circadian phase under specific inpatient conditions and can be continuously monitored by means of a rectal thermistor; ambulatory outpatient or inpatient CBT is not an appropriate circadian phase marker [17]. Participants typically have no trouble tolerating this approach to CBT. Skin temperature, by contrast, has not been proven to be an accurate measure of circadian phase.

In protocols that require frequent blood sampling, placement of an indwelling intravenous (IV) line can facilitate sampling during wake and sleep episodes. The IV setup allows for blood sampling from within or outside the room, so that blood sampling during sleep episodes does not disturb the participant. The exact time the blood sample is collected (rather than the scheduled time) should be recorded. This is extremely important for studies involving hormones whose secretion varies in a circadian and/or pulsatile manner.

Urine samples can be collected approximately every 2–3 h while the participant is awake, before and after sleep episodes, and after spontaneous voids. Saliva can be collected by having the participant spit into a test tube. The exact time the sample is collected (rather than the scheduled time) should be noted.

Sleep Deprivation and Sleep Restriction Protocols

Sleep deprivation and sleep restriction can be conducted in different ways, each of which may affect both experimental results and inferences made about the impact of sleep on functional outcomes. For example, the choice of timing of the habitual sleep and sleep deprivation/restriction are important. The timing of baseline (presleep loss intervention) sleep episodes should be relative to the individuals' habitual sleep time. If an individual's habitual sleep times (as established during the 1–2 weeks prior to the inpatient study, as recommended above) are 2–10 am, then an experimentally imposed sleep episode beginning at 10 pm will likely have a marked sleep latency simply because it differs so greatly from the habitual sleep pattern and therefore may not be appropriate as "baseline" for comparison conditions. For sleep restriction methods, consider whether to start the sleep episode late, end the sleep episode early or both, depending on the importance of the pattern of light exposure, sleep latency, and other factors affected.

During the "extra" wake time associated with sleep deprivation/restriction protocols, the environment and activities should be considered. The light levels in the room and from electronic devices should be relatively low, so as to not shift the circadian pacemaker [18, 19]. Interaction with other individuals or entertainment media should be relatively stress-free. For example, we recommend no intense discussions and only G-, PG-, or PG13-rated movies, TV shows, or games, since those with other ratings are designed to elicit strong emotions that may impact sleep and/or physiological measurements.

Protocols involving manipulation of selective sleep stages can provide insights into the relative importance of specific aspects of sleep. These require trained personnel to score the sleep stage in "real time" and then intervene when criteria are met (e.g., 1 epoch of N3 sleep). The possibility of false positives (i.e., intervention when the stage did not occur) or false negatives (i.e., lack of intervention when the stage did occur) should be accounted for when the sleep recording is rescored later. The choice of intervention (e.g., spoken participant name or gradual increase in noise level) should be considered, as the response to generic stimuli may differ from responses to "high-valence" stimuli (such as the participant's name or the sound of a baby crying). Also note that indirect effects of sleep perturbations may occur. For example, NREM sleep deprivation is often associated with substantial REM sleep deprivation since REM sleep tends to occur only after a NREM sleep. In addition, slow wave sleep (N3) deprivation may be accompanied by increases in stage N1, N2, and arousal index. Thus, it should consider that indirect effects may plausibly be causally related to conclusions attributed solely to the primary intervention.

Analysis Considerations

Consultation with a statistician is crucial given the diversity of measurements, longitudinal aspects, correlated data streams, and other considerations that impact study design and analysis. Careful consideration of these issues will ensure appropriate statistical power with the number of participants to be enrolled and the metrics to be collected. Immediately after each data set is collected, checking for errors, inconsistencies, missing data, and other potential questions should be performed to identify problems rapidly and implement changes if necessary. Performing such checks during the study, rather than waiting until the end of the study (after all participants have been enrolled), allows the opportunity to resolve any discovered issues and quickly implement necessary changes. Statistician involvement throughout the study, and after all primary data are collected and analyzed, is crucial to ensure that planned statistical tests are appropriate. Common errors are to apply statistics (e.g., mean and standard deviation) that assume a statistically normal (e.g., Gaussian) distribution inappropriately, such as to data (1) that do not fit that distribution or (2) with too few data points, or (3) that are not independent (e.g. multiple observations from each individual).

Conclusion

This chapter outlines suggestions for conducting sleep deprivation and restriction experiments in an inpatient experimental setting. Given the amount of time and resources required to conduct inpatient sleep experiments, it is critical to control for the many factors that may affect results to ensure that the obtained data are robust and reliable.

References

1. Cohen DA, Wang W, Wyatt JK, Kronauer RE, Dijk DJ, Czeisler CA, et al. Uncovering residual effects of chronic sleep loss on human performance. Sci Transl Med. 2010;2(14):14ra13.
2. Aeschbach D, Matthews JR, Postolache TT, Jackson MA, Giesen HA, Wehr TA. Dynamics of the human EEG during prolonged wakefulness: evidence for frequency-specific circadian and homeostatic influences. Neurosci Lett. 1997;239(2–3):121–4.
3. Cajochen C, Wyatt JK, Czeisler CA, Bonikowska M, Dijk DJ. Non-linear interaction between the circadian and homeostatic modulation of slow eye movements (SEMs) during wakefulness in humans. J Sleep Res. 2000;9:58.
4. Pavlova MK, Duffy JF, Shea SA. Polysomnographic respiratory abnormalities in asymptomatic individuals. Sleep. 2008;31(2):241–8.
5. Bianchi MT, Wang W, Klerman E. Sleep misperception in healthy adults: implications for insomnia diagnosis. J Clin Sleep Med. 2012;8(5):547–54.
6. Harvey AG, Tang NK. (Mis)perception of sleep in insomnia: a puzzle and a resolution. Psychol Bull. 2012;138(1):77–101.
7. Van Dongen HPA, Baynard MD, Maislin G, Dinges DF. Systematic interindividual differences in neurobehavioral impairment from sleep loss: evidence of trait-like differential vulnerability. Sleep. 2004;27:423–33.
8. Leproult R, Colecchia EF, Berardi AM, Stickgold R, Kosslyn SM, Van Cauter E. Individual differences in subjective and objective alertness during sleep deprivation are stable and unrelated. Am J Physiol Regul Integr Comp Physiol. 2003;284:R280–90.
9. Frey DJ, Badia P, Wright Jr KP. Inter- and intra-individual variability in performance near the circadian nadir during sleep deprivation. J Sleep Res. 2004;13(4):305–15.
10. Iber C, Ancoli-Israel S, Chesson A, Quan SF. The AASM manual for the scoring of sleep and associated events: rules, terminology and technical specifications, vol. 1. Westchester, IL: American Academy of Sleep Medicine; 2007.
11. Cajochen C, Wyatt JK, Czeisler CA, Dijk DJ. Separation of circadian and wake duration-dependent modulation of EEG activation during wakefulness. Neuroscience. 2002;114(4):1047–60.
12. Kunz MA. Estimation of sleep and wake from wrist actigraphy: a validation study using sleep and wake quantified from ambulatory polysomnography [dissertation]. Boston, MA: Boston University; 2004.
13. Kushida CA, Chang A, Gadkary C, Guilleminault C, Carrillo O, Dement WC. Comparison of actigraphic, polysomnographic, and subjective assessment of sleep parameters in sleep-disordered patients. Sleep Med. 2001;2:389–96.
14. Natale V, Plazzi G, Martoni M. Actigraphy in the assessment of insomnia: a quantitative approach. Sleep. 2009;32(6):767–71.
15. Ancoli-Israel S, Cole R, Alessi C, Chambers M, Moorcroft W, Pollak CP. The role of actigraphy in the study of sleep and circadian rhythms. Sleep. 2003;26(3):342–92.
16. Stone KL, Ancoli-Israel S. Actigraphy. In: Kryger MH, Roth T, Dement WC, editors. Principles and practices of sleep medicine, vol. 5. Philadelphia, PA: Elsevier; 2010. p. 1668–75.
17. Klerman EB, Lee Y, Czeisler CA, Kronauer RE. Linear demasking techniques are unreliable for estimating the circadian phase of ambulatory temperature data. J Biol Rhythms. 1999;14(4):260–74.
18. Chang A, Aeschbach D, Duffy JF, Czeisler CA. Impact of evening use of light-emitting electronic readers on circadian timing and sleep latency. Sleep. 2012;35:A206.
19. Duffy JF, Czeisler CA. Effect of light on human circadian physiology. Sleep Med Clin. 2009;4:165–77.

Imaging Sleep and Sleep Deprivation

4

Thien Thanh Dang-Vu

Introduction

Earlier brain imaging studies of sleep resorted to positron emission tomography (PET) to characterize neural activity at the systems level during rapid-eye-movement (REM) sleep and non-REM (NREM) sleep [1, 2]. PET shows the regional distribution of compounds labeled with positron-emitting isotopes. The most frequently used in sleep research were oxygen-15-labeled water ($H_2{}^{15}O$), which is a marker of regional cerebral blood flow (rCBF), and 18-F fluorodeoxyglucose (^{18}FDG), a marker of regional brain glucose metabolism (cerebral metabolic rate of glucose, CMRGlu). PET studies allowed comparison of brain activity between REM sleep or NREM sleep and wakefulness. Functional magnetic resonance imaging (fMRI) was subsequently used to assess brain responses associated with phasic events within sleep stages [3, 4]. This technique, which relies on the measurement of the blood-oxygen-level-dependent (BOLD) signal, benefits from a better spatial and temporal resolution compared to PET, which allowed capturing the neural correlates of transient events such as NREM sleep oscillations. PET and fMRI studies identified brain responses underlying sleep stages and sleep oscillations in healthy volunteers, therefore bringing an essential contribution to sleep physiology.

Lack of sleep is highly prevalent in our modern societies, and bears many deleterious consequences. For instance, it is known that sleep deprivation constitutes one of the major causes of vehicle accidents [5, 6]. Sleep deprivation can be associated with specific disorders of sleep (e.g., sleep apnea, insomnia), psychological (e.g., anxiety), or medical conditions. But it can also be present in otherwise healthy populations, due to nightly exposure to noisy environments, irregular schedules associated with work shifts, or lack of sleep hygiene. Given the wide clinical impact of sleep deprivation, numerous studies attempted to describe its cognitive and behavioral effects. In this perspective, neuroimaging was used to report the alterations of brain function associated with the effects of experimentally induced sleep deprivation on waking performances. These studies, which mainly resorted to PET and fMRI, brought important insight into the neural mechanisms of (mis)adaptation to sleep deprivation.

The aim of this chapter is therefore to provide the reader with a brief overview of neuroimaging contribution to the physiology of sleep and sleep deprivation. The focus will be on neuroimaging studies conducted either during sleep or during wakefulness after sleep deprivation, in healthy volunteers. There is extensive literature on the relationships between sleep and memory

T.T. Dang-Vu, M.D., Ph.D. (✉)
Department of Exercise Science, Center for Studies in Behavioral Neurobiology, Concordia University, Montreal, QC, Canada
e-mail: tt.dangvu@concordia.ca

M.T. Bianchi (ed.), *Sleep Deprivation and Disease: Effects on the Body, Brain and Behavior*, DOI 10.1007/978-1-4614-9087-6_4, © Springer Science+Business Media New York 2014

consolidation, and the use of neuroimaging in this context, but this topic exceeds the scope of the present chapter. Several review articles provide comprehensive discussion on that topic [4, 7–10]. Finally, neither will we discuss the abundant literature about neuroimaging in specific disorders of sleep, which has been extensively reviewed elsewhere [11, 12].

Functional Neuroimaging of Sleep

Neuroimaging of Sleep Stages

PET studies compared CMRGlu or rCBF between NREM sleep or REM sleep and wakefulness.

NREM sleep consistently displayed decreased perfusion or metabolism in brainstem, thalamus, basal forebrain, basal ganglia, and cerebellum [2, 13–17]. At the cortical level, decreases were found in associative cortices, in particular in prefrontal and anterior cingulate cortex, as well as in the precuneus. Only one PET study found relative increases in glucose metabolism during NREM sleep, notably in the hippocampus [18]. Decreases of brain activity during NREM sleep were interpreted as reflecting the disengagement of structures involved in arousal and vigilance, and the homeostatic recovery of cortical areas that are the most active during wakefulness. Hippocampal recruitment during NREM sleep is in line with other studies suggesting a reprocessing and consolidation of declarative memories during this sleep stage [8, 19]. Early fMRI studies conducted during sleep confirmed the localized decreases in brain responses during NREM sleep compared to wakefulness [20, 21].

During REM sleep, both regional increases and decreases of brain activity were observed with PET [14, 22–25]. Increases of rCBF or CMRGlu were located in structures involved in REM sleep generation: pons, thalamus, and basal forebrain. In addition, increases were also observed in limbic structures (amygdala, hippocampus, anterior cingulate cortex) and in temporo-occipital cortex, possibly underlying the high emotional load and the predominantly visual content of dreams, respectively [26–28]. Decreases were noted in associative areas of the dorsolateral prefrontal cortex, posterior cingulate gyrus, precuneus, and inferior parietal cortex, possibly underlying essential characteristics of the dream report, such as the lack of insight, the temporo-spatial distortion, the inability to control the flow of events in dreams, and the amnesia at awakening [25].

Neuroimaging of Sleep Oscillations

Sleep stages are defined by spontaneous neural rhythms that organize sleep microarchitecture.

During NREM sleep, brain activity is shaped by coalescent brain oscillations, which were found to be produced by complex thalamo-cortical interactions in animals [29]. During lighter stages of NREM sleep (mostly stage N2), these brain waves consist of spindles, which are waxing-and-waning oscillations at a frequency of 11–15 Hz, and detectable on the human electroencephalogram (EEG). When NREM sleep deepens, spindles on the EEG are progressively replaced by large-amplitude (>75 μV) low-frequency (0.5–4 Hz) waves, which are termed slow waves or slow oscillations [30].

PET studies attempted to describe the neural correlates of these waves in humans, through simultaneous recordings of PET and EEG during sleep in healthy volunteers. While a direct assessment of brain activations associated with the occurrence of these waves was precluded by the limited temporal resolution of the technique, PET still allowed correlations of brain perfusion with measures of EEG spectral power (e.g., spectral power in the spindle frequency band as an indirect marker of spindle events). Using this method, a study reported a negative correlation between EEG spectral power in the spindle band (12–15Hz) and rCBF in the thalamus bilaterally [31]. Likewise, slow waves were also studied with PET by correlating rCBF with EEG power in the slow wave frequency band (slow wave activity, SWA; 1.5–4 Hz). Negative correlations were observed between SWA and rCBF mostly in the ventromedial prefrontal cortex, but also in the basal forebrain, putamen, insula, posterior cingulate gyrus, and precuneus [32]. These results indicated the prominently cortical nature of this rhythm, with initiation sites consistently located in frontal and insular cortices, in line with previous EEG studies [33–36]. It is important to emphasize the negative pattern of correlation found with both spindles and slow waves, which might suggest that these rhythms are produced as a result of localized decreases of brain activities. The explanation should however take into account the limited temporal resolution of PET, which averages rCBF values across the entire scanning time (>1 min). Given the alternation of neuronal hyperpolarization and depolarization phases occurring with sleep oscillations [29], this negative correlation might be due to a more prominent effect of hyperpolarization periods over depolarization phases on brain perfusion, therefore masking the intense neuronal discharges possibly underlying spindle and slow wave generation.

In order to address these limitations in the interpretation of findings, further functional neuroimaging studies resorted to fMRI simultaneously recorded with EEG during nighttime sleep in young healthy participants. Indeed, given its superior temporal (and spatial) resolution, fMRI allowed to directly study the brain activations associated with the occurrence of spindle and slow wave events during the first NREM sleep cycle. In these studies, sleep oscillations were automatically detected offline on EEG recordings after correction of artifacts induced by the scanner [37, 38]. Functional MRI analysis of sleep spindles then revealed the brain areas in which BOLD responses were consistently associated with detected spindle events compared to the baseline NREM sleep brain activity. Increased brain responses were associated with spindles in the thalamus, in agreement with thalamic involvement in spindle generation [39], as well as in the anterior cingulate cortex, insula, and superior temporal gyrus [40] (Fig. 4.1a). Likewise, fMRI studies of sleep identified neural structures consistently associated with detected slow waves above NREM sleep baseline activity. Enhanced BOLD responses were found with slow waves in the inferior and medial frontal gyrus, in line with the frontal predominance of slow waves, as well as in the parahippocampal gyrus, precuneus, posterior cingulate cortex, brainstem, and cerebellum [41] (Fig. 4.1b). Both fMRI studies demonstrated the persistence of phasic increases of brain activity during NREM sleep, beyond the baseline decrease found in previous studies of NREM sleep. In addition, these results highlighted the crucial brain areas involved in the generation of NREM sleep rhythms, and therefore in the induction and stabilization of NREM sleep. The recruitment of these networks during NREM sleep oscillations has important implications for the understanding of sleep functions. For instance, the activation of hippocampal and parahippocampal areas during NREM sleep oscillations provides further evidence for a role of sleep in memory consolidation, and the importance of sleep oscillations in this process [42].

A major behavioral criterion defining sleep is the lack of responsiveness to external stimulation. While it is commonly believed that the brain is isolated from the environment during sleep, there is some evidence for a persistence of neural responsiveness to stimuli such as sounds during sleep [43]. Recent fMRI studies further evaluated this question by studying the effects of NREM sleep oscillations on the processing of sounds during sleep. In these studies, young healthy volunteers were recorded with simultaneous EEG/fMRI during sleep, while pure tones ("beep") were randomly presented through headphones. Offline categorization of tones classified sounds according to their occurrence outside or within detected spindles. The study showed that tones presented during NREM sleep outside spindles activated the primary auditory cortex and thalamus, along with additional activations in the brainstem, cerebellum, middle frontal gyrus, precuneus, and posterior cingulate gyrus [44]. This observation confirmed the persistence of thalamo-cortical reactivity to external stimulation during NREM sleep. Importantly, the study found that sounds presented within spindles did not elicit any consistent activation in the thalamus and primary auditory cortex. Instead, only a small area in the brainstem (possibly including the nuclei of the lateral lemniscus) was activated with tones during spindles, which is in line with the concept

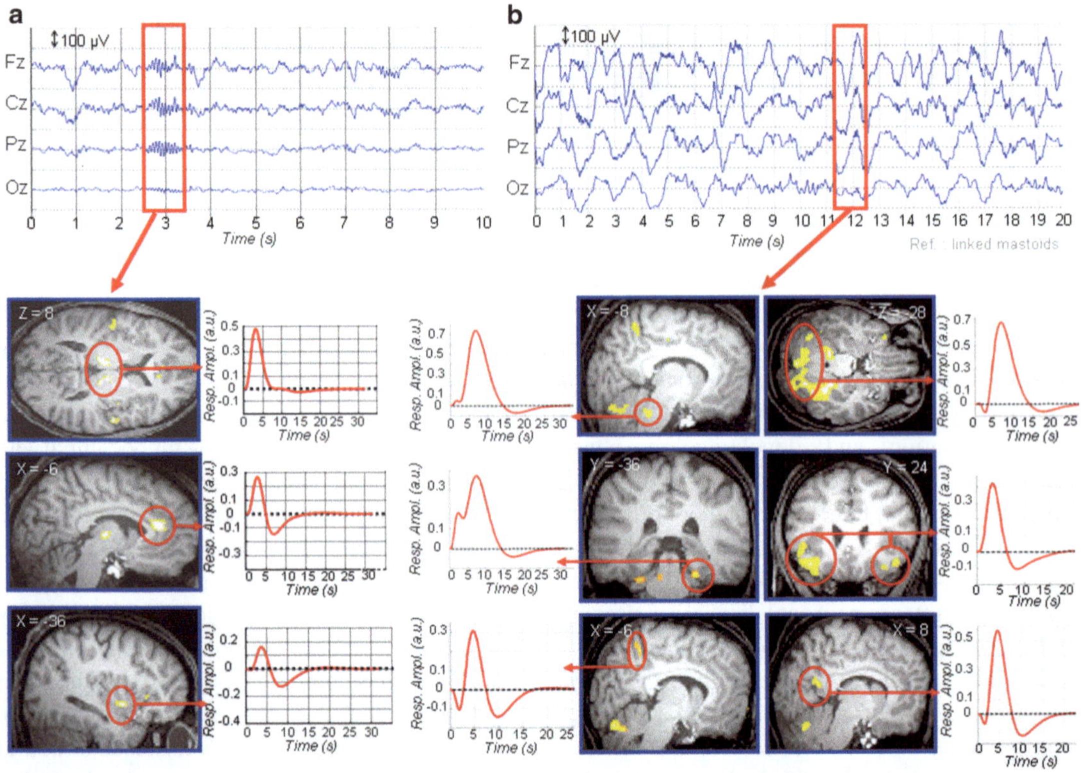

Fig. 4.1 Neural correlates of NREM sleep oscillations as evidenced by fMRI. (**a**) fMRI correlates of spindles. The *upper panel* shows a (stage 2) NREM sleep epoch depicting a typical spindle on scalp EEG recording. Brain activity is estimated for each detected spindle compared to the baseline brain activity of NREM sleep. The *lower left panels* show the significant brain responses associated with spindles ($P<0.05$, corrected for multiple comparisons on a volume of interest), including the thalamus, anterior cingulate cortex, and insula (from *top* to *bottom*) [40]. Functional results are displayed on an individual structural image (display at $P<0.001$, uncorrected), at different levels of the *x*, *y*, and *z* axes as indicated for each section. The *lower right panels* show the time course (in seconds) of fitted response amplitudes (in arbitrary units) during spindles in the corresponding *circled* brain area. All responses consist in regional increases of brain activity. (**b**) fMRI correlates of slow waves. The *upper panel* shows a (stage 4) NREM sleep epoch depicting typical slow waves on scalp EEG recording. Brain activity is estimated for each detected slow wave compared to the baseline brain activity of NREM sleep. The *lower panels* show the significant brain responses associated with slow waves ($P<0.05$, corrected for multiple comparisons on a volume of interest), including the brainstem, cerebellum, parahippocampal gyrus, inferior frontal gyrus, precuneus, and posterior cingulate gyrus (from *left* to *right* and *top* to *bottom*) [41]. Functional results are displayed on an individual structural image (display at $P<0.001$, uncorrected), at different levels of the *x*, *y*, and *z* axes as indicated for each section. The *lower side panels* show the time course (in seconds) of fitted response amplitudes (in arbitrary units) during slow wave in the corresponding *circled* brain area. All responses consist in regional increases of brain activity (reprinted from Dang-Vu [4] and adapted from Schabus [40] and Dang-Vu [41]. Copyright (2007, 2008) National Academy of Sciences, USA)

of a thalamic filtering of external information during sleep spindles (Fig. 4.2). By reducing the consistency of transmission of sensory information to the cortex, spindles contribute to isolate the cortex from the environment, therefore preserving sleep stability. The finding is in line with data showing that individuals with a higher density of spindles are less likely to be disturbed by various types of noises during NREM sleep compared to those with a lower spindle density [45]. Recent fMRI data also show that the phase of the slow wave affects the neural processing of sounds presented during NREM sleep [46]. Therefore brain oscillations not only shape brain activity patterns

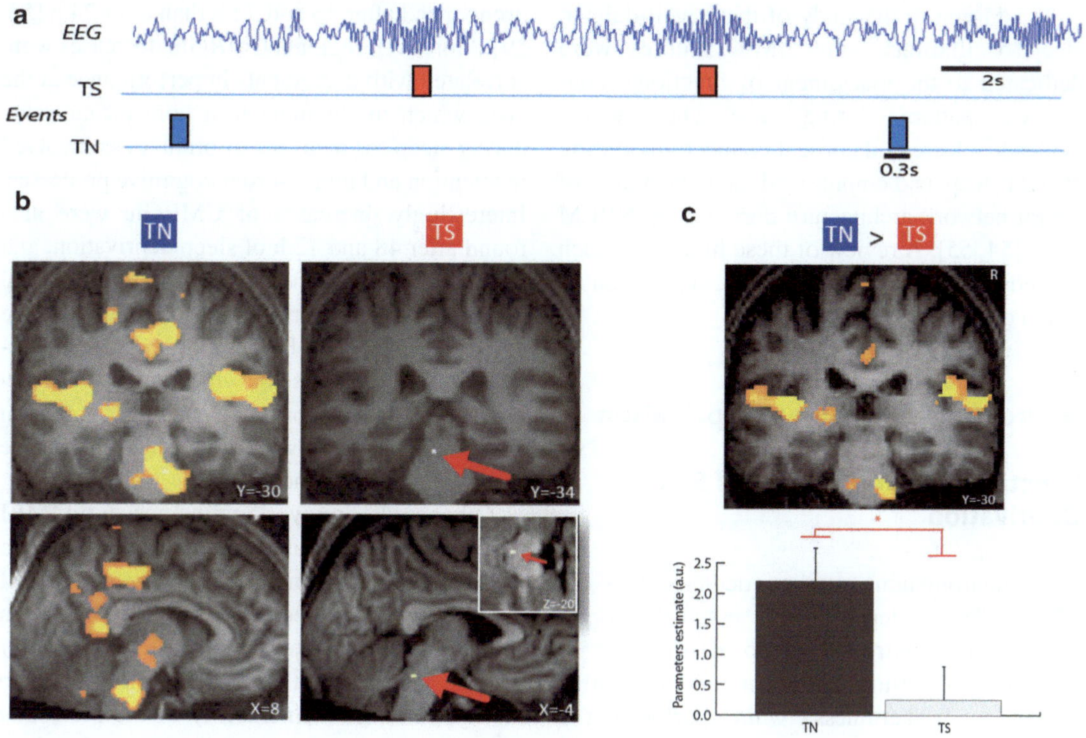

Fig. 4.2 Spindles and the processing of auditory information during NREM sleep. (**a**) Tones were categorized according to their occurrence during NREM sleep stages N2–N3 within spindles (TS, *red squares*) or outside spindles (TN, *blue squares*). (**b**) The *left panels* show the brain activations associated with tones presented during NREM sleep in the absence of spindles (TN), including the primary auditory cortex, thalamus, brainstem, cerebellum, precuneus, and posterior cingulate gyrus. The *right panels* show the brain activations associated with tones presented within spindles (TS), confined to a small area of the brainstem (see *arrow* and *inset*). Brain responses were significant at $P<0.05$, corrected for multiple comparisons on a volume of interest. (**c**) The *top panel* shows the brain responses significantly associated with TN, as compared to TS. The *bottom panel* shows the mean parameter estimates (arbitrary units ± SEM) for TN and TS in the primary auditory cortex (*$P<0.05$). Larger responses were observed for TN as compared to TS in this area (Reprinted from Dang-Vu [3] and adapted from Dang-Vu [44]. Copyright (2011) National Academy of Sciences, USA)

during NREM sleep but also strongly modulate the interactions between the sleeping brain and the environment.

During REM sleep, phasic activity is mainly constituted by ocular saccades (rapid eye movements) on the electrooculogram. In cats, these saccades were shown associated with electrical potentials recorded in many parts of the brain, particularly in the pons, lateral geniculate bodies of the thalamus, and occipital cortex, which explains their name as ponto-geniculo-occipital (PGO) waves [47–50]. Functional neuroimaging allowed to noninvasively verify their existence in humans. A PET study assessed the correlations between brain perfusion and density of rapid eye movements during REM sleep in young healthy volunteers: positive correlations were found in the lateral geniculate bodies and in the occipital cortex [51]. Two fMRI studies confirmed this result by showing that the occurrence of rapid eye movements was associated with increased BOLD response in the thalamus, occipital cortex, and pons during REM sleep [52, 53]. By consistently demonstrating the recruitment of key structures for PGO waves with rapid eye movements, these studies provide strong evidence for the phasic modulation of brain activity by oscillations similar to PGO waves in human REM sleep.

In addition to the study of these well-defined sleep oscillations, other fMRI studies were dedicated to the assessment of functional connectivity patterns during sleep. These works evidenced decreased cortical connectivity during NREM sleep, and emphasized the local nature of neural network architecture during deep NREM sleep [54, 55]. A review of these findings, which exceeds the scope of the present chapter, can be found elsewhere [56].

Neuroimaging of Sleep Deprivation

Functional Neuroimaging of Sleep Deprivation

Most neuroimaging studies dedicated to the effects of sleep deprivation assessed the consequences of controlled sleep deprivation in experimental settings on brain function during subsequent wakefulness, while performing a variety of cognitive tasks. Interestingly, these studies—conducted on healthy volunteers—showed that the effects of sleep deprivation on brain activity were quite heterogeneous when examining different cognitive functions.

Early studies investigated brain responses to attentional tasks following sleep deprivation. For instance, an ^{18}FDG PET study assessed the effects of 32 h of sleep deprivation on brain glucose metabolism during a visual vigilance test [57]. Relative decreases of CMRGlu were observed in the temporal lobes and increases were noted in the visual cortex. In addition, reduced performance to the vigilance test was correlated with decreased CMRGlu in the thalamus, basal ganglia, and limbic structures.

The majority of neuroimaging studies of sleep deprivation involved working memory tasks. Using a task that combined attention with working memory and arithmetic processing, another ^{18}FDG PET study examined CMRGlu during wakefulness after different duration of sleep deprivation (24, 48, and 72 h, respectively). A decrease of CMRGlu was observed during task performance in the prefrontal cortex and thalamus after sleep deprivation, and this decline was more pronounced after 48 and 72 h than after 24 h [58, 59]. Moreover, regional CMRGlu decreases were correlated with decrements in performance at the task, which might indicate a homeostatic need during sleep for recovery of brain areas involved in attention and higher-order cognitive processes. Interestingly, increases of CMRGlu were also found after 48 and 72 h of sleep deprivation, and localized in visual and motor areas (e.g., lateral superior occipital cortices, lingual and fusiform gyri, anterior cerebellum, primary and supplementary motor cortices), which might be interpreted as compensatory mechanisms to maintain alertness and cognitive performance in the face of extended wakefulness [59].

Other studies on working memory used fMRI protocols. Using a task similar to the one from the PET study (arithmetic processing), an fMRI report found decreased brain responses mainly in prefrontal areas during practice of the task after 35 h of sleep deprivation [60], in agreement with the hypothesized vulnerability of the prefrontal cortex to sleep deprivation [61]. However, various fMRI studies testing different aspects of working memory found different patterns of brain activations. Resorting to a delayed-match-to-sample task, an fMRI study found decreased brain responses in distributed cortical areas including temporal, parietal, and occipital structures, correlated with task performance decreases, after 48 h of sleep deprivation [62]. The same group also conducted a similar study on the effects of 48 h of sleep deprivation, using this time a nonverbal recognition working memory task [63]. Decreased cortical brain responses were found in cerebellum, fusiform gyrus, precuneus, and temporal areas, in relationship with memory performance deterioration. Closer to the results of the PET study, another example of fMRI study found decreased activations in several areas of the prefrontal (left dorsolateral, right ventrolateral) and parietal (posterior) cortices during practice of the Sternberg working memory task after 30 h of sleep deprivation [64].

Several studies also assessed the consequences of sleep deprivation on verbal learning. In one of these studies, 35 h of sleep deprivation induced a higher activation of prefrontal and parietal cortices, despite a worse performance and more severe sleepiness in the sleep-deprived condition [65]. Interestingly, in the same study, higher activity in the prefrontal cortex after sleep deprivation positively correlated with subjective sleepiness, possibly reflecting compensation for the enhanced homeostatic drive for sleep. Increased activity in the parietal lobes on the other hand was associated with a better performance on the verbal learning task, possibly indicating compensatory changes to preserve an optimal learning performance when challenged by sleep deprivation. Similar activations and correlations were found by the same group (35 h of sleep deprivation) with a paradigm combining verbal learning and arithmetic tasks [66].

Beyond the effects of sleep deprivation on specific cognitive domains, functional neuroimaging studies also investigated the modulation of brain responses after sleep deprivation by the level of difficulty or complexity of a task. For instance, it was found that increasing task difficulty in a logical reasoning paradigm induced larger responses in several cortical areas (inferior parietal, inferior frontal, and dorsolateral prefrontal), and induced new responses in others (anterior cingulate, temporal) after 35 h of sleep deprivation [67]. In a verbal working memory task, increasing task complexity led to a larger activation in the dorsolateral prefrontal cortex after 24 h of sleep deprivation [68]. The same group additionally showed the differential vulnerability of different cortical regions to the combined effect of sleep deprivation and working memory task difficulty/load [69]. Taken together, increased brain responses have been interpreted as compensatory mechanisms to confront high task demands when sleep-deprived.

Several fMRI articles were interested in looking at the differential vulnerability of individuals to sleep deprivation. These works have indeed demonstrated that brain responses to sleep deprivation for the same task are not homogeneous across participants. One of these studies divided subjects into two groups according to their performance at a working memory task after 30 h of sleep deprivation: a "resilient" group and a "vulnerable" group, the latter displaying the worst performances after sleep deprivation [70]. In the resilient group, distributed cortical activations were found (dorsolateral and ventrolateral prefrontal, supplementary motor area, posterior parietal) during practice of task after sleep deprivation, whereas only the dorsolateral prefrontal cortex was found activated in the vulnerable group. The differential activations might reflect different abilities to recruit compensatory neural responses in the face of sleep deprivation. The patterns of brain activation after sleep deprivation therefore depend on individual vulnerability to sleep deprivation. Further studies found that this differential vulnerability to sleep deprivation could be predicted by task-induced brain responses already after a normal night of sleep. Indeed, it was observed with fMRI that activity in the left frontal and parietal cortex during practice of a working memory task after normal sleep negatively correlated with performance decline from normal sleep to 24 h of sleep deprivation [71]. When looking at brain responses across conditions, the same group found that working memory task performance decline correlated with the decrease of task-induced left parietal activation from normal sleep to sleep deprivation, suggesting that parietal activation constitutes a biomarker of individual resilience to sleep deprivation [72].

Functional neuroimaging studies have described the early effects of sleep deprivation on brain activity during practice of different cognitive tasks. The most striking feature emerging from these findings is the extremely important heterogeneity of neural activation patterns affected by sleep deprivation. Both decreases and increases in brain responses were found, and correlated with deterioration of behavioral performance after sleep deprivation. Localization of the neural structures affected by sleep deprivation was also highly variable, encompassing prefrontal, parietal, but also temporo-occipital structures. Interpretation of these results thus remains speculative, and includes various hypotheses ranging from homeostatic needs for regional brain recovery (resulting in a failure to efficiently perform cognitive tasks) to compensatory mechanisms attempting to maintain (sub)optimal cognitive

a

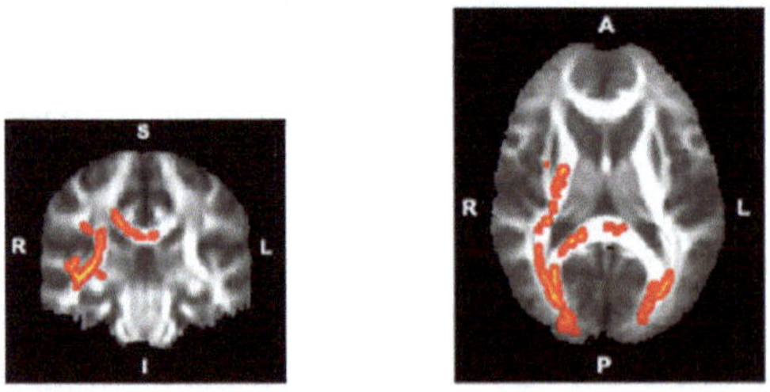

Region	Vulnerability Group VUL FA	NON FA	pearson correlation
Posterior limb of internal capsule	0.68	0.70	0.56
Retrolenticular part of internal capsule	0.61	0.64	0.45
Superior corona radiata	0.48	0.50	0.34
Posterior cornona radiata	0.48	0.51	0.49
Forceps major	0.66	0.70	0.6
Corticospinal tract	0.62	0.63	0.39
Posterior thalamic radiation	0.64	0.66	0.49
Superior longitudinal fasciculus	0.51	0.53	0.45
Genu of CC	0.71	0.74	0.52
Body of CC	0.62	0.65	0.26
Splenium of SS	0.80	0.83	0.39
Mean FA	0.62	0.64	p < .05

b

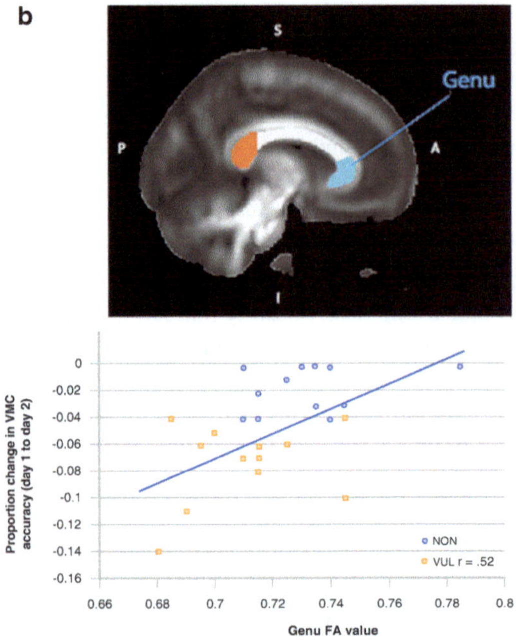

Fig. 4.3 (**a**) Coronal and axial brain slice from the whole brain tract-based spatial statistics (TBSS) results, highlighting regions that showed greater fractional anisotropy (FA) in subjects less vulnerable to sleep deprivation (NON) compared to those more vulnerable to sleep deprivation (VUL) ($P<0.01$, corrected). Table of mean FA values for the extracted pathways of interest and their correlations with percent change in visual-motor control (VMC) accuracy between days 1 and 2. (**b**) From *top* to *bottom* is one sagittal slice showing the three regions of the corpus callosum (CC) that were analyzed for FA differences. Graph showing the correlation between the FA values extracted from the genu of the CC and the proportion change in VMC accuracy between days 1 and 2 (Reprinted from Rocklage [75] with permission)

function. Possible explanations for discrepancies between studies include task-dependent effects (given the high diversity of tasks used in these studies), the different levels of complexity and difficulty of the tasks, and the variable duration of sleep deprivation between studies. Importantly, these studies have also emphasized the individual vulnerability of subjects to sleep deprivation, and the possibility of predicting this vulnerability with functional neuroimaging prior to sleep deprivation. Finally, the precise mechanisms responsible for the deterioration of cognitive performance after sleep deprivation still remain debated. Existing functional neuroimaging data however suggest that sleep deprivation primarily affects "lower-level" processes (e.g., visual attention), which in turn impact on "higher-level" functions required for the completion of complex cognitive tasks [73, 74]. Further studies are needed to confirm this hypothesis.

Structural Neuroimaging and Sleep Deprivation

Recent data interestingly showed that not only brain function but also brain anatomy contributes to the effects of sleep deprivation. In particular, it was shown that modifications of white matter tracts, predominantly in the right hemisphere, could be observed between subjects less vulnerable to sleep deprivation and those more vulnerable [75]. In this report, vulnerability to sleep deprivation was assessed by performance at a simple visuo-motor control task conducted before and after 24 h of sleep deprivation. This finding suggests that the organization of white matter tracts might affect one's cognitive vulnerability to sleep deprivation (Fig. 4.3). The study opens new perspectives for the investigation of the neural mechanisms of sleep deprivation, using structural neuroimaging.

Conclusions

Neuroimaging has brought seminal contributions to the field of sleep research. In this chapter, we showed that imaging could be used to identify brain areas that are consistently recruited during different stages of sleep and in association with various neural oscillations of sleep. These studies characterized the neural structures involved in sleep regulation and functions in humans, and demonstrated the intense brain activations taking place even during deep sleep. Neuroimaging also evidenced the changes in brain function and structure when confronted to sleep deprivation. These data emphasized the neural structures and pathways affected by the lack of sleep during wakefulness. In addition, they demonstrated the possibility of predicting the individual vulnerability to sleep deprivation, by identifying specific functional and anatomical neural patterns. Few neuroimaging studies have investigated the effects of pharmacological (e.g., central stimulants [76], acetylcholinesterase inhibitors [77]) and non-pharmacological (e.g., transcranial magnetic stimulation [78]) interventions on the sleep-deprived brain, and this promising area deserves further investigation.

Acknowledgements Dr. Dang-Vu receives research support from the Canadian Institutes of Health Research (CIHR), the Fonds de Recherche du Québec - Santé (FRQ-S), the Natural Sciences and Engineering Research Council of Canada (NSERC), the Sleep Research Society, the Petro-Canada Young Innovators Awards Program, and Concordia University.

References

1. Dang Vu TT, Desseilles M, Peigneux P, Laureys S, Maquet P. Sleep and sleep states: PET activation patterns. In: Squire LR, editor. Encyclopedia of neuroscience. Oxford: Academic; 2009. p. 955–61.
2. Maquet P. Functional neuroimaging of normal human sleep by positron emission tomography. J Sleep Res. 2000;9(3):207–31.
3. Dang-Vu TT. Neuronal oscillations in sleep: insights from functional neuroimaging. Neuromolecular Med. 2012;14(3):154–67.
4. Dang-Vu TT, Schabus M, Desseilles M, Sterpenich V, Bonjean M, Maquet P. Functional neuroimaging insights into the physiology of human sleep. Sleep. 2010;33(12):1589–603.
5. Horne JA, Reyner LA. Sleep related vehicle accidents. BMJ. 1995;310(6979):565–7.
6. Mitler MM, Carskadon MA, Czeisler CA, Dement WC, Dinges DF, Graeber RC. Catastrophes, sleep, and public policy: consensus report. Sleep. 1988; 11(1):100–9.
7. Dang-Vu TT, Desseilles M, Peigneux P, Maquet P. A role for sleep in brain plasticity. Pediatr Rehabil. 2006;9(2):98–118.
8. Diekelmann S, Born J. The memory function of sleep. Nat Rev Neurosci. 2010;11(2):114–26.
9. Maquet P. The role of sleep in learning and memory. Science. 2001;294(5544):1048–52.
10. Peigneux P, Laureys S, Delbeuck X, Maquet P. Sleeping brain, learning brain. The role of sleep for memory systems. Neuroreport. 2001;12(18):A111–24.
11. Dang-Vu TT, Desseilles M, Petit D, Mazza S, Montplaisir J, Maquet P. Neuroimaging in sleep medicine. Sleep Med. 2007;8(4):349–72.
12. Desseilles M, Dang-Vu T, Schabus M, Sterpenich V, Maquet P, Schwartz S. Neuroimaging insights into the pathophysiology of sleep disorders. Sleep. 2008; 31(6):777–94.
13. Maquet P, Degueldre C, Delfiore G, Aerts J, Peters JM, Luxen A, et al. Functional neuroanatomy of human slow wave sleep. J Neurosci. 1997;17(8):2807–12.
14. Braun AR, Balkin TJ, Wesenten NJ, Carson RE, Varga M, Baldwin P, et al. Regional cerebral blood flow throughout the sleep-wake cycle. An H2(15)O PET study. Brain. 1997;120(Pt 7):1173–97.
15. Kajimura N, Uchiyama M, Takayama Y, Uchida S, Uema T, Kato M, et al. Activity of midbrain reticular formation and neocortex during the progression of human non-rapid eye movement sleep. J Neurosci. 1999;19(22):10065–73.
16. Andersson JL, Onoe H, Hetta J, Lidstrom K, Valind S, Lilja A, et al. Brain networks affected by synchronized sleep visualized by positron emission tomography. J Cereb Blood Flow Metab. 1998;18(7):701–15.
17. Maquet P, Dive D, Salmon E, Sadzot B, Franco G, Poirrier R, et al. Cerebral glucose utilization during sleep-wake cycle in man determined by positron emission tomography and [18F]2-fluoro-2-deoxy-D-glucose method. Brain Res. 1990;513(1):136–43.
18. Nofzinger EA, Buysse DJ, Miewald JM, Meltzer CC, Price JC, Sembrat RC, et al. Human regional cerebral glucose metabolism during non-rapid eye movement sleep in relation to waking. Brain. 2002;125(Pt 5):1105–15.
19. Peigneux P, Laureys S, Fuchs S, Collette F, Perrin F, Reggers J, et al. Are spatial memories strengthened in the human hippocampus during slow wave sleep? Neuron. 2004;44(3):535–45.
20. Czisch M, Wehrle R, Kaufmann C, Wetter TC, Holsboer F, Pollmacher T, et al. Functional MRI

during sleep: BOLD signal decreases and their electrophysiological correlates. Eur J Neurosci. 2004; 20(2):566–74.
21. Kaufmann C, Wehrle R, Wetter TC, Holsboer F, Auer DP, Pollmacher T, et al. Brain activation and hypothalamic functional connectivity during human non-rapid eye movement sleep: an EEG/fMRI study. Brain. 2006;129(Pt 3):655–67.
22. Maquet P, Peters J, Aerts J, Delfiore G, Degueldre C, Luxen A, et al. Functional neuroanatomy of human rapid-eye-movement sleep and dreaming. Nature. 1996;383(6596):163–6.
23. Nofzinger EA, Mintun MA, Wiseman M, Kupfer DJ, Moore RY. Forebrain activation in REM sleep: an FDG PET study. Brain Res. 1997;770(1–2):192–201.
24. Maquet P, Laureys S, Peigneux P, Fuchs S, Petiau C, Phillips C, et al. Experience-dependent changes in cerebral activation during human REM sleep. Nat Neurosci. 2000;3(8):831–6.
25. Maquet P, Ruby P, Maudoux A, Albouy G, Sterpenich V, Dang-Vu T, et al. Human cognition during REM sleep and the activity profile within frontal and parietal cortices: a reappraisal of functional neuroimaging data. Prog Brain Res. 2005;150:219–27.
26. Dang Vu TT, Schabus M, Desseilles M, Schwartz S, Maquet P. Neuroimaging of REM sleep and dreaming. In: McNamara P, Barrett D, editors. The new science of dreaming. Westport: Praeger; 2007. p. 95–113.
27. Dang-Vu TT, Desseilles M, Albouy G, Darsaud A, Gais S, Rauchs G, et al. Dreaming: a neuroimaging view. Swiss Arch Neurol Psychiatr. 2005;156(8):415–25.
28. Schwartz S, Maquet P. Sleep imaging and the neuropsychological assessment of dreams. Trends Cogn Sci. 2002;6(1):23–30.
29. Steriade M, McCarley RW. Brain control of wakefulness and sleep. New York: Springer; 2005.
30. Iber C, Ancoli-Israel S, Chesson AL, Quan SF. The AASM manual for the scoring of sleep and associated events. Westchester: American Academy of Sleep Medicine; 2007.
31. Hofle N, Paus T, Reutens D, Fiset P, Gotman J, Evans AC, et al. Regional cerebral blood flow changes as a function of delta and spindle activity during slow wave sleep in humans. J Neurosci. 1997;17(12):4800–8.
32. Dang-Vu TT, Desseilles M, Laureys S, Degueldre C, Perrin F, Phillips C, et al. Cerebral correlates of delta waves during non-REM sleep revisited. Neuroimage. 2005;28(1):14–21.
33. Massimini M, Huber R, Ferrarelli F, Hill S, Tononi G. The sleep slow oscillation as a traveling wave. J Neurosci. 2004;24(31):6862–70.
34. Murphy M, Riedner BA, Huber R, Massimini M, Ferrarelli F, Tononi G. Source modeling sleep slow waves. Proc Natl Acad Sci U S A. 2009;106(5):1608–13.
35. Finelli LA, Borbely AA, Achermann P. Functional topography of the human nonREM sleep electroencephalogram. Eur J Neurosci. 2001;13(12):2282–90.
36. Happe S, Anderer P, Gruber G, Klosch G, Saletu B, Zeitlhofer J. Scalp topography of the spontaneous K-complex and of delta-waves in human sleep. Brain Topogr. 2002;15(1):43–9.
37. Leclercq Y, Balteau E, Dang-Vu T, Schabus M, Luxen A, Maquet P, et al. Rejection of pulse related artefact (PRA) from continuous electroencephalographic (EEG) time series recorded during functional magnetic resonance imaging (fMRI) using constraint independent component analysis (cICA). Neuroimage. 2009;44(3):679–91.
38. Srivastava G, Crottaz-Herbette S, Lau KM, Glover GH, Menon V. ICA-based procedures for removing ballistocardiogram artifacts from EEG data acquired in the MRI scanner. Neuroimage. 2005;24(1):50–60.
39. Steriade M, Domich L, Oakson G, Deschenes M. The deafferented reticular thalamic nucleus generates spindle rhythmicity. J Neurophysiol. 1987;57(1):260–73.
40. Schabus M, Dang-Vu TT, Albouy G, Balteau E, Boly M, Carrier J, et al. Hemodynamic cerebral correlates of sleep spindles during human non-rapid eye movement sleep. Proc Natl Acad Sci U S A. 2007; 104(32):13164–9.
41. Dang-Vu TT, Schabus M, Desseilles M, Albouy G, Boly M, Darsaud A, et al. Spontaneous neural activity during human slow wave sleep. Proc Natl Acad Sci U S A. 2008;105(39):15160–5.
42. Bergmann TO, Molle M, Diedrichs J, Born J, Siebner HR. Sleep spindle-related reactivation of category-specific cortical regions after learning face-scene associations. Neuroimage. 2012;59(3):2733–42.
43. Portas CM, Krakow K, Allen P, Josephs O, Armony JL, Frith CD. Auditory processing across the sleep-wake cycle: simultaneous EEG and fMRI monitoring in humans. Neuron. 2000;28(3):991–9.
44. Dang-Vu TT, Bonjean M, Schabus M, Boly M, Darsaud A, Desseilles M, et al. Interplay between spontaneous and induced brain activity during human non-rapid eye movement sleep. Proc Natl Acad Sci U S A. 2011;108(37):15438–43.
45. Dang-Vu TT, McKinney SM, Buxton OM, Solet JM, Ellenbogen JM. Spontaneous brain rhythms predict sleep stability in the face of noise. Curr Biol. 2010;20(15):R626–7.
46. Schabus M, Dang-Vu TT, Heib DP, Boly M, Desseilles M, Vandewalle G, et al. The fate of incoming stimuli during NREM sleep is determined by spindles and the phase of the slow oscillation. Front Neurol. 2012;3:40.
47. Jouvet M, Michel F. Corrélations electromyographiques du sommeil chez le Chat décortiqué et mésencéphalique chronique. C R Soc Biol. 1959; 153:422–5.
48. Mikiten TH, Niebyl PH, Hendley CD. EEG desynchronization during behavioral sleep associated with spike discharges from the thalamus of the cat. Fed Proc. 1961;20:327.
49. Mouret J, Jeannerod M, Jouvet M. L'activite electrique du systeme visuel au cours de la phase paradoxale du sommeil chez le chat. J Physiol Paris. 1963;55:305–6.

50. Hobson JA. L'activité electrique du cortex et du thalamus au cours du sommeil désynchronisé chez le chat. C R Soc Biol. 1964;158:2131–5.
51. Peigneux P, Laureys S, Fuchs S, Delbeuck X, Degueldre C, Aerts J, et al. Generation of rapid eye movements during paradoxical sleep in humans. Neuroimage. 2001;14(3):701–8.
52. Wehrle R, Czisch M, Kaufmann C, Wetter TC, Holsboer F, Auer DP, et al. Rapid eye movement-related brain activation in human sleep: a functional magnetic resonance imaging study. Neuroreport. 2005;16(8):853–7.
53. Miyauchi S, Misaki M, Kan S, Fukunaga T, Koike T. Human brain activity time-locked to rapid eye movements during REM sleep. Exp Brain Res. 2009;192(4):657–67.
54. Larson-Prior LJ, Power JD, Vincent JL, Nolan TS, Coalson RS, Zempel J, et al. Modulation of the brain's functional network architecture in the transition from wake to sleep. Prog Brain Res. 2011;193:277–94.
55. Spoormaker VI, Schroter MS, Gleiser PM, Andrade KC, Dresler M, Wehrle R, et al. Development of a large-scale functional brain network during human non-rapid eye movement sleep. J Neurosci. 2010; 30(34):11379–87.
56. Duyn JH. EEG-fMRI methods for the study of brain networks during sleep. Front Neurol. 2012;3:100.
57. Wu JC, Gillin JC, Buchsbaum MS, Hershey T, Hazlett E, Sicotte N, et al. The effect of sleep deprivation on cerebral glucose metabolic rate in normal humans assessed with positron emission tomography. Sleep. 1991;14(2):155–62.
58. Thomas M, Sing H, Belenky G, Holcomb H, Mayberg H, Dannals R, et al. Neural basis of alertness and cognitive performance impairments during sleepiness. I. Effects of 24 h of sleep deprivation on waking human regional brain activity. J Sleep Res. 2000;9(4): 335–52.
59. Thomas ML, Sing HC, Belenky G, Holcomb HH, Mayberg HS, Dannals RF, et al. Neural basis of alertness and cognitive performance impairments during sleepiness. II. Effects of 48 and 72 hours of sleep deprivation on waking human regional brain activity. Thalamus Relat Syst. 2003;2:199–229.
60. Drummond SP, Brown GG, Stricker JL, Buxton RB, Wong EC, Gillin JC. Sleep deprivation-induced reduction in cortical functional response to serial subtraction. Neuroreport. 1999;10(18):3745–8.
61. Horne JA. Human sleep, sleep loss and behaviour. Implications for the prefrontal cortex and psychiatric disorder. Br J Psychiatry. 1993;162:413–9.
62. Habeck C, Rakitin BC, Moeller J, Scarmeas N, Zarahn E, Brown T, et al. An event-related fMRI study of the neurobehavioral impact of sleep deprivation on performance of a delayed-match-to-sample task. Brain Res Cogn Brain Res. 2004; 18(3):306–21.
63. Bell-McGinty S, Habeck C, Hilton HJ, Rakitin B, Scarmeas N, Zarahn E, et al. Identification and differential vulnerability of a neural network in sleep deprivation. Cereb Cortex. 2004;14(5):496–502.
64. Mu Q, Nahas Z, Johnson KA, Yamanaka K, Mishory A, Koola J, et al. Decreased cortical response to verbal working memory following sleep deprivation. Sleep. 2005;28(1):55–67.
65. Drummond SP, Brown GG, Gillin JC, Stricker JL, Wong EC, Buxton RB. Altered brain response to verbal learning following sleep deprivation. Nature. 2000;403(6770):655–7.
66. Drummond SP, Gillin JC, Brown GG. Increased cerebral response during a divided attention task following sleep deprivation. J Sleep Res. 2001;10(2):85–92.
67. Drummond SP, Brown GG, Salamat JS, Gillin JC. Increasing task difficulty facilitates the cerebral compensatory response to total sleep deprivation. Sleep. 2004;27(3):445–51.
68. Chee MW, Choo WC. Functional imaging of working memory after 24 hr of total sleep deprivation. J Neurosci. 2004;24(19):4560–7.
69. Choo WC, Lee WW, Venkatraman V, Sheu FS, Chee MW. Dissociation of cortical regions modulated by both working memory load and sleep deprivation and by sleep deprivation alone. Neuroimage. 2005;25(2):579–87. Research Support, Non-U.S. Gov't.
70. Mu Q, Mishory A, Johnson KA, Nahas Z, Kozel FA, Yamanaka K, et al. Decreased brain activation during a working memory task at rested baseline is associated with vulnerability to sleep deprivation. Sleep. 2005;28(4):433–46.
71. Chee MW, Chuah LY, Venkatraman V, Chan WY, Philip P, Dinges DF. Functional imaging of working memory following normal sleep and after 24 and 35 h of sleep deprivation: correlations of fronto-parietal activation with performance. Neuroimage. 2006;31(1):419–28.
72. Lim J, Choo WC, Chee MW. Reproducibility of changes in behaviour and fMRI activation associated with sleep deprivation in a working memory task. Sleep. 2007;30(1):61–70.
73. Chee MW, Chuah YM. Functional neuroimaging and behavioral correlates of capacity decline in visual short-term memory after sleep deprivation. Proc Natl Acad Sci U S A. 2007;104(22):9487–92.
74. Chuah LY, Chee MW. Functional neuroimaging of sleep deprived healthy volunteers and persons with sleep disorders: a brief review. Ann Acad Med Singapore. 2008;37(8):689–94.
75. Rocklage M, Williams V, Pacheco J, Schnyer DM. White matter differences predict cognitive vulnerability to sleep deprivation. Sleep. 2009;32(8):1100–3.
76. Thomas RJ, Kwong K. Modafinil activates cortical and subcortical sites in the sleep-deprived state. Sleep. 2006;29(11):1471–81.
77. Chuah LY, Chong DL, Chen AK, Rekshan III WR, Tan JC, Zheng H, et al. Donepezil improves episodic memory in young individuals vulnerable to the effects of sleep deprivation. Sleep. 2009;32(8):999–1010.
78. Luber B, Stanford AD, Bulow P, Nguyen T, Rakitin BC, Habeck C, et al. Remediation of sleep-deprivation-induced working memory impairment with fMRI-guided transcranial magnetic stimulation. Cereb Cortex. 2008;18(9):2077–85.

Part III

Sleep and the Brain

Sleep Deprivation and Neurological Diseases

5

Matt T. Bianchi

Overview of the Two Most Common Sleep Disorders: Sleep Apnea and Insomnia

Several recent reviews have highlighted comorbidity between sleep disorders and neurological disorders [1–9]. We will begin by taking a broad view of sleep deprivation to include insufficient sleep as well as common sleep disturbances of insomnia and sleep apnea. Sleep apnea is a common disorder characterized by recurrent respiratory pauses during sleep. Most sleep apnea is obstructive in nature, referring to the recurrent collapse of airway soft tissue that occludes air flow during sleep. Respiratory pauses induce a cascade of events, most notably episodic hypoxia and sleep fragmentation. Untreated sleep apnea is associated with increased cardiovascular and cerebrovascular morbidity and mortality, which may be reversed with treatment [10]. In addition, daytime sleepiness and fatigue impact overall quality of life, as well as risk for motor vehicle accidents [11]. As described in this chapter, treatment of sleep disorders has some evidence in certain neurological conditions, but in the absence of high-quality evidence in this population, the extensive literature on the importance of sleep in health and performance is a compelling motivation to consider evaluation and treatment of sleep disorders in the individual with neurological compromise.

The overall prevalence of sleep apnea in adults depends on the diagnostic criteria and the population demographics [12]. The commonly cited single digit prevalence values stem from older literature, while the more recent and generally higher prevalence data invokes the current apnea–hypopnea index (AHI) cutoff value of 5 events per hour (assuming snoring or a sleep-related symptom is also present) [13]. Comparing prevalence in subpopulations such as those with neurological disorders is complicated by the use of different sleep apnea definitions (such as AHI cutoff values of 5, 10, 15, or even higher, or if sleepiness is required). Furthermore, drawing inferential relationships regarding the presence and severity of sleep apnea is complicated by the one-night snapshot provided by polysomnography (PSG) data—which does not take into account night-to-night variability, sleep stages, or body position, all of which can impact the summary AHI metric (see [14] and references therein).

The most common risk factors are obesity, older age, male sex, and "crowded" airway anatomy. Snoring and sleepiness are classic symptoms, but these are neither sensitive nor specific for sleep apnea. Although it has been suggested that patient identification is fairly simple on clinical grounds [12], the reality is that the major sleep apnea risk factors contribute only a minority of the risk, making clinical prediction challenging. For example, the most widely used screening

M.T. Bianchi, M.D., Ph.D., M.M.Sc. (✉)
Division of Sleep Medicine, Department of Neurology, Massachusetts General Hospital, Boston, MA, USA
e-mail: mtbianchi@partners.org

M.T. Bianchi (ed.), *Sleep Deprivation and Disease: Effects on the Body, Brain and Behavior*,
DOI 10.1007/978-1-4614-9087-6_5, © Springer Science+Business Media New York 2014

questionnaires have insufficient sensitivity and specificity to actually be useful in screening, especially for very high or very low risk populations [15]. In particular, when administered in populations with higher than average sleep apnea prevalence, a negative screening result does not sufficiently lower the risk of disease, as I have shown using Bayesian inference [15]. In contrast, objective testing is too costly for large-scale screening ($400–$1,500 for a single night test). Intermediate tests, such as home pulse-oximetry, are insensitive and not cost-effective [16]. Even overall clinical impression has weak predictive value [17]. Given the challenges of linking symptoms and classical presentations (obesity, snoring, pickwickian appearance) with the presence and/or severity of sleep apnea, one can use the following dual philosophy to motivate testing: (a) the elevated pretest probability of sleep apnea in many neurological disorders and (b) the potential impact of treating occult apnea in the vulnerable neurological patient.

Among the available treatments for sleep apnea, the gold standard is considered to be continuous positive airway pressure, or CPAP (although see references [18, 19]), delivered through any of many mask interface options. Second line options for those who do not tolerate CPAP (~30 % of patients) include dental positioning appliances, or surgery on the palate or mandible. Conservative measures have shown some promise, such as positional therapy (avoiding supine sleep) and weight loss, but adherence remains a challenge and therefore these methods are not considered therapeutic options in isolation. Furthermore, there is a great deal of variability in the degree of position dependence which limits the population for which positional therapy is relevant, and there is also variability between sleep apnea severity and obesity, with only a minority of the variance in severity being associated with BMI (see references [14, 20], and references therein).

Insomnia is highly prevalent in adults, being chronic and/or severe in 10 % or more, and is of particular relevance to the neurological patient [5, 21]. The nosology of insomnia is an ongoing discussion, which complicates research efforts—not only because of varied definitions but also because of overlap of subtypes within individuals [22]. Just as there are many contributing and perpetuating factors to insomnia in the general population, a multidisciplinary approach to evaluation of insomnia is important in neurology. Treatment of insomnia is challenging in the general population for several reasons, including the mismatch between objective measures of sleep–wake duration and patient reports, as well as cultural beliefs regarding the "normal" duration and continuity of sleep. Patients may self-medicate with over-the-counter agents, or they may obtain hypnotic agents from providers. Sleep hygiene education is an important first step, as some patients may not recognize the potential impact of napping, caffeine, light, late meals, or other behaviors on the quality and quantity of their sleep. The time in bed relative to the individual's sleep capacity should be explored in order to determine whether a sleep restriction intervention may be helpful. Patients may respond to the fragmented or interrupted sleep by increasing the time in bed, which may have the paradoxical consequence of enhancing fragmentation of sleep because the biological sleep capacity cannot fill the time spent in bed. Comparative studies have shown that more structured behavioral interventions, such as cognitive behavioral therapy for insomnia (CBT-I), are at least as effective as hypnotic therapy, and of course lack drug-related adverse effects [23]. Identifying by history and treating contributing factors such as mood, pain, nocturia, and motor symptoms may improve sleep quality. To the extent possible, reducing medications that may cause insomnia should be considered, but because such medications may be providing benefits (such as certain antidepressants, beta blockers, and cholinesterase inhibitors), the risk–benefit balance should be considered.

Despite the common use of pharmacological sleep-aids in those reporting insomnia, there is a growing literature pertaining to the risks of these agents. Also, medication side effects are increasingly concerning with advancing age, including drug interactions, impact on memory, fall risk, and paradoxical effects (benzos, antihistamines, neuroleptics) [5, 24], which may be even more pertinent in the neurological patient. Over-the-counter agents such as melatonin, valerian, or herbal teas can be trialed but the evidence basis is sparse. Also, melatonin drug interactions (including with coumadin) should be noted. Importantly, many over-the-counter sleep-aids contain antihistamines such as diphenhydramine, which may not be recognized by patients perusing "PM" versions of common analgesics or advertised sleep-aids claiming to employ herbal formulations but also include the antihistamine. Balancing the risks and benefits of sleep medications, especially in the neurological patient, is not straightforward, and should be made on a patient-by-patient basis.

Stroke

Cerebrovascular disease has been linked to sleep apnea as both a cause and a consequence. The majority of stroke is ischemic; although ischemic and hemorrhagic stroke have different mechanisms and implications, not all sleep-related studies separate these subtypes. From the perspective of neurological injury, the presence or severity of sleep apnea has not been clearly associated with the location of the stroke [25], but isolated cases have reported brainstem infarct and sleep apnea (especially central apnea). From the perspective of sleep, associations with stroke risk have been suggested for sleep duration [4], periodic limb movements [26], as well as sleep apnea [27]. Sleep disorders such as sleep apnea are themselves independently associated with risk factors that are also relevant for stroke risk, such as age, male sex, and obesity. Medical comorbidities that are associated with sleep apnea are also associated with stroke, such as hypertension and diabetes.

A large meta-analysis has confirmed a high prevalence of sleep apnea in patients with a history of recent stroke or TIA [27]; for the included studies, most PSGs were done within 1 month of the neurological event. The prevalence of mild sleep apnea (AHI>5) was 72 %, while the prevalence of AHI>20 was 38 %. Only 7 % were categorized as primary central apnea. These severity and prevalence values may be underestimates because most studies excluded patients who could not consent or who had major comorbidities, and of course patients who did not survive their stroke were not studied. In another recent meta-analysis examining sleep apnea as a risk factor for future stroke, it was shown that sleep apnea conferred greater than twofold increase in incident stroke [28]. The risk was proportional to the severity of sleep apnea. Other work has suggested central apnea events conferred specific stroke risk in the elderly, whereas obstructive apnea index, arousal index, and oxygenation metrics did not [29].

Treatment of OSA in stroke patients may have multiple potential benefits. Untreated sleep apnea is associated with hypertension, atrial fibrillation, and cardiac disease—all of which may impact stroke risk. Treating sleep apnea may directly reduce stroke risk conferred by autonomic fluctuations, cardiac arrhythmias, and hypoxemia, as well as indirectly through improvements in associated stroke risk factors. Treating sleep apnea in the patient with sleepiness may improve quality of life as well. Investigation of sleep apnea through PSG has been recommended for all stroke survivors in an extensive review of the literature associating stroke with sleep apnea [2]. Treatment benefit seems a reasonable expectation based on indirect reasoning, and promising data has been reported in regard to CPAP compliance and neurological recovery [30–39], even when initiated in the acute setting [40] (but see [41]). Sham-controlled CPAP treatment trials may be feasible in this population [42], but clearly there is great heterogeneity among stroke survivors in terms of potential barriers to compliance, which has been quite poor in some studies [43], and the complexities of treating sleep apnea in this population should not be taken lightly [44].

Shift work has been associated with a very small (4 %) increase in stroke risk per 5 years of shift work, but only after 30 years of shift work after adjusting for other risk factors [45]. Similarly small absolute risk increase was reported in a large meta-analysis of stroke and myocardial infarction in shift work (although mortality was not associated with shift work) [46]. In a recent large meta-analysis, both short and long self-reported sleep durations were associated with increased risk of cardiovascular and cerebrovascular events [47], in the "U-shaped" relationship so commonly encountered in epidemiological studies linking sleep duration to morbidity and mortality [48, 49]. Short self-reported sleep duration (<6 h) was marginally significantly associated with 15 % increase in stroke risk, while long self-reported sleep duration (>8–9 h) carried a larger relative risk of 1.65, compared to a reference category of 7–8 h [47]. In one interesting study, short sleep (<7.5 h) was associated with increased risk of incident stroke only in individuals with MRI evidence of existing silent stroke [50].

Epilepsy

The relationship between sleep and circadian rhythms with epilepsy and its pharmacotherapy has long been of interest clinically [51–54]. Sleep disturbance is such a well-known risk factor for lowering seizure threshold that for decades neurologists have employed deprivation as a clinical tool to trigger seizures. Sleep deprivation has been shown to increase inter-ictal hyperexcitability [55], but a recent study of patients with focal epilepsy suggested that the group assigned to sleep deprivation during their inpatient long-term EEG monitoring did not differ from the non-deprived group in seizure frequency [56].

Sleep disturbance is a more common complaint in patients with epilepsy than in the general population [57, 58]. Sleep apnea, RLS, insomnia, parasomnia, and narcolepsy may occur in epilepsy patients [59]. Complaints of sleepiness or fatigue are common in patients with epilepsy, and these nonspecific symptoms may be attributed to the epilepsy or to side effects of anticonvulsant medications [54]; but they may also relate to occult sleep apnea. Sleep disturbance contributes to decreased quality of life in general [60] as well as specifically in epilepsy patients [57]. Patients with epilepsy may report poor sleep or sleep deprivation as a factor influencing their seizure frequency and/or seizure control. However, there is limited evidence regarding whether insomnia treatment improves seizure control.

Undiagnosed sleep apnea in this population may represent a potentially treatable contributor to two major patient concerns, poor seizure control and daytime fatigue. A recent review of the literature indicates a high prevalence of undiagnosed sleep apnea [54]. In studies ranging in size from $n=13$ to $n=283$, the prevalence of sleep apnea ranged from 33 to 80 %, with moderate to severe apnea present in 15–25 % of epilepsy patients. The most important aspect of comorbid sleep apnea in epilepsy patients is that treating sleep apnea can improve quality of life, daytime symptoms, and even seizure control [54, 61–63]. Whether sleep apnea preceded and sensitized one to develop incident epilepsy, or whether the pathophysiology of epilepsy (or its pharmacotherapy) predisposes one to develop sleep apnea, remains an open question.

Neurodegenerative Disorders

It may be useful to conceptualize neurodegenerative disorders according to their proposed molecular pathology, including in their association with sleep disorders [7, 64]. Diseases linked to tau abnormalities (tauopathies) include Alzheimer's disease (AD), progressive supranuclear palsy (PSP), Corticobasal degeneration (CBD), and fronto-temporal dementia (FTD), while those linked to synuclein abnormalities (synucleinopathies) include Parkinson's disease (PD), Lewy body dementia (LBD), and multiple system atrophy (MSA). Degenerative disorders affecting motor and cognitive systems may manifest sleep pathology either as a primary pathology of the disease or through indirect mechanisms. For example, degeneration of brainstem nuclei involved in sleep as well as respiration and motor control have been implicated [65]. REM behavior disorder (RBD), in which dreams are physically enacted in the setting of loss of the normal REM-related muscle atonia, has been associated with degeneration of brainstem centers involved in REM sleep [66, 67]. Sleep fragmentation and insomnia have also been described in neurodegeneration, although causality remains poorly understood. It is likely that certain disease-related factors such as motor manifestations and nocturia contribute to insomnia in addition to primary brain pathology effects. Age and age-related medical problems are associated with sleep apnea, although again there may be more direct links as well.

Parkinson's Disease

Subjective sleep complaints are common in survey/inventory-based studies of patients with PD [68–70]. These complaints span a variety of problems, including fatigue, sleep maintenance difficulties, leg motor symptoms, and dream enactment—all of which may have major impact on neurological function and quality of life in this population [7, 71]. The cited studies show variable relationships with disease severity and/or duration, as well as medication regimens. PD with dementia has been shown to have greater daytime sleepiness as measured by ESS scores, but there were no CSF orexin differences seen [72]. From the insomnia standpoint, as has been shown for non-neurological populations, PD patients may demonstrate sleep–wake misperception, as they showed subjective overestimation of sleep latency (by 15 min), and underestimation of total sleep time (by over 1 h) [73] compared to objective measurements.

Sleep benefit (less motor symptomatology upon awakening) has been reported in a third to half of PD patients [74, 75]. Interestingly, improved motor function has been reported following a night of sleep deprivation in PD patients [76]. However, other studies have shown a more variable effect among patients. The effect of total and partial sleep deprivation was tested on motor function and, while a subset showed improved motor function with partial deprivation, the group as a whole showed no effect, suggesting individual variability in the impact of acute sleep loss [77].

In terms of sleep factors that may predict future development of PD, self-reported long sleep duration has been associated with increased PD risk in epidemiological studies, while self-reported short sleep duration and shift work was associated with lower risk [78]. However, as with any study based on self-reported habitual sleep duration, caution is needed regarding interpretation of the associations, and in particular regarding the implication that altering sleep duration might impact future morbidity risk. For example, one would not want to interpret these results to imply that shift work or sleep restriction is causally protective against future PD, and thus suggest them as preventative measures. Such interventions might carry other risks, not to mention questions of feasibility. However, association studies may suggest interesting hypotheses to test from a mechanistic standpoint. In another survey study, Gao et al. reported an association of reported daytime napping with increased PD risk, and also noted a U-shaped risk relationship with nocturnal self-reported sleep duration in prevalence analysis [79]. One cannot tease apart whether napping reflects sleepiness from PD-related sleep disturbance or fatigue, and is simply a marker of disease, versus the possibility that naps themselves somehow contribute to future PD risk. Moreover, the self-reported sleep durations, especially the U-shaped relationship, carry much unresolved uncertainty not only with regard to mechanism but also in regard to factors such as the lack of objective sleep metrics, the common discrepancy between subjective and objective metrics when both are available, the challenges pertaining to uncontrolled confounding medical associations with high or low self-reported sleep durations, and the unmeasured night-to-night variability in sleep duration.

Sleepiness and fatigue are multifactorial in PD, and may result from sleep fragmentation and insomnia, occult sleep apnea, disturbance from RBD, comorbid depression, and dopaminergic agents. Sleep apnea has been reported in different studies to have either similar prevalence to matched controls or increased prevalence. For example, Young et al. reported in a small study (<20 subjects) that mild and severe PD cases had similar objective PSG metrics, including indices of fragmentation, and that the AHI mean values were normal in both groups [80]. Both groups had elevated PLMS metrics. In contrast, several other groups reported elevated AHI values in similarly small studies of 10–45 patients [72, 81–84]. PLMS and RBD were also prevalent in these cohorts.

Interestingly, in one study, the prevalence of sleep apnea in PD patients with and without concomitant sleepiness was 27 %, while that in a control population was higher at 40 %—however, the controls consisted of patients admitted to rule out venous thrombo-embolism [85]. The authors concluded based on the prevalence in this study design that "sleep apnea does not seem to be a clinically relevant issue in PD." A similar case–control study reported that the mean AHI (12/h) was similar in PD as in matched controls; the prevalence of AHI>5 was 49 % in PD versus a striking 66 % in controls [86]. Another study used the Sleep Heart Health Study as a historical control, and found similar prevalence of sleep apnea in their cohort of PD patients, and the AHI was not correlated with BMI, snoring, or sleepiness [87].

These comparative prevalence studies are instructive in several respects. First, when investigating the prevalence of sleep apnea in a population, the choice of the control population matters, not simply for matching based on key features (age, sex, BMI), but also in terms of that population's pretest probability of sleep apnea [85], and how the control population was measured (home studies, in the case of reference [87]). A sleep apnea prevalence in the control population of 40 % in Cohen de Cock is quite high, perhaps because those individuals admitted to rule out venous thrombo-embolism are not representative of the general population. Second, and perhaps more importantly, even if ideally matched controls showed an identical sleep apnea prevalence as PD patients, it does not follow that sleep apnea in PD patients is clinically irrelevant. For example, patients with neurological compromise may be more sensitive to perturbations of sleep, may have altered disease natural history if sleep apnea is comorbid, and may have decreased quality of life. Clearly one must separate the question of whether sleep apnea risk is increased in PD (or any neurological illness) from the question of whether sleep apnea is impacting the general or neurological health of the individual.

The standard of care is to treat sleep apnea with AHI>5 if sleep-related symptoms are present, and to treat those with AHI>15 regardless of symptoms [13]. This is based in part on studies suggesting that symptoms and morbidity are associated with severity. However, one could argue that the standard should be even more aggressive among populations with neurological dysfunction, who may be more vulnerable to challenges such as sleep apnea that disrupt sleep. The question of whether or not sleep apnea is more prevalent in PD patients is certainly of interest from a mechanistic and epidemiological perspective. From the patient care perspective, sleep apnea can be considered a potentially reversible contributor to health and quality of life, whether it is present incidentally or causally.

When deciding whether to test for sleep apnea in this (or any) population, it is also important to note that the relationship of the Epworth score and AHI is poor, and even BMI (a major risk factor) explains only a minority of risk in this disease with multifactorial pathogenic mechanisms, as discussed earlier. Approximately half of patients with even severe sleep apnea will have no sleepiness based on subjective and objective metrics [88]. The dissociation of symptoms and disease severity may reflect our crude measures of sleep apnea severity and the challenges in quantifying sleepiness, in addition to individual differences in vulnerability to sleep disturbances. The weak correlation of symptoms and routine clinical metrics with the presence or severity of sleep apnea suggests that testing decisions may be driven by a Bayesian strategy, that is, based on prevalence studies instead of exclusively considering (unreliable) clinical clues. A conservative approach is to recognize that the medical morbidity associated with untreated sleep apnea is linked to the objective metrics, and thus the lack of symptoms or traditional risk factors should not dissuade clinicians from testing PD patients for potentially treatable sleep disturbances including sleep apnea, PLMS, and RBD.

Multiple System Atrophy

Sleep complaints including sleepiness and insomnia are common in the MSA population for a variety of reasons, similar to the situation in PD patients [89–91]. Also like the PD population, there is increased prevalence of RBD in the MSA population [92]. Sleep can be fragmented in these patients [93], with or without concomitant sleep apnea. Sleep apnea is of particular concern in MSA patients, because of associations with nocturnal stridor which may be related to mortality in this population. There is increased prevalence of sleep apnea in MSA patients, ranging from 30 to >90 % of patients studied with PSG [94–97]. In some cases primary central apnea (periodic breathing) was found, but mainly obstructions were evident. Also of note, as has been shown in general populations [20], there was little relationship of the sleep apnea metrics with Epworth Sleepiness scores. Dissociation of patient-report and objective findings is also of concern regarding stridor, which may be more evident on PSG than by history [64], which adds to the motivation to perform PSG in this population.

Treatment with CPAP is indicated in MSA patients with sleep apnea. Although compliance is (not unexpectedly) related to baseline motor dysfunction in this population [98], CPAP treatment may improve nocturnal stridor [99, 100] as well as symptoms in those who tolerate it [98, 101]. However, in the experimental setting of propofol-induced "sleep," it was reported that positive airway pressure may not alleviate obstruction in certain MSA patients characterized by floppy epiglottis, and in some individuals obstructions could actually be worsened by CPAP [102]. It is important to note also that compliance with CPAP, even among those who tolerate and adapt to treatment, is rarely 100 %, such that surgical interventions have been discussed in the these patients with nocturnal stridor given the potential risks of acute respiratory failure. However, even surgery can carry unexpected risk, as central apnea has been reported to emerge following tracheostomy in MSA [103].

Alzheimer's Disease

Sleep-related symptoms are commonly associated with cognitive impairment of a variety of neurological causes [104]. AD is the most common cause of dementia in older adults, and is commonly associated with sleep disturbance of various sorts [105–108]. It has been suggested, perhaps not surprisingly, that increased sleep fragmentation correlated with cognitive impairment, while more mild cognitive findings were associated with more preserved architecture [109]. Insomnia symptoms in particular have also been linked to decreased cognitive function in older adults. One longitudinal study showed that insomnia symptoms conferred a 50 % risk of cognitive decline at 3 years, but no association was seen in women [110]. Another study showed greater than twofold increase in risk of development of new diagnosis of AD with baseline insomnia over a 7-year follow-up [111]. Like other medical illness linked to sleep duration, there is data suggesting that long sleep duration also confers risk, as shown by a large 3-year study in which short (<5 h) and long (>9 h) self-reported daily total sleep durations were associated with new AD diagnosis, but only the long duration group remained significant (greater than twofold) in the adjusted model [112]. In another study, cross-sectional associations between insomnia symptoms and cognitive performance were seen in older women, although there was no prediction of incident cognitive decline over the 2-year follow-up prospective portion [113].

Treatments targeting sleep disturbance should favor non-pharmacological strategies whenever possible, given the vulnerability of older adults to adverse effects of sedative and/or hypnotic agents [114]. These can include sleep–wake schedule management (such as avoiding excessive napping, keeping regular wake-times, and sleep restriction therapy), as well as cognitive behavioral therapy in those able to participate. Interestingly, a randomized controlled trial of melatonin failed to improve actigraphy-scored sleep durations in AD patients, although the lower dose (which was sustained release) was associated with improved caregiver ratings of patient sleep [115]. Another trial utilizing a combination of morning bright light and night-time melatonin in a nursing home setting showed improved daytime metrics (less napping, increased actigraphy-based activity level), but no change in nocturnal sleep in AD patients [116].

Sleep apnea has been linked to memory and cognition impairments in non-demented populations [1, 117], and thus it is not unreasonable to consider sleep apnea as a potentially reversible contributor in patients with cognitive impairment or dementia [118]. Early studies showed a high prevalence of sleep apnea in older individuals [119], including correlations between sleep apnea and cognitive impairments [120–123] and daytime (but not night time) agitation [120], although one of these studies showed similar prevalence of sleep apnea in non-demented controls in their small series [121]. Several metrics of sleep apnea severity were correlated with cognitive status in older women enrolled in the Study of Osteoporotic Fractures, as measured by the mini mental status exam, and the relationship was more prominent in those harboring the epsilon4 allele of apolipoprotein E on genetic testing [124]. In a longitudinal analysis of ~5 % of this cohort studied with in-home PSG, 35 % had an AHI over 15/h (using a 3 % desaturation criteria for hypopnea). In the ~5-year follow-up window, non-demented individuals with sleep apnea had an adjusted odds ratio of 1.8 for incident transition to mild cognitive impairment or dementia [125]. Other PSG metrics were not predictive, such as total sleep time, arousal index, time spent under 90 % oxygen saturation, or wake after sleep onset.

However, not all studies support the association of sleep apnea and cognitive function. For example, two recent cross-sectional studies tested 700–800 older adults each, and, while they found high prevalence of sleep apnea (50–70 %) [126, 127], neither study found significant associations of sleep apnea with cognitive performance testing.

The most important question regarding the association of sleep apnea with cognitive function and dementia is whether interventions to resolve sleep apnea improve neurocognitive performance. CPAP has been shown to be tolerated by many AD patients, and adherence was inversely related to depressive symptomatology [128]. Subjective symptom improvement was seen in a randomized controlled trial of community dwelling mild to moderate AD patients, using the Epworth Sleepiness score as the outcome [129]. Objective improvements after CPAP initiation have been reported in some measures of cognitive performance [130] as well as PSG-derived metrics of sleep architecture and fragmentation in mild to moderate AD [131]. In an extension study of this randomized trial reporting improved sleep architecture, improved mood and slowed deterioration was observed in those patients who adhered to CPAP therapy over the 1-year follow-up [132].

Other Neurodegenerative Disorders

Although symptoms of sleep disturbance are common in patients with Huntington's disease [133–136], objective PSG studies in this population consist of mainly small case series. RBD has been reported, as well as sleep apnea [137] but the evidence is mixed with some studies showing no breathing problems [138–140]. There are limited reports of sleep complaints and/or PSG studies for LBD [141, 142], CBD [143], OPCA [144, 145], and the spinocerebellar ataxias [146–149]. As discussed above, the clinical rationale to evaluate and treat neurological patients is arguably independent of whether disorders such as sleep apnea occur at a higher than baseline prevalence, mainly because of the potential benefit of treatment at the individual level.

Neuromuscular Weakness

Sleep disturbance from a symptom standpoint is highly prevalent in patients with amyotrophic lateral sclerosis (ALS), and includes complaints of onset and maintenance insomnia, nocturia, muscle cramps, and restless legs [150]. As respiratory dysfunction is a key component of the motor deterioration in this population, it is important to note that nocturnal BiPAP improves quality of life in ALS patients and improves survival in the subset without severe bulbar weakness [151]. The presence of sleep apnea in this population would not be surprising, but the literature on prevalence is mixed (though most studies have been small). Several studies have indicated that sleep apnea is present in 15 to >70 % ALS patients using home and lab testing strategies in patients at different stages of disease progression [150, 152–159], while some have reported no significant sleep apnea [160]. Some of these studies reported central/mixed apnea, but it is unclear if simple muscle weakness gives the appearance of diminished effort rather than a mechanism linked to classic central apnea (such as chemoreceptor dysfunction). It is important to note that some of these studies showed that sleep apnea may occur in ALS patients even in the absence of respiratory abnormalities during routine waking testing commonly performed in the course of clinical evaluation (but see [161]). Diaphragmatic pacing has actually been shown to improve both sleep apnea and sleep fragmentation [162].

Myasthenia gravis (MG) is another disorder characterized by muscular weakness in which sleep apnea is an important clinical consideration. Indeed, sleep apnea has been reported in 20–75 % of stable MG patients in different (generally small) case series reports, one of which interestingly showed resolution of sleep apnea in two thirds of those who underwent thymectomy [163–166]. The severity of sleep apnea was reported not to correlate with respiratory weakness in one small study in which 4 of 19 stable MG subjects had sleep apnea [167]. Little is known from the literature about the impact of sleep apnea treatment upon neurological function in MG patients [168].

Sleep apnea has been reported in patients with myotonic dystrophy [169, 170]. Neither of these studies, in which 55–94 % of patients had sleep apnea, showed clear relationship of the nocturnal breathing with daytime symptoms or sleepiness. A minority of cases had central apnea.

Sleep apnea has not been associated, in limited studies, with acute demyelinating neuropathy [171], although subjective sleep disturbance is common in this population [172].

Multiple Sclerosis

Sleep complaints and daytime fatigue are common in MS patients, and the etiology is likely multifactorial [173]. The data is mixed regarding whether there is increased prevalence of sleep apnea in this population [8]. Recent work however suggests increased risk [174], in particular among those with brainstem lesions [175]. RLS and insomnia are also associated with MS, and represent further points of intervention that may augment quality of life. Objective PSG findings suggestive of sleep fragmentation and/or sleep apnea have been associated with the mental but not physical component summary scores [176]. Decreased sleep efficiency, and elevated PLMS (particularly in those with brainstem lesions), has been reported as well [177]. Little is known about casual relationships that could link primary sleep disorders with subsequent risk of MS, although mechanisms of inflammation and immune function are potential links. In one epidemiological study, MS risk was associated with a history of shift work, in particular at least 3 years duration before the age of 20 [178].

Other Neurological Disorders

Like many other pathologies, pain and headache have bidirectional relationship with sleep, in that they can impact sleep, and sleep disturbance of various types may be risk factors for the development and chronicity of headache and pain [179–181]. Sleep disturbances such as insomnia and shift work are associated with headache acutely and may also contribute to development of chronic headache [182]. Sleep duration has also been studied, and those with self-reported short sleep have increased migraine frequency [183]. The data linking headache subtypes to sleep apnea has been mixed, with some authors reporting no relationship [184], while others reported improvement in headache with sleep apnea treatment [185]. Investigation of potentially reversible causes of sleep disturbance, such as occult sleep apnea, seems reasonable especially in chronic or refractory headache cases.

Among patients utilizing chronic opiates for pain, or partial agonists for treatment of opiate dependence, the subtype of sleep apnea characterized by central and/or complex apnea may occur. Complex apnea refers to the emergence of central apnea upon the delivery of positive airway pressure (especially BiPAP), and while the presence of central apnea may be predictive of this response to pressure therapy, this can occur even if the baseline sleep apnea seems to be obstructive in nature. This worsening of apnea with treatment is felt to be related to chemoreceptor dysfunction and resulting alteration of CO_2-based apnea threshold responses. Effective treatment for central/complex apnea can be initiated with adaptive servoventilation techniques in this population [186] and more generally any individual demonstrating complex apnea.

There are case reports of respiratory abnormalities associated with brainstem gliomas. It is unknown whether sleep disturbance represents a risk factor for central nervous system malignancies. However, it is likely that sleep disorders could exacerbate clinical symptoms associated with brain tumors and their treatments. For example, seizures are a common manifestation of CNS malignancy, and sleep apnea may contribute to seizure vulnerability or effectiveness of pharmacotherapy, though this remains to be tested. Adjunctive steroid treatment may cause insomnia and thus impair daytime functioning, a situation that can be further complicated by underlying primary sleep disorder such as sleep apnea, which may also worsen with steroid-associated weight gain.

Idiopathic intracranial hypertension, or psuedotumor cerebri, has been associated with sleep apnea, both at the symptom level [187], and on formal PSG testing in one study that showed an elevated prevalence of 70 % (21 out of 30 patients) [188]. Treatment may be associated with improved outcomes [189].

Most sleep disorders found in the general population are also reported in the TBI population, with the most common symptoms involving insomnia and fatigue [190–193]. A recent meta-analysis of sleep disturbance, including PSG findings, in patients with TBI increased prevalence of a variety of sleep complaints including insomnia as well as 25–50 % with sleep apnea [194]. In a study of combat soldiers with TBI, over 50 % had insomnia, and 35 % had sleep apnea based on AHI > 5 and clinical criteria [195]. Sleep disorders are quite common in active duty military, with over 50 % having sleep apnea in a cohort referred for PSG [195]; 30 % had an AHI value >10, and elevated PLMS was also seen, but neither of these findings correlated with Global Assessment of Functioning scores [196]. Physiological markers of fragmentation (decreased efficiency, increased stage N1 sleep) may occur in those with TBI. Although treatment studies are in their infancy, one recent study showed that resolution of a variety of sleep disorders (sleep apnea, PLMS, narcolepsy) did not correlate with sleep-related symptoms or neurocognitive test scores.

Prion disorders, not surprisingly, have significant impact on sleep physiology, and the interested reader is directed to recent reviews [197–199]. Sleep disruption related to the intensive care unit environment (independent of the illness requiring admission) is of increasing interest, as reviewed recently [200–203].

Conclusion

The growing literature is increasingly informing our understanding of the relationships between sleep disorders and neurological disorders, in particular sleep apnea and insomnia. The prevailing trend is that there are likely bidirectional mechanistic links. However, it is arguable that even if the risk of disorders such as sleep apnea is not specifically elevated in a given neurological population, evaluation and treatment may indirectly have positive impact. Sleep-related symptoms are common among patients and also reported by caregivers of those with cognitive impairment. However, serious sleep disorders such as sleep apnea may not manifest specific symptoms, or the vague symptoms of fatigue or sleepiness may be attributed to other causes especially in the neurological patient. Sleep-related symptoms may not reach the forefront of symptom reporting during clinical evaluations because of more pressing issues of neurological dysfunction. From a practical standpoint, however, it is critical to consider that sleep disturbance is generally treatable, and thus evaluation and treatment in the vulnerable neurological patient seems a reasonable approach. Characterizing the mechanisms by which treatment can improve symptoms or even the underlying disease process (or plasticity related to recovery) remains of high importance for future research.

References

1. Lal C, Strange C, Bachman D. Neurocognitive impairment in obstructive sleep apnea. Chest. 2012;141(6):1601–10.
2. Hermann DM, Bassetti CL. Sleep-related breathing and sleep–wake disturbances in ischemic stroke. Neurology. 2009;73(16):1313–22.
3. Culebras A, Kelly JJ. Sleep disorders and neuromuscular diseases. Rev Neurol Dis. 2008;5(3):153–8.
4. Palma JA, Urrestarazu E, Iriarte J. Sleep loss as risk factor for neurologic disorders: a review. Sleep Med. 2013;14(3):229–36.
5. Mayer G, Jennum P, Riemann D, Dauvilliers Y. Insomnia in central neurologic diseases–occurrence and management. Sleep Med Rev. 2011;15(6):369–78.
6. Tsai JC. Neurological and neurobehavioral sequelae of obstructive sleep apnea. NeuroRehabilitation. 2010;26(1):85–94.
7. Chokroverty S. Sleep and neurodegenerative diseases. Semin Neurol. 2009;29(4):446–67.
8. Brass SD, Duquette P, Proulx-Therrien J, Auerbach S. Sleep disorders in patients with multiple sclerosis. Sleep Med Rev. 2010;14(2):121–9.
9. Autret A, Lucas B, Mondon K, et al. Sleep and brain lesions: a critical review of the literature and additional new cases. Neurophysiol Clin. 2001;31(6): 356–75.
10. Budhiraja R, Budhiraja P, Quan SF. Sleep-disordered breathing and cardiovascular disorders. Respir Care. 2010;55(10):1322–32. discussion 1330-1322.
11. Tregear S, Reston J, Schoelles K, Phillips B. Obstructive sleep apnea and risk of motor vehicle crash: systematic review and meta-analysis. J Clin Sleep Med. 2009;5(6):573–81.
12. Kapur VK. Obstructive sleep apnea: diagnosis, epidemiology, and economics. Respir Care. 2010; 55(9):1155–67.
13. Epstein LJ, Kristo D, Strollo Jr PJ, et al. Clinical guideline for the evaluation, management and long-term care of obstructive sleep apnea in adults. J Clin Sleep Med. 2009;5(3):263–76.
14. Eiseman NA, Westover MB, Ellenbogen JM, Bianchi MT. The impact of body posture and sleep stages on sleep apnea severity in adults. J Clin Sleep Med. 2012;8(6):655–6A.
15. Bianchi MT. Screening for obstructive sleep apnea: Bayes weighs in. Open Sleep J. 2009;2:56–9.
16. Epstein LJ, Dorlac GR. Cost-effectiveness analysis of nocturnal oximetry as a method of screening for sleep apnea-hypopnea syndrome. Chest. 1998; 113(1):97–103.
17. Skomro RP, Kryger MH. Clinical presentations of obstructive sleep apnea syndrome. Prog Cardiovasc Dis. 1999;41(5):331–40.
18. Boyd SB, Walters AS. Effectiveness of treatment apnea-hypopnea index: a mathematical estimate of the true apnea-hypopnea index in the home setting. J Oral Maxillofac Surg. 2013;71(2):351–7.
19. Ravesloot MJ, de Vries N. Reliable calculation of the efficacy of non-surgical and surgical treatment of obstructive sleep apnea revisited. Sleep. 2011; 34(1):105–10.
20. Eiseman NA, Westover MB, Mietus JE, Thomas RJ, Bianchi MT. Classification algorithms for predicting sleepiness and sleep apnea severity. J Sleep Res. 2012;21(1):101–12.
21. Roth T. Insomnia: definition, prevalence, etiology, and consequences. J Clin Sleep Med. 2007;3(5 Suppl):S7–10.
22. Edinger JD, Krystal AD. Subtyping primary insomnia: is sleep state misperception a distinct clinical entity? Sleep Med Rev. 2003;7(3):203–14.
23. Edinger JD, Means MK. Cognitive-behavioral therapy for primary insomnia. Clin Psychol Rev. 2005;25(5):539–58.
24. Ioachimescu OC, El-Solh AA. Pharmacotherapy of insomnia. Expert Opin Pharmacother. 2012; 13(9):1243–60.
25. Sandberg O, Franklin KA, Bucht G, Gustafson Y. Sleep apnea, delirium, depressed mood, cognition, and ADL ability after stroke. J Am Geriatr Soc. 2001;49(4):391–7.
26. Walters AS, Rye DB. Review of the relationship of restless legs syndrome and periodic limb movements in sleep to hypertension, heart disease, and stroke. Sleep. 2009;32(5):589–97.
27. Johnson KG, Johnson DC. Frequency of sleep apnea in stroke and TIA patients: a meta-analysis. J Clin Sleep Med. 2010;6(2):131–7.
28. Loke YK, Brown JW, Kwok CS, Niruban A, Myint PK. Association of obstructive sleep apnea with risk

of serious cardiovascular events: a systematic review and meta-analysis. Circ Cardiovasc Qual Outcomes. 2012;5(5):720–8.
29. Munoz R, Duran-Cantolla J, Martinez-Vila E, et al. Central sleep apnea is associated with increased risk of ischemic stroke in the elderly. Acta Neurol Scand. 2012;126(3):183–8.
30. Bravata DM, Concato J, Fried T, et al. Auto-titrating continuous positive airway pressure for patients with acute transient ischemic attack: a randomized feasibility trial. Stroke. 2010;41(7):1464–70.
31. Bravata DM, Concato J, Fried T, et al. Continuous positive airway pressure: evaluation of a novel therapy for patients with acute ischemic stroke. Sleep. 2011;34(9):1271–7.
32. Ryan CM, Bayley M, Green R, Murray BJ, Bradley TD. Influence of continuous positive airway pressure on outcomes of rehabilitation in stroke patients with obstructive sleep apnea. Stroke. 2011;42(4):1062–7.
33. Benbir G, Karadeniz D. A pilot study of the effects of non-invasive mechanical ventilation on the prognosis of ischemic cerebrovascular events in patients with obstructive sleep apnea syndrome. Neurol Sci. 2012;33(4):811–8.
34. Parra O, Sanchez-Armengol A, Bonnin M, et al. Early treatment of obstructive apnoea and stroke outcome: a randomised controlled trial. Eur Respir J. 2011;37(5):1128–36.
35. Martinez-Garcia MA, Galiano-Blancart R, Roman-Sanchez P, Soler-Cataluna JJ, Cabero-Salt L, Salcedo-Maiques E. Continuous positive airway pressure treatment in sleep apnea prevents new vascular events after ischemic stroke. Chest. 2005;128(4):2123–9.
36. Scala R, Turkington PM, Wanklyn P, Bamford J, Elliott MW. Acceptance, effectiveness and safety of continuous positive airway pressure in acute stroke: a pilot study. Respir Med. 2009;103(1):59–66.
37. Sandberg O, Franklin KA, Bucht G, Eriksson S, Gustafson Y. Nasal continuous positive airway pressure in stroke patients with sleep apnoea: a randomized treatment study. Eur Respir J. 2001;18(4):630–4.
38. Wessendorf TE, Wang YM, Thilmann AF, Sorgenfrei U, Konietzko N, Teschler H. Treatment of obstructive sleep apnoea with nasal continuous positive airway pressure in stroke. Eur Respir J. 2001;18(4):623–9.
39. Broadley SA, Jorgensen L, Cheek A, et al. Early investigation and treatment of obstructive sleep apnoea after acute stroke. J Clin Neurosci. 2007; 14(4):328–33.
40. Minnerup J, Ritter MA, Wersching H, et al. Continuous positive airway pressure ventilation for acute ischemic stroke: a randomized feasibility study. Stroke. 2012;43(4):1137–9.
41. Palombini L, Guilleminault C. Stroke and treatment with nasal CPAP. Eur J Neurol. 2006;13(2):198–200.
42. Brown DL, Chervin RD, Kalbfleisch JD, et al. Sleep apnea treatment after stroke (SATS) trial: is it feasible? J Stroke Cerebrovasc Dis. 2011. [Epub ahead of print]
43. Hsu CY, Vennelle M, Li HY, Engleman HM, Dennis MS, Douglas NJ. Sleep-disordered breathing after stroke: a randomised controlled trial of continuous positive airway pressure. J Neurol Neurosurg Psychiatry. 2006;77(10):1143–9.
44. Tomfohr LM, Hemmen T, Natarajan L, et al. Continuous positive airway pressure for treatment of obstructive sleep apnea in stroke survivors: what do we really know? Stroke. 2012;43(11):3118–23.
45. Brown DL, Feskanich D, Sanchez BN, Rexrode KM, Schernhammer ES, Lisabeth LD. Rotating night shift work and the risk of ischemic stroke. Am J Epidemiol. 2009;169(11):1370–7.
46. Vyas MV, Garg AX, Iansavichus AV, et al. Shift work and vascular events: systematic review and meta-analysis. BMJ. 2012;345:e4800.
47. Cappuccio FP, Cooper D, D'Elia L, Strazzullo P, Miller MA. Sleep duration predicts cardiovascular outcomes: a systematic review and meta-analysis of prospective studies. Eur Heart J. 2011;32(12): 1484–92.
48. Bliwise DL, Young TB. The parable of parabola: what the U-shaped curve can and cannot tell us about sleep. Sleep. 2007;30(12):1614–5.
49. Cappuccio FP, D'Elia L, Strazzullo P, Miller MA. Sleep duration and all-cause mortality: a systematic review and meta-analysis of prospective studies. Sleep. 2010;33(5):585–92.
50. Eguchi K, Hoshide S, Ishikawa S, Shimada K, Kario K. Short sleep duration is an independent predictor of stroke events in elderly hypertensive patients. J Am Soc Hypertens. 2010;4(5):255–62.
51. Loddenkemper T, Lockley SW, Kaleyias J, Kothare SV. Chronobiology of epilepsy: diagnostic and therapeutic implications of chrono-epileptology. J Clin Neurophysiol. 2011;28(2):146–53.
52. Bazil CW. Nocturnal seizures and the effects of anticonvulsants on sleep. Curr Neurol Neurosci Rep. 2008;8(2):149–54.
53. Herman ST, Walczak TS, Bazil CW. Distribution of partial seizures during the sleep–wake cycle: differences by seizure onset site. Neurology. 2001;56(11):1453–9.
54. van Golde EG, Gutter T, de Weerd AW. Sleep disturbances in people with epilepsy; prevalence, impact and treatment. Sleep Med Rev. 2011;15(6):357–68.
55. Badawy RA, Curatolo JM, Newton M, Berkovic SF, Macdonell RA. Sleep deprivation increases cortical excitability in epilepsy: syndrome-specific effects. Neurology. 2006;67(6):1018–22.
56. Malow BA, Passaro E, Milling C, Minecan DN, Levy K. Sleep deprivation does not affect seizure frequency during inpatient video-EEG monitoring. Neurology. 2002;59(9):1371–4.
57. de Weerd A, de Haas S, Otte A, et al. Subjective sleep disturbance in patients with partial epilepsy: a questionnaire-based study on prevalence and impact on quality of life. Epilepsia. 2004;45(11): 1397–404.

58. Khatami R, Zutter D, Siegel A, Mathis J, Donati F, Bassetti CL. Sleep–wake habits and disorders in a series of 100 adult epilepsy patients—a prospective study. Seizure. 2006;15(5):299–306.
59. Manni R, Terzaghi M. Comorbidity between epilepsy and sleep disorders. Epilepsy Res. 2010;90(3):171–7.
60. Leger D, Scheuermaier K, Philip P, Paillard M, Guilleminault C. SF-36: evaluation of quality of life in severe and mild insomniacs compared with good sleepers. Psychosom Med. 2001;63(1):49–55.
61. Malow BA, Foldvary-Schaefer N, Vaughn BV, et al. Treating obstructive sleep apnea in adults with epilepsy: a randomized pilot trial. Neurology. 2008; 71(8):572–7.
62. Hollinger P, Khatami R, Gugger M, Hess CW, Bassetti CL. Epilepsy and obstructive sleep apnea. Eur Neurol. 2006;55(2):74–9.
63. Vendrame M, Auerbach S, Loddenkemper T, Kothare S, Montouris G. Effect of continuous positive airway pressure treatment on seizure control in patients with obstructive sleep apnea and epilepsy. Epilepsia. 2011;52(11):e168–71.
64. Gaig C, Iranzo A. Sleep-disordered breathing in neurodegenerative diseases. Curr Neurol Neurosci Rep. 2012;12(2):205–17.
65. Fuller PM, Gooley JJ, Saper CB. Neurobiology of the sleep–wake cycle: sleep architecture, circadian regulation, and regulatory feedback. J Biol Rhythms. 2006;21(6):482–93.
66. Gagnon JF, Postuma RB, Mazza S, Doyon J, Montplaisir J. Rapid-eye-movement sleep behaviour disorder and neurodegenerative diseases. Lancet Neurol. 2006;5(5):424–32.
67. Iranzo A, Santamaria J, Tolosa E. The clinical and pathophysiological relevance of REM sleep behavior disorder in neurodegenerative diseases. Sleep Med Rev. 2009;13(6):385–401.
68. Partinen M. Sleep disorder related to Parkinson's disease. J Neurol. 1997;244(4 Suppl 1):S3–6.
69. Kumar S, Bhatia M, Behari M. Sleep disorders in Parkinson's disease. Mov Disord. 2002;17(4): 775–81.
70. Factor SA, McAlarney T, Sanchez-Ramos JR, Weiner WJ. Sleep disorders and sleep effect in Parkinson's disease. Mov Disord. 1990;5(4):280–5.
71. Gunn DG, Naismith SL, Lewis SJ. Sleep disturbances in Parkinson disease and their potential role in heterogeneity. J Geriatr Psychiatry Neurol. 2010;23(2):131–7.
72. Compta Y, Santamaria J, Ratti L, et al. Cerebrospinal hypocretin, daytime sleepiness and sleep architecture in Parkinson's disease dementia. Brain. 2009;132(Pt 12):3308–17.
73. Happe S, Klosch G, Lorenzo J, et al. Perception of sleep: subjective versus objective sleep parameters in patients with Parkinson's disease in comparison with healthy elderly controls. Sleep perception in Parkinson's disease and controls. J Neurol. 2005;252(8):936–43.
74. Currie LJ, Bennett Jr JP, Harrison MB, Trugman JM, Wooten GF. Clinical correlates of sleep benefit in Parkinson's disease. Neurology. 1997;48(4):1115–7.
75. Merello M, Hughes A, Colosimo C, Hoffman M, Starkstein S, Leiguarda R. Sleep benefit in Parkinson's disease. Mov Disord. 1997;12(4):506–8.
76. Reist C, Sokolski KN, Chen CC, Coskinas E, Demet EM. The effect of sleep deprivation on motor impairment and retinal adaptation in Parkinson's disease. Prog Neuropsychopharmacol Biol Psychiatry. 1995;19(3):445–54.
77. Hogl B, Peralta C, Wetter TC, Gershanik O, Trenkwalder C. Effect of sleep deprivation on motor performance in patients with Parkinson's disease. Mov Disord. 2001;16(4):616–21.
78. Chen H, Schernhammer E, Schwarzschild MA, Ascherio A. A prospective study of night shift work, sleep duration, and risk of Parkinson's disease. Am J Epidemiol. 2006;163(8):726–30.
79. Gao J, Huang X, Park Y, et al. Daytime napping, nighttime sleeping, and Parkinson disease. Am J Epidemiol. 2011;173(9):1032–8.
80. Young A, Home M, Churchward T, Freezer N, Holmes P, Ho M. Comparison of sleep disturbance in mild versus severe Parkinson's disease. Sleep. 2002;25(5):573–7.
81. Dhawan V, Dhoat S, Williams AJ, et al. The range and nature of sleep dysfunction in untreated Parkinson's disease (PD). A comparative controlled clinical study using the Parkinson's disease sleep scale and selective polysomnography. J Neurol Sci. 2006;248(1–2):158–62.
82. Wetter TC, Trenkwalder C, Gershanik O, Hogl B. Polysomnographic measures in Parkinson's disease: a comparison between patients with and without REM sleep disturbances. Wien Klin Wochenschr. 2001;113(7–8):249–53.
83. Wetter TC, Collado-Seidel V, Pollmacher T, Yassouridis A, Trenkwalder C. Sleep and periodic leg movement patterns in drug-free patients with Parkinson's disease and multiple system atrophy. Sleep. 2000;23(3):361–7.
84. Baumann C, Ferini-Strambi L, Waldvogel D, Werth E, Bassetti CL. Parkinsonism with excessive daytime sleepiness—a narcolepsy-like disorder? J Neurol. 2005;252(2):139–45.
85. Cochen De Cock V, Abouda M, Leu S, et al. Is obstructive sleep apnea a problem in Parkinson's disease? Sleep Med. 2010;11(3):247–52.
86. Yong MH, Fook-Chong S, Pavanni R, Lim LL, Tan EK. Case control polysomnographic studies of sleep disorders in Parkinson's disease. PLoS One. 2011;6(7):e22511.
87. Trotti LM, Bliwise DL. No increased risk of obstructive sleep apnea in Parkinson's disease. Mov Disord. 2010;25(13):2246–9.
88. Gottlieb DJ, Whitney CW, Bonekat WH, et al. Relation of sleepiness to respiratory disturbance index: the Sleep Heart Health Study. Am J Respir Crit Care Med. 1999;159(2):502–7.

89. Ghorayeb I, Yekhlef F, Chrysostome V, Balestre E, Bioulac B, Tison F. Sleep disorders and their determinants in multiple system atrophy. J Neurol Neurosurg Psychiatry. 2002;72(6):798–800.
90. Moreno-Lopez C, Santamaria J, Salamero M, et al. Excessive daytime sleepiness in multiple system atrophy (SLEEMSA study). Arch Neurol. 2011; 68(2):223–30.
91. Ghorayeb I, Bioulac B, Tison F. Sleep disorders in multiple system atrophy. J Neural Transm. 2005; 112(12):1669–75.
92. Plazzi G, Corsini R, Provini F, et al. REM sleep behavior disorders in multiple system atrophy. Neurology. 1997;48(4):1094–7.
93. Nam H, Hong YH, Kwon HM, Cho J. Does multiple system atrophy itself affect sleep structure? Neurologist. 2009;15(5):274–6.
94. Vetrugno R, Provini F, Cortelli P, et al. Sleep disorders in multiple system atrophy: a correlative video-polysomnographic study. Sleep Med. 2004; 5(1):21–30.
95. Guo XY, Cao B, Lei F, et al. Clinical and polysomnographic features of patients with multiple system atrophy in Southwest China. Sleep Breath. 2013. Apr 6. [Epub ahead of print]
96. Shimohata T, Shinoda H, Nakayama H, et al. Daytime hypoxemia, sleep-disordered breathing, and laryngopharyngeal findings in multiple system atrophy. Arch Neurol. 2007;64(6):856–61.
97. Shimohata T, Nakayama H, Tomita M, Ozawa T, Nishizawa M. Daytime sleepiness in Japanese patients with multiple system atrophy: prevalence and determinants. BMC Neurol. 2012;12:130.
98. Ghorayeb I, Yekhlef F, Bioulac B, Tison F. Continuous positive airway pressure for sleep-related breathing disorders in multiple system atrophy: long-term acceptance. Sleep Med. 2005;6(4):359–62.
99. Iranzo A, Santamaria J, Tolosa E. Continuous positive air pressure eliminates nocturnal stridor in multiple system atrophy. Barcelona Multiple System Atrophy Study Group. Lancet. 2000;356(9238):1329–30.
100. Iranzo A, Santamaria J, Tolosa E, et al. Long-term effect of CPAP in the treatment of nocturnal stridor in multiple system atrophy. Neurology. 2004;63(5): 930–2.
101. Iranzo A. Management of sleep-disordered breathing in multiple system atrophy. Sleep Med. 2005; 6(4):297–300.
102. Shimohata T, Tomita M, Nakayama H, Aizawa N, Ozawa T, Nishizawa M. Floppy epiglottis as a contraindication of CPAP in patients with multiple system atrophy. Neurology. 2011;76(21):1841–2.
103. Jin K, Okabe S, Chida K, et al. Tracheostomy can fatally exacerbate sleep-disordered breathing in multiple system atrophy. Neurology. 2007;68(19):1618–21.
104. Guarnieri B, Adorni F, Musicco M, et al. Prevalence of sleep disturbances in mild cognitive impairment and dementing disorders: a multicenter Italian clinical cross-sectional study on 431 patients. Dement Geriatr Cogn Disord. 2012;33(1):50–8.
105. Vitiello MV, Bliwise DL, Prinz PN. Sleep in Alzheimer's disease and the sundown syndrome. Neurology. 1992;42(7 Suppl 6):83–93. discussion 93-84.
106. Vitiello MV, Poceta JS, Prinz PN. Sleep in Alzheimer's disease and other dementing disorders. Can J Psychol. 1991;45(2):221–39.
107. Vitiello MV, Prinz PN. Alzheimer's disease. Sleep and sleep/wake patterns. Clin Geriatr Med. 1989; 5(2):289–99.
108. Vitiello MV, Prinz PN, Williams DE, Frommlet MS, Ries RK. Sleep disturbances in patients with mild-stage Alzheimer's disease. J Gerontol. 1990; 45(4):M131–8.
109. Moe KE, Vitiello MV, Larsen LH, Prinz PN. Symposium: cognitive processes and sleep disturbances: sleep/wake patterns in Alzheimer's disease: relationships with cognition and function. J Sleep Res. 1995;4(1):15–20.
110. Cricco M, Simonsick EM, Foley DJ. The impact of insomnia on cognitive functioning in older adults. J Am Geriatr Soc. 2001;49(9):1185–9.
111. Osorio RS, Pirraglia E, Aguera-Ortiz LF, et al. Greater risk of Alzheimer's disease in older adults with insomnia. J Am Geriatr Soc. 2011;59(3):559–62.
112. Benito-Leon J, Bermejo-Pareja F, Vega S, Louis ED. Total daily sleep duration and the risk of dementia: a prospective population-based study. Eur J Neurol. 2009;16(9):990–7.
113. Tworoger SS, Lee S, Schernhammer ES, Grodstein F. The association of self-reported sleep duration, difficulty sleeping, and snoring with cognitive function in older women. Alzheimer Dis Assoc Disord. 2006;20(1):41–8.
114. David R, Zeitzer J, Friedman L, et al. Non-pharmacologic management of sleep disturbance in Alzheimer's disease. J Nutr Health Aging. 2010; 14(3):203–6.
115. Singer C, Tractenberg RE, Kaye J, et al. A multicenter, placebo-controlled trial of melatonin for sleep disturbance in Alzheimer's disease. Sleep. 2003;26(7):893–901.
116. Dowling GA, Burr RL, Van Someren EJ, et al. Melatonin and bright-light treatment for rest-activity disruption in institutionalized patients with Alzheimer's disease. J Am Geriatr Soc. 2008;56(2): 239–46.
117. Sanchez AI, Martinez P, Miro E, Bardwell WA, Buela-Casal G. CPAP and behavioral therapies in patients with obstructive sleep apnea: effects on daytime sleepiness, mood, and cognitive function. Sleep Med Rev. 2009;13(3):223–33.
118. Bliwise DL. Is sleep apnea a cause of reversible dementia in old age? J Am Geriatr Soc. 1996;44(11):1407–9.
119. Ancoli-Israel S, Kripke DF, Klauber MR, Mason WJ, Fell R, Kaplan O. Sleep-disordered breathing in community-dwelling elderly. Sleep. 1991; 14(6):486–95.
120. Gehrman PR, Martin JL, Shochat T, Nolan S, Corey-Bloom J, Ancoli-Israel S. Sleep-disordered breathing

and agitation in institutionalized adults with Alzheimer disease. Am J Geriatr Psychiatry. 2003; 11(4):426–33.
121. Smallwood RG, Vitiello MV, Giblin EC, Prinz PN. Sleep apnea: relationship to age, sex, and Alzheimer's dementia. Sleep. 1983;6(1):16–22.
122. Erkinjuntti T, Partinen M, Sulkava R, Telakivi T, Salmi T, Tilvis R. Sleep apnea in multiinfarct dementia and Alzheimer's disease. Sleep. 1987; 10(5):419–25.
123. Ancoli-Israel S, Klauber MR, Butters N, Parker L, Kripke DF. Dementia in institutionalized elderly: relation to sleep apnea. J Am Geriatr Soc. 1991; 39(3):258–63.
124. Spira AP, Blackwell T, Stone KL, et al. Sleep-disordered breathing and cognition in older women. J Am Geriatr Soc. 2008;56(1):45–50.
125. Yaffe K, Laffan AM, Harrison SL, et al. Sleep-disordered breathing, hypoxia, and risk of mild cognitive impairment and dementia in older women. JAMA. 2011;306(6):613–9.
126. Sforza E, Roche F, Thomas-Anterion C, et al. Cognitive function and sleep related breathing disorders in a healthy elderly population: the SYNAPSE study. Sleep. 2010;33(4):515–21.
127. Foley DJ, Masaki K, White L, Larkin EK, Monjan A, Redline S. Sleep-disordered breathing and cognitive impairment in elderly Japanese–American men. Sleep. 2003;26(5):596–9.
128. Ayalon L, Ancoli-Israel S, Stepnowsky C, et al. Adherence to continuous positive airway pressure treatment in patients with Alzheimer's disease and obstructive sleep apnea. Am J Geriatr Psychiatry. 2006;14(2):176–80.
129. Chong MS, Ayalon L, Marler M, et al. Continuous positive airway pressure reduces subjective daytime sleepiness in patients with mild to moderate Alzheimer's disease with sleep disordered breathing. J Am Geriatr Soc. 2006;54(5):777–81.
130. Ancoli-Israel S, Palmer BW, Cooke JR, et al. Cognitive effects of treating obstructive sleep apnea in Alzheimer's disease: a randomized controlled study. J Am Geriatr Soc. 2008;56(11):2076–81.
131. Cooke JR, Ancoli-Israel S, Liu L, et al. Continuous positive airway pressure deepens sleep in patients with Alzheimer's disease and obstructive sleep apnea. Sleep Med. 2009;10(10):1101–6.
132. Cooke JR, Ayalon L, Palmer BW, et al. Sustained use of CPAP slows deterioration of cognition, sleep, and mood in patients with Alzheimer's disease and obstructive sleep apnea: a preliminary study. J Clin Sleep Med. 2009;5(4):305–9.
133. Videnovic A, Leurgans S, Fan W, Jaglin J, Shannon KM. Daytime somnolence and nocturnal sleep disturbances in Huntington disease. Parkinsonism Relat Disord. 2009;15(6):471–4.
134. Hansotia P, Wall R, Berendes J. Sleep disturbances and severity of Huntington's disease. Neurology. 1985;35(11):1672–4.
135. Goodman AO, Barker RA. How vital is sleep in Huntington's disease? J Neurol. 2010; 257(6):882–97.
136. Myers RH, Sax DS, Schoenfeld M, et al. Late onset of Huntington's disease. J Neurol Neurosurg Psychiatry. 1985;48(6):530–4.
137. Goodman AO, Rogers L, Pilsworth S, et al. Asymptomatic sleep abnormalities are a common early feature in patients with Huntington's disease. Curr Neurol Neurosci Rep. 2011;11(2):211–7.
138. Cuturic M, Abramson RK, Vallini D, Frank EM, Shamsnia M. Sleep patterns in patients with Huntington's disease and their unaffected first-degree relatives: a brief report. Behav Sleep Med. 2009;7(4):245–54.
139. Arnulf I, Nielsen J, Lohmann E, et al. Rapid eye movement sleep disturbances in Huntington disease. Arch Neurol. 2008;65(4):482–8.
140. Bollen EL, Den Heijer JC, Ponsioen C, et al. Respiration during sleep in Huntington's chorea. J Neurol Sci. 1988;84(1):63–8.
141. Boeve BF, Silber MH, Ferman TJ, et al. REM sleep behavior disorder and degenerative dementia: an association likely reflecting Lewy body disease. Neurology. 1998;51(2):363–70.
142. Grace JB, Walker MP, McKeith IG. A comparison of sleep profiles in patients with dementia with lewy bodies and Alzheimer's disease. Int J Geriatr Psychiatry. 2000;15(11):1028–33.
143. Roche S, Jacquesson JM, Destee A, Defebvre L, Derambure P, Monaca C. Sleep and vigilance in corticobasal degeneration: a descriptive study. Neurophysiol Clin. 2007;37(4):261–4.
144. Kneisley LW, Rederich GJ. Nocturnal stridor in olivopontocerebellar atrophy. Sleep. 1990;13(4):362–8.
145. Chokroverty S, Sachdeo R, Masdeu J. Autonomic dysfunction and sleep apnea in olivopontocerebellar degeneration. Arch Neurol. 1984;41(9):926–31.
146. Boesch SM, Frauscher B, Brandauer E, Wenning GK, Poewe W, Hogl B. Restless legs syndrome and motor activity during sleep in spinocerebellar ataxia type 6. Sleep Med. 2006;7(6):529–32.
147. Velazquez-Perez L, Voss U, Rodriguez-Labrada R, et al. Sleep disorders in spinocerebellar ataxia type 2 patients. Neurodegener Dis. 2011;8(6):447–54.
148. Tuin I, Voss U, Kang JS, et al. Stages of sleep pathology in spinocerebellar ataxia type 2 (SCA2). Neurology. 2006;67(11):1966–72.
149. D'Abreu A, Franca Jr M, Conz L, et al. Sleep symptoms and their clinical correlates in Machado-Joseph disease. Acta Neurol Scand. 2009;119(4):277–80.
150. Lo Coco D, Mattaliano P, Spataro R, Mattaliano A, La Bella V. Sleep–wake disturbances in patients with amyotrophic lateral sclerosis. J Neurol Neurosurg Psychiatry. 2011;82(8):839–42.
151. Bourke SC, Tomlinson M, Williams TL, Bullock RE, Shaw PJ, Gibson GJ. Effects of non-invasive ventilation on survival and quality of life in patients

with amyotrophic lateral sclerosis: a randomised controlled trial. Lancet Neurol. 2006;5(2):140–7.
152. Ferguson KA, Strong MJ, Ahmad D, George CF. Sleep-disordered breathing in amyotrophic lateral sclerosis. Chest. 1996;110(3):664–9.
153. David WS, Bundlie SR, Mahdavi Z. Polysomnographic studies in amyotrophic lateral sclerosis. J Neurol Sci. 1997;152 Suppl 1:S29–35.
154. Atalaia A, De Carvalho M, Evangelista T, Pinto A. Sleep characteristics of amyotrophic lateral sclerosis in patients with preserved diaphragmatic function. Amyotroph Lateral Scler. 2007;8(2):101–5.
155. Bourke SC, Shaw PJ, Gibson GJ. Respiratory function vs sleep-disordered breathing as predictors of QOL in ALS. Neurology. 2001;57(11):2040–4.
156. Lyall RA, Donaldson N, Polkey MI, Leigh PN, Moxham J. Respiratory muscle strength and ventilatory failure in amyotrophic lateral sclerosis. Brain. 2001;124(Pt 10):2000–13.
157. Kimura K, Tachibana N, Kimura J, Shibasaki H. Sleep-disordered breathing at an early stage of amyotrophic lateral sclerosis. J Neurol Sci. 1999; 164(1):37–43.
158. Tsara V, Serasli E, Steiropoulos P, Tsorova A, Antoniadou M, Zisi P. Respiratory function in amyotrophic lateral sclerosis patients. The role of sleep studies. Hippokratia. 2010;14(1):33–6.
159. de Carvalho M, Costa J, Pinto S, Pinto A. Percutaneous nocturnal oximetry in amyotrophic lateral sclerosis: periodic desaturation. Amyotroph Lateral Scler. 2009;10(3):154–61.
160. Arnulf I, Similowski T, Salachas F, et al. Sleep disorders and diaphragmatic function in patients with amyotrophic lateral sclerosis. Am J Respir Crit Care Med. 2000;161(3 Pt 1):849–56.
161. Carratu P, Cassano A, Gadaleta F, et al. Association between low sniff nasal-inspiratory pressure (SNIP) and sleep disordered breathing in amyotrophic lateral sclerosis: preliminary results. Amyotroph Lateral Scler. 2011;12(6):458–63.
162. Gonzalez-Bermejo J, Morelot-Panzini C, Salachas F, et al. Diaphragm pacing improves sleep in patients with amyotrophic lateral sclerosis. Amyotroph Lateral Scler. 2012;13(1):44–54.
163. Amino A, Shiozawa Z, Nagasaka T, et al. Sleep apnoea in well-controlled myasthenia gravis and the effect of thymectomy. J Neurol. 1998;245(2):77–80.
164. Stepansky R, Weber G, Zeitlhofer J. Sleep apnea and cognitive dysfunction in myasthenia gravis. Acta Med Austriaca. 1997;24(3):128–31.
165. Nicolle MW, Rask S, Koopman WJ, George CF, Adams J, Wiebe S. Sleep apnea in patients with myasthenia gravis. Neurology. 2006;67(1):140–2.
166. Quera-Salva MA, Guilleminault C, Chevret S, et al. Breathing disorders during sleep in myasthenia gravis. Ann Neurol. 1992;31(1):86–92.
167. Prudlo J, Koenig J, Ermert S, Juhasz J. Sleep disordered breathing in medically stable patients with myasthenia gravis. Eur J Neurol. 2007;14(3):321–6.
168. Naseer S, Kolade VO, Idrees S, Naseer S, Chandra A. Improvement in ocular myasthenia gravis during CPAP therapy for sleep apnea. Tenn Med. 2012; 105(9):33–4.
169. Pincherle A, Patruno V, Raimondi P, et al. Sleep breathing disorders in 40 Italian patients with myotonic dystrophy type 1. Neuromuscul Disord. 2012;22(3):219–24.
170. Kiyan E, Okumus G, Cuhadaroglu C, Deymeer F. Sleep apnea in adult myotonic dystrophy patients who have no excessive daytime sleepiness. Sleep Breath. 2010;14(1):19–24.
171. Koeppen S, Kraywinkel K, Wessendorf TE, et al. Long-term outcome of Guillain-Barre syndrome. Neurocrit Care. 2006;5(3):235–42.
172. Karkare K, Sinha S, Taly AB, Rao S. Prevalence and profile of sleep disturbances in Guillain-Barre syndrome: a prospective questionnaire-based study during 10 days of hospitalization. Acta Neurol Scand. 2013;127(2):116–23.
173. Penner I, Calabrese P. Managing fatigue: clinical correlates, assessment procedures and therapeutic strategies. Int MS J. 2010;17(1):28–34.
174. Kaminska M, Kimoff RJ, Benedetti A, et al. Obstructive sleep apnea is associated with fatigue in multiple sclerosis. Mult Scler. 2012;18(8):1159–69.
175. Braley TJ, Segal BM, Chervin RD. Sleep-disordered breathing in multiple sclerosis. Neurology. 2012; 79(9):929–36.
176. Trojan DA, Kaminska M, Bar-Or A, et al. Polysomnographic measures of disturbed sleep are associated with reduced quality of life in multiple sclerosis. J Neurol Sci. 2012;316(1–2):158–63.
177. Ferini-Strambi L, Filippi M, Martinelli V, et al. Nocturnal sleep study in multiple sclerosis: correlations with clinical and brain magnetic resonance imaging findings. J Neurol Sci. 1994;125(2):194–7.
178. Hedstrom AK, Akerstedt T, Hillert J, Olsson T, Alfredsson L. Shift work at young age is associated with increased risk for multiple sclerosis. Ann Neurol. 2011;70(5):733–41.
179. Moldofsky H. Sleep and pain. Sleep Med Rev. 2001;5(5):385–96.
180. Alberti A. Headache and sleep. Sleep Med Rev. 2006;10(6):431–7.
181. Jennum P, Jensen R. Sleep and headache. Sleep Med Rev. 2002;6(6):471–9.
182. Rains JC, Poceta JS. Sleep-related headaches. Neurol Clin. 2012;30(4):1285–98.
183. Kelman L, Rains JC. Headache and sleep: examination of sleep patterns and complaints in a large clinical sample of migraineurs. Headache. 2005;45(7): 904–10.
184. Neau JP, Paquereau J, Bailbe M, Meurice JC, Ingrand P, Gil R. Relationship between sleep apnoea syndrome, snoring and headaches. Cephalalgia. 2002;22(5):333–9.
185. Johnson KG, Ziemba AM, Garb JL. Improvement in headaches with continuous positive airway pressure

for obstructive sleep apnea: a retrospective analysis. Headache. 2013;53(2):333–43.
186. Ramar K, Ramar P, Morgenthaler TI. Adaptive servoventilation in patients with central or complex sleep apnea related to chronic opioid use and congestive heart failure. J Clin Sleep Med. 2012;8(5):569–76.
187. Fraser JA, Bruce BB, Rucker J, et al. Risk factors for idiopathic intracranial hypertension in men: a case-control study. J Neurol Sci. 2010;290(1–2):86–9.
188. Thurtell MJ, Bruce BB, Rye DB, Newman NJ, Biousse V. The Berlin questionnaire screens for obstructive sleep apnea in idiopathic intracranial hypertension. J Neuroophthalmol. 2011;31(4):316–9.
189. Lee AG, Golnik K, Kardon R, Wall M, Eggenberger E, Yedavally S. Sleep apnea and intracranial hypertension in men. Ophthalmology. 2002;109(3):482–5.
190. Viola-Saltzman M, Watson NF. Traumatic brain injury and sleep disorders. Neurol Clin. 2012;30(4):1299–312.
191. Castriotta RJ, Murthy JN. Sleep disorders in patients with traumatic brain injury: a review. CNS Drugs. 2011;25(3):175–85.
192. Castriotta RJ, Wilde MC, Lai JM, Atanasov S, Masel BE, Kuna ST. Prevalence and consequences of sleep disorders in traumatic brain injury. J Clin Sleep Med. 2007;3(4):349–56.
193. Ponsford JL, Ziino C, Parcell DL, et al. Fatigue and sleep disturbance following traumatic brain injury—their nature, causes, and potential treatments. J Head Trauma Rehabil. 2012;27(3):224–33.
194. Mathias JL, Alvaro PK. Prevalence of sleep disturbances, disorders, and problems following traumatic brain injury: a meta-analysis. Sleep Med. 2012;13(7):898–905.
195. Collen J, Orr N, Lettieri CJ, Carter K, Holley AB. Sleep disturbances among soldiers with combat-related traumatic brain injury. Chest. 2012;142(3):622–30.
196. Verma A, Anand V, Verma NP. Sleep disorders in chronic traumatic brain injury. J Clin Sleep Med. 2007;3(4):357–62.
197. Montagna P. Fatal familial insomnia: a model disease in sleep physiopathology. Sleep Med Rev. 2005;9(5):339–53.
198. Montagna P, Gambetti P, Cortelli P, Lugaresi E. Familial and sporadic fatal insomnia. Lancet Neurol. 2003;2(3):167–76.
199. Parkes JD. Genetic factors in human sleep disorders with special reference to Norrie disease, Prader-Willi syndrome and Moebius syndrome. J Sleep Res. 1999;8 Suppl 1:14–22.
200. Elliott R, McKinley S, Cistulli P. The quality and duration of sleep in the intensive care setting: an integrative review. Int J Nurs Stud. 2011;48(3):384–400.
201. Figueroa-Ramos MI, Arroyo-Novoa CM, Lee KA, Padilla G, Puntillo KA. Sleep and delirium in ICU patients: a review of mechanisms and manifestations. Intensive Care Med. 2009;35(5):781–95.
202. Hardin KA. Sleep in the ICU: potential mechanisms and clinical implications. Chest. 2009;136(1):284–94.
203. Drouot X, Cabello B, d'Ortho MP, Brochard L. Sleep in the intensive care unit. Sleep Med Rev. 2008;12(5):391–403.

Sleep Deprivation and Psychiatric Disorders

6

Matt T. Bianchi and Maren Nyer

Introduction

Adequate quantity and quality of sleep is fundamental to psychological and psychiatric stability. Sleep loss has been associated with psychological status in healthy subjects undergoing experimental sleep deprivation [1]. Negative impact on mood scales has been reported with both sleep deprivation and sleep fragmentation protocols in healthy adults [2]. Interestingly, acute sleep deprivation may have differential impact on healthy individuals compared to patients with depression, wherein mood may transiently improve. Symptoms of sleep disturbance and/or non-refreshing sleep are common components of many psychiatric disorders. The term sleep disturbance most typically refers to insomnia, and thus we begin with an overview of insomnia, emphasizing the challenges in characterizing this complex constellation of symptoms and presentations. Insomnia may be reported as a subjective complaint involving difficulty with initiation of sleep, maintaining sleep throughout the night, and/or awakening earlier than intended. Objective data is not required for either the psychiatric or sleep medicine diagnostic criteria for insomnia or its subtypes, and indeed laboratory polysomnography (PSG) is not routinely indicated in the evaluation of patients with insomnia [3, 4]. Instead, the diagnosis is made by the subjective clinical history, including the diagnostic subtype varieties such as primary, psychophysiological, or secondary to other causes. Despite this reliance on self-report for the diagnosis of insomnia, it is important to be aware of a particular phenomenon in some patients called paradoxical, misperception, or subjective insomnia [5]. This is defined by a mismatch between objective measures and the subjective reporting of the insomnia sleep complaint: when PSG and subjective data are available, the sleep latency can be overestimated, and the total sleep time (TST) can be underestimated, compared to objective measures. While there is increasing evidence that this mismatch occurs along a spectrum of severity [6–10], the strict diagnostic criteria used for paradoxical insomnia require extreme underestimation of TST in otherwise normal sleep, and thus its prevalence is estimated at only 5 % in the diagnostic manual of sleep disorders [11]. However, the occurrence of some degree of mismatch may be much more common.

Although objective measures are not routinely indicated for insomnia [3], performing PSG allows one to describe the degree of misperception between the objective and subjective aspects of a patient's sleep disturbance. Treatment response, whether via pharmacological or behavioral

M.T. Bianchi, M.D., Ph.D., M.M.Sc. (✉)
Division of Sleep Medicine, Department of Neurology, Massachusetts General Hospital, Boston, MA, USA
e-mail: mtbianchi@partners.org

M. Nyer, Ph.D.
Depression and Clinical Research Program, Department of Psychiatry, Massachusetts General Hospital, Boston, MA, USA

M.T. Bianchi (ed.), *Sleep Deprivation and Disease: Effects on the Body, Brain and Behavior*, DOI 10.1007/978-1-4614-9087-6_6, © Springer Science+Business Media New York 2014

interventions, is also based on subjective clinical report, and thus the issue of mismatch (subjective perception of sleep improvement relative to objective measures) arises in the management/treatment phase, as well as the diagnostic phase for patients with insomnia. Understanding the degree of mismatch via objective sleep measurement might assist in management of insomnia among those with misperception. For example, among patients choosing pharmacotherapy for insomnia, the risk–benefit discussion should include, among other things, some estimate of the medical severity of the insomnia, which is most recently linked to objective sleep duration [12]. In addition, and perhaps most interestingly, feedback provided to reassure patients that they are sleeping more than they perceive may be of clinical benefit [13, 14]. If further trials confirm that feedback using objective home sleep monitoring is effective, such non-pharmacological strategies may enjoy important benefits over pharmacotherapy, which has been increasingly linked to adverse outcomes [15–20]. However, these epidemiological association studies have their own limitations [21, 22]. Structured risk–benefit balance is challenging in the domain of pharmacotherapy – a motivating factor to actively pursue non-pharmacological interventions to expand the already proven options of cognitive behavioral therapy [23, 24].

The majority of epidemiological reports of insomnia prevalence and links to other medical and psychiatric problems are primarily based on subjective reports (with some exceptions [25, 26]). As there is a growing literature describing the prevalence of mismatch between objective and subjective metrics of sleep, some caution is required when interpreting epidemiological links with self-reported insomnia symptoms and/or sleep durations. In other words, within a group of individuals felt to be "similar" in that they all report 5 h of sleep per night due to insomnia, there may be a spectrum of objective sleep durations on objective testing. Because of the potential for misperception, this apparently homogenous group may differ in objective measures of sleep duration, thus introducing "noise" into the epidemiological literature. Thus, epidemiological studies run the risk of diminished or falsely negative associations of insomnia and clinically relevant morbidity. For example, subjective–objective mismatch may occur across the spectrum of insomnia diagnostic subtypes, thus decreasing the power to identify associations that have objective underlying mechanisms that can be identified through physiological, serologic, or other forms of testing. These underlying mechanisms may have important implications for guiding appropriate interventions for insomnia.

There is additional potential for inconsistency in self-reported sleep depending on when an individual is asked to report the duration of sleep. For example, comparing the self-reported sleep durations obtained in the morning (referring to the prior night), with a retrospective self-reported summary of the previous week of sleep, individuals who underestimated their sleep duration on the morning diary entries showed a greater underestimation in their 1-week-later retrospective self-report [27]. In other words, patient self-report appears to become increasingly discordant with objective measures over time. This has important implications for the clinical evaluation of insomnia patients, who may report on even longer durations of weeks or months, with the possibility of what may be considered a meta-misperception of their sleep–wake patterns. Clinical practice often involves having patients record a daily diary of their sleep, which may mitigate some of this exaggeration effect.

The altered perception of sleep–wake times among those with insomnia may actually have a biological basis, which may be distinct from the biology of objective sleep disturbance. For review of this intriguing phenomenon, the reader is directed to the excellent summary by Harvey and Tang [5]. Several groups have proposed contributing factors associated with subjective–objective mismatch in insomnia. Altered time perception has been proposed as a mechanism, meaning that there is a primary issue of altered perception of time, and this time misperception may not be specific for only wakefulness and may extend to sleep time perception as well. However, some studies do not support a primary time perception issue [27, 28]. Psychological factors have been investigated, including personality types and mood symptoms [9, 29–31]. Objective physiological correlates include hyperarousal mechanisms [32], alpha–delta pattern of NREM sleep EEG [33], and the cyclic alternating pattern [34]. Our recent efforts to link sleep stages, arousal index, or sleep fragmentation showed no clear relationship with the degree of mismatch in a clinical cohort [10]. This included a machine learning approach (Naïve Bayes Classifier) to use a collection of demographic and PSG characteristics to predict mismatch, emphasizing the complexity of this problem. We also reported that subjective–objective mismatch was distinct for sleep latency (overestimated in insomnia) and for wake after sleep onset (WASO; underestimated in insomnia), an additional reminder of the complexity of a process that patients and providers alike may implicitly assume to be straightforward. Thus, the mismatch that may occur between subjective and objective sleep–wake times can differentially impact wake time depending on context (sleep onset versus within-sleep-period awakenings), in addition to overall sleep duration.

It should also be noted that occult sleep disorders may be comorbid with insomnia, such as obstructive sleep apnea (OSA) [35, 36], which cannot be reliably excluded with screening inventories [37]. This is an important topic of clinical relevance, given that the literature has been interpreted to conclude that PSG is not indicated for evaluation of mood disorders; this is based in part on the question of whether sleep physiology (such as REM latency) might be considered supportive data for making the psychiatric diagnosis. Instead, one could consider PSG evaluation for occult OSA as a potential treatable contributor to sleep and/or mood symptoms. Thus, it is arguable that some patients with insomnia should undergo objective testing for the dual purpose of gaining insight into the degree of mismatch and identifying potentially treatable comorbid conditions. An additional consideration is that certain more commonly used pharmacological treatments for insomnia among patients with mood disorders (such as benzodiazepines) carry a potential risk of worsening breathing in sleep, and thus one would not want to overlook the possibility of occult sleep apnea.

Anxiety and Depression

It is perhaps not surprising that epidemiological associations have been reported between insomnia and mood symptoms or disorders [38–42]. Sleep complaints, especially disturbed or nonrefreshing sleep, are part of the diagnostic criteria for mood disorders, and thus correlation is expected based on the clinical definitions alone. However, the question of causality between sleep disturbance and mood disorders/symptoms is difficult to answer for several reasons, as has been discussed previously [43–45]. There is likely to be shared pathophysiology between insomnia and mood disorders, such that each can impact the other; there may also be shared risk factors or common biological pathways that contribute to both. Also, the temporal order of symptom appearance has been shown in both directions, namely that insomnia may precede mood complaints, or may appear after or with the onset of a mood disorder. It is likely that several mechanistic links are possible, and teasing them apart, especially within the context of the mainly subjective measures of sleep, remains challenging due to the mismatch between objective and subjective sleep reports. When both insomnia and a mood disorder or symptoms are present, it is not always the case that insomnia is secondary to the mood disorder, and thus treatment should not simply focus on the psychiatric arena in hopes of indirectly resolving the insomnia [46–48]. Despite the overlap between sleep disturbance (such as insomnia or OSA) and psychiatric disorders, it may be that one or the other aspect of the clinical presentation may dominate the diagnostic and treatment strategies. It is thus important to explore sleep and psychiatric symptoms in concert when evaluating a patient with either one of these complaints.

Studies in Which Insomnia Precedes Mood Symptoms

Several studies have shown that sleep complaints are associated with increased future risk of psychiatric disorders. A meta-analysis of risk factors for incident depression in older adults reported that over 50 % of the risk for future development of depression was associated with insomnia complaints [49]. Perlis has reported an increased risk of incident depression among older adults with baseline insomnia [50]. In a 1-year study of over 10,000 adults, baseline insomnia in those without psychiatric diagnoses predicted incident depression [42]. In a 20-year study of young adults, Buysse reported that 17–50 % of individuals with insomnia episodes of at least 2 weeks in duration later developed major depression [51].

In a large survey study of adults assessed at baseline and at 10-year follow-up, Neckelmann et al. reported that baseline insomnia increased risk of incident anxiety disorder (OR 1.6), but the association was even stronger for those reporting insomnia only at the 10-year time point (OR 3.4) or at both the entry and the 10-year time points (OR 4.9) [52]. Intervening time courses were not assessed, but the presence of insomnia at both time points suggests that chronic or recurrent insomnia has a greater association than transient insomnia for incident anxiety. This study also investigated associations with depression, but found it was only associated with insomnia at the 10-year follow-up point (OR 1.8), though not with prior insomnia or persistent (both time points) insomnia.

Breslau et al. showed in a longitudinal study that individuals reporting insomnia had a higher prevalence of depression—and those with both insomnia and sleepiness had even further comorbid depression [53]. Baseline insomnia also predicted a variety of incident psychiatric diagnoses at follow-up, including anxiety and substance abuse. Yokoyama et al. showed greater incident depression with sleep onset difficulties, but not other sub-categories of insomnia—i.e., sleep maintenance or early morning awakening [54]. Further research into insomnia phenotyping [55–57] may be useful to establish epidemiological associations; however, it may prove challenging to gather large enough sample sizes to achieve adequate statistical power to test multiple insomnia sub-categories.

Studies in Which Mood Symptoms Precede Insomnia

Other studies have shown that baseline psychiatric symptoms or disorders are associated with incident insomnia. LeBlanc reported that insomnia was associated with concurrent symptoms of anxiety and depression, whereas incident insomnia was associated with prior reports of pain, poor self-rated health, positive insomnia family history, and previous insomnia [58]. Singareddy reported that incident insomnia was predicted by mental health (including depression) [59]. Salo also showed increased incidence of insomnia in patients with depression—and also, interestingly, with sleep medication which predicted subsequent depression independent of insomnia symptoms [60]. Similarly, Kripke has reported an association between hypnotic use and depression [61]. Bi-directional influences (in terms of the temporal order of insomnia and mood symptoms) have been noted in another epidemiological prospective study [62], and in a 1-year longitudinal study of nearly 5,000 adults, bi-directional associations between sleep and psychiatric symptoms were reported [63]. Baseline anxiety, depression, and pain symptoms predicted incident insomnia at follow-up, and baseline insomnia was associated with incident anxiety, depression, and pain symptoms at follow-up. In that study, persistent insomnia (evident at both time points) was associated with advanced age. Insomnia may be a perpetuating factor in cases of persistent or relapsing depression [64, 65]. Depression has also been associated with persistent insomnia [26].

Treatment of Concomitant Insomnia and Depression

There is great interest in multimodal treatment strategies for patients in whom depression and insomnia coexist. For example, it has been reported that sleep complaints are among the most common in patients under remission from depression using an SSRI [66], although in that study relapse was not predicted by this finding. Establishing a causal relationship by clinical history may or may not be critical for treatment planning in the patient with both diagnoses. Alternatively, if the history suggests a clear temporal order of insomnia after mood symptoms, one might opt for a trial of mood treatment (medication or behavioral) to determine if the insomnia would resolve with mood improvement. Choice of antidepressant agent may consider the sleep complaints, with more activating agents possibly chosen in the patient with hypersomnia (after ruling out primary causes), while sedating antidepressants might hold dual benefit for a patient with concurrent insomnia.

Recent randomized controlled studies suggest the utility of concomitant treatment of sleep and depression, whether pharmacologically [47, 48, 67–70] or with behavioral therapy [71]. Importantly, it was shown that elective hypnotic use was not prevalent in follow-up of a combined drug therapy trial, and that subjective sleep benefits persisted after hypnotic discontinuation [68].

In summary, the collection of epidemiological studies cited above suggests a complex interplay between sleep disorders, especially insomnia, and depression and anxiety. It is likely that bi-directional mechanisms exist, such that in patients presenting with either a sleep disorder or a mood disorder, treatment of one may reduce future risk of development of the other, or improve the symptoms of the other if concomitantly present. Much work remains to test this exciting hypothesis more broadly.

Other Sleep Disorders Linked to Mood Symptoms

Fatigue and/or sleepiness is weakly associated with sleep apnea presence or severity, and when present in the psychiatric population they are arguably even less specific [72], making the clinical screening for sleep apnea even more challenging than it already is [37]. For example, the Epworth Sleepiness scale, despite its wide use, shows minimal relation to the presence or severity of OSA [73, 74]. Depression has also been associated with sleep apnea in clinical populations, with depression rates between 7 % to over 60 % of OSA patients, and the relationship may be stronger in women than in men [72, 75, 76]. Depressed mood could indirectly increase OSA risk, perhaps through weight gain. In a study of patients with major depression and comorbid insomnia, more than a third had an AHI >15 on PSG testing [36]. In a large-scale study of over one million medical records, Sharafkhaneh showed increased prevalence of anxiety, depression, and PTSD in the United States Veterans with OSA, although in this study the prevalence of OSA was somewhat low at 2.9 % [77]. Although the literature is inconsistent in cross-sectional studies of OSA and depression [72], in a prospective study, the risk of incident depression was linked to the severity of OSA at baseline [78].

Treatment of OSA may have positive mood impact on patients with comorbid depression, in addition the improvements in quality of life and sleepiness reported in general [79], although the placebo potential in this setting should not be overlooked [80]. Although some recent work showed no improvement in mood after CPAP treatment, important limitations exist, including that the outcome mood measures were only after 2 or 3 weeks of follow-up [81, 82]. It is possible, on the converse perspective, that treating depression could indirectly improve OSA by increasing motivation, since interventions such as weight loss and adherence to CPAP require ongoing patient effort [83].

It is also worth noting that insomnia and OSA are frequently comorbid [35], thus potentially further increasing the risk of mood symptoms. There is less data linking other sleep disorders with mood symptoms. In a large 6-year follow-up study of the Nurses Health Study (over 50,000 women), Li showed that baseline self-report of physician-diagnosed restless legs syndrome (RLS) was associated with incident diagnoses of depression (relative risk of 1.5) [84].

Role of Sleep Testing for Patients with Mood Disorders

As mentioned earlier, in general, isolated mood symptoms are not considered to be an independent indication for PSG. However, there are several arguments to be made for objective investigation of sleep in patients with mood disorders. For example, comorbid insomnia is common, and understanding potential contributors to insomnia such as periodic limb movements of sleep, occult OSA, and misperception all require formal testing to evaluate. Even in the psychiatric patient without significant sleep complaints, occult OSA may be present, as it can be asymptomatic by objective and subjective evaluations of sleepiness [73, 85, 86]. As emphasized above, predicting OSA is not straightforward based on the clinical history and symptoms alone. Discovering occult OSA in a patient with psychiatric symptoms may however be an important therapeutic opportunity, and thus it is important to consider this possibility. The relationship of "classic" OSA features (e.g., obesity, snoring) with the presence and severity of OSA is only modest, so the practitioner should not be falsely reassured by the absence of common markers of OSA—e.g., normal BMI and absence of snoring or sleepiness—when considering whether to evaluate for OSA.

Sleep and Bipolar Disorder

Sleep complaints are also common in patients with bipolar disorder, during manic as well as depressed phases [87]. Insomnia is associated with mania, and while this may be described as decreased sleep need, the experience can be distressing. In some patients, increasing insomnia symptoms may be an antecedent stimulus for switching to a manic phase [88], and therapeutic sleep deprivation has been associated with increased probability of manic symptoms [89]. However, more recent data suggests that acute deprivation coupled with bright light and phase advance chronotherapy yielded longer duration (7 weeks) improvements in mood [90]. There is only sparse data regarding OSA and bipolar disorder, consisting mainly of case reports and preliminary studies of clinical screening [91, 92].

Posttraumatic Stress Disorder

Patients with posttraumatic stress disorder (PTSD) have been shown to have objective impairments of sleep architecture, for example, by actigraphy [93] and by PSG [94–97]. This population may also show discrepancies between subjective sleep reports and objective measures, as is commonly seen with patients reporting insomnia. However, at least one study showed accurate match between subjective and actigraphic TST reporting in PTSD [98]. However, in that study, sleep latency and WASO were misestimated in all subjects, with or without PTSD, while controls overestimated TST compared to actigraphy. OSA has also been observed at higher prevalence in PTSD [95, 99], emphasizing the importance of objective evaluation of sleep in this population.

A 2007 meta-analysis of studies using PSG to evaluate PTSD patients suggested that the disorder is associated with increased amounts of stage N1 sleep, and decreased amounts of stage N3 sleep. In addition, age, sex, and comorbid depression were suggested to modulate PTSD-related sleep physiology. REM density (eye movement frequency during REM sleep) was also found to be increased in PTSD. These results are important because such factors may differ among studies and thus contribute to heterogeneity in the literature of PTSD and sleep [97]. van Liempt showed that PTSD patients had twice as many night-time awakenings in the early portion of PSG recording, and decreased GH levels despite similar amounts of slow wave sleep by absolute minutes and percentage of TST [100]. Using a bed sensor over multiple nights, Woodward and colleagues showed autonomic dysfunction among those with PTSD, as well as increased time in bed and increased TST (as estimated by the bed monitor, not PSG) [101]. Ulmer and colleagues similarly showed autonomic dysfunction in the form of altered blood pressure regulation (baroreceptor sensitivity) linked to sleep fragmentation in women with PTSD [102].

Comorbidity between PTSD and substance use, as well as prescription medication use, makes the evaluation of sleep physiology a challenge since illicit drugs, alcohol, over-the-counter, and prescription medications may all have effects on sleep as measured by PSG. Nevertheless, deciphering sleep changes is central to the development, natural history, and treatment response of PTSD. In addition, it is possible that preexisting sleep abnormalities or sleep disorders may make certain individuals who experience trauma more vulnerable to the development of PTSD. Finally, further research is needed to establish whether treatment to optimize sleep will also improve PTSD symptomatology. Despite these uncertainties, it is worth emphasizing that insomnia and OSA warrant treatment independent of PTSD, and thus it would seem reasonable to pursue evaluation and management of such sleep disorders in the PTSD population.

Schizophrenia and Sleep

Sleep disorders are common in those with schizophrenia and sleep disturbance is among the most common symptoms of the disorder. It is reported that between 30 and 80 % of patients with schizophrenia have some form of sleep and circadian rhythm disruption (SCRD) [103]. In fact, in a community sample of older adults with schizophrenia, sleep improvements were ranked among the highest needs of treatment [104]. Objectively measured sleep disturbances in schizophrenia include reductions in TST, increased sleep latency, reduced REM sleep density and REM sleep latency, decreased sleep efficiency, and reduced slow wave sleep [105]. The most significant subjective sleep impairments are reported to be insomnia, as characterized by difficulty initiating and maintaining sleep [106].

It is possible that side effects of antipsychotic medications play a role in sleep disturbance in this population. However, this seems unlikely as sleep disturbance commonly precedes the onset of Schizophrenia and the disturbance of SCRD is observed in both medicated and un-medicated patients with Schizophrenia. Furthermore, patients with schizophrenia treated with antipsychotics demonstrate improvements in sleep physiology—i.e., atypical antipsychotics have been associated with improved sleep efficiency and increased TST and slow wave sleep [103, 107].

Suicidality and Sleep

Sleep disorders and/or disturbed sleep have been linked to suicidality—with studies investigating suicidal ideation, suicide attempts, and completed suicides. Of note, sleep disturbance is a common and disruptive class of symptoms across psychiatric disorders, often listed in the actual diagnostic criteria. Understanding sleep complaints among psychiatric patients at risk for suicide may increase the potential to intervene against suicidality in vulnerable individuals. Most of the evidence reports associations of suicidality with sleep disturbance, but much less is known regarding whether the sleep disturbance is a reliable predictor of future suicidality [108].

Sleep complaints appear to be common in epidemiological studies of attempted suicide. In a study of 100 emergency room patients who had survived a serious suicide attempt, although the presence of a specific plan was not predictive of the suicide attempt, insomnia symptoms were among several predictive symptoms. Specifically, 92 % reported at least one insomnia symptom (onset or maintenance problems) while 46 % reported "global" insomnia (onset and maintenance) [109]. In another study of 165 suicide attempters, sleep disturbance was common: onset insomnia (73 %), maintenance insomnia (69 %), and early morning awakening (58 %) [110].

The National Comorbidity Survey Replication (a large representative sample) found that sleep problems (i.e., difficulty initiating sleep, maintaining sleep, early morning awakening) were associated with increased risk of suicidality—that is, suicidal ideation and plans or attempts (OR=4.2–9.1) [111]. Most notably, this relationship remained even after controlling for mental health diagnoses, such as depression, anxiety disorders, and substance abuse. This study also found that different aspects of sleep disturbance were associated with different forms of suicidal behavior. For example, difficulty initiating sleep predicted suicidal ideation and planning, while problems maintaining sleep predicted suicidal ideation and suicide attempt. Total insomnia scores and early morning awakening were predicting for suicidal ideation, planning, and suicide attempt—all three forms of measured suicidal dimensions. The association of insomnia symptoms and suicidality has also been described in other countries: a large-scale Korean survey reported an association between decreased sleep time and increased suicidal ideation in women [112].

With regard to treatment, identification and intervention of sleep disturbance and/or disorders may be useful for the prevention and treatment of suicidality in psychiatric disorders, but much work is required to further explore this area.

Conclusion

Sleep disturbance clearly plays a fundamental role in psychiatric disorders. Although the mechanistic links are complex and incompletely understood, sleep problems represent a potential point of intervention in this population. Whether addressing concomitant insomnia with behavioral or pharmacological strategies, or screening for treatable primary disorders such as sleep apnea, the opportunity for intervention is within reach during routine clinical care. With recent technological advances for measuring sleep, there will be increasing opportunity to monitor sleep on a longitudinal basis, providing important objective data to complement the largely symptom-driven clinical practice. For example, novel autonomic metrics have recently been shown useful in characterizing sleep disturbance in depression [113]. From diagnostic phenotyping to treatment monitoring to relapse prediction, sleep physiology continues to offer important windows into psychopathology.

References

1. Kahn-Greene ET, Killgore DB, Kamimori GH, Balkin TJ, Killgore WD. The effects of sleep deprivation on symptoms of psychopathology in healthy adults. Sleep Med. 2007;8(3):215–21.
2. Stepanski EJ. The effect of sleep fragmentation on daytime function. Sleep. 2002;25(3):268–76.
3. Chesson Jr A, Hartse K, Anderson WM, et al. Practice parameters for the evaluation of chronic insomnia. An American Academy of Sleep Medicine report. Standards of Practice Committee of the American Academy of Sleep Medicine. Sleep. 2000;23(2):237–41.
4. Littner M, Hirshkowitz M, Kramer M, et al. Practice parameters for using polysomnography to evaluate insomnia: an update. Sleep. 2003;26(6):754–60.
5. Harvey AG, Tang NK. (Mis)perception of sleep in insomnia: a puzzle and a resolution. Psychol Bull. 2012;138(1):77–101.
6. Edinger JD, Fins AI. The distribution and clinical significance of sleep time misperceptions among insomniacs. Sleep. 1995;18(4):232–9.
7. Manconi M, Ferri R, Sagrada C, et al. Measuring the error in sleep estimation in normal subjects and in patients with insomnia. J Sleep Res. 2010;19(3): 478–86.
8. Semler CN, Harvey AG. Misperception of sleep can adversely affect daytime functioning in insomnia. Behav Res Ther. 2005;43(7):843–56.
9. Vanable PA, Aikens JE, Tadimeti L, Caruana-Montaldo B, Mendelson WB. Sleep latency and duration estimates among sleep disorder patients: variability as a function of sleep disorder diagnosis, sleep history, and psychological characteristics. Sleep. 2000;23(1):71–9.
10. Bianchi MT, Williams KL, McKinney S, Ellenbogen JM. The subjective–objective mismatch in sleep perception among those with insomnia and sleep apnea. J Sleep Res. 2013;22(5):557–68.
11. International Classification of Sleep Disorders. Diagnostic & coding manual. 2nd ed. Westchester, NY: American Academy of Sleep Medicine; 2005.
12. Vgontzas AN, Fernandez-Mendoza J, Liao D, Bixler EO. Insomnia with objective short sleep duration: the most biologically severe phenotype of the disorder. Sleep Med Rev. 2013;17(4):241–54.
13. Tang NK, Harvey AG. Correcting distorted perception of sleep in insomnia: a novel behavioural experiment? Behav Res Ther. 2004;42(1):27–39.
14. Tang NK, Harvey AG. Altering misperception of sleep in insomnia: behavioral experiment versus verbal feedback. J Consult Clin Psychol. 2006; 74(4):767–76.
15. Kripke DF, Langer RD, Kline LE. Hypnotics' association with mortality or cancer: a matched cohort study. BMJ Open. 2012;2(1):e000850.

16. Panneman MJ, Goettsch WG, Kramarz P, Herings RM. The costs of benzodiazepine-associated hospital-treated fall Injuries in the EU: a Pharmo study. Drugs Aging. 2003;20(11):833–9.
17. Herings RM, Stricker BH, de Boer A, Bakker A, Sturmans F. Benzodiazepines and the risk of falling leading to femur fractures. Dosage more important than elimination half-life. Arch Intern Med. 1995; 155(16):1801–7.
18. Dealberto MJ, McAvay GJ, Seeman T, Berkman L. Psychotropic drug use and cognitive decline among older men and women. Int J Geriatr Psychiatry. 1997;12(5):567–74.
19. Hemmelgarn B, Suissa S, Huang A, Boivin JF, Pinard G. Benzodiazepine use and the risk of motor vehicle crash in the elderly. JAMA. 1997;278(1): 27–31.
20. Lader M. Benzodiazepines revisited–will we ever learn? Addiction. 2011;106(12):2086–109.
21. Bianchi MT, Thomas RJ, Ellenbogen JM. Hypnotics and mortality risk. J Clin Sleep Med. 2012;8(4): 351–2.
22. Verster JC, Roth T. Blood drug concentrations of benzodiazepines correlate poorly with actual driving impairment. Sleep Med Rev. 2013;17(2):153–9.
23. Benca RM. Consequences of insomnia and its therapies. J Clin Psychiatry. 2001;62 Suppl 10:33–8.
24. Morgenthaler T, Kramer M, Alessi C, et al. Practice parameters for the psychological and behavioral treatment of insomnia: an update. An American academy of sleep medicine report. Sleep. 2006;29(11):1415–9.
25. Kripke DF, Langer RD, Elliott JA, Klauber MR, Rex KM. Mortality related to actigraphic long and short sleep. Sleep Med. 2011;12(1):28–33.
26. Vgontzas AN, Fernandez-Mendoza J, Bixler EO, et al. Persistent insomnia: the role of objective short sleep duration and mental health. Sleep. 2012; 35(1):61–8.
27. Fichten CS, Creti L, Amsel R, Bailes S, Libman E. Time estimation in good and poor sleepers. J Behav Med. 2005;28(6):537–53.
28. Rioux I, Tremblay S, Bastien CH. Time estimation in chronic insomnia sufferers. Sleep. 2006;29(4): 486–93.
29. Bonnet MH, Arand DL. Physiological activation in patients with sleep state misperception. Psychosom Med. 1997;59(5):533–40.
30. Edinger JD, Fins AI, Glenn DM, et al. Insomnia and the eye of the beholder: are there clinical markers of objective sleep disturbances among adults with and without insomnia complaints? J Consult Clin Psychol. 2000;68(4):586–93.
31. Rosa RR, Bonnet MH. Reported chronic insomnia is independent of poor sleep as measured by electroencephalography. Psychosom Med. 2000;62(4):474–82.
32. Bonnet MH, Arand DL. Hyperarousal and insomnia: state of the science. Sleep Med Rev. 2010;14(1):9–15.
33. Martinez D, Breitenbach TC, Lenz Mdo C. Light sleep and sleep time misperception—relationship to alpha–delta sleep. Clin Neurophysiol. 2010; 121(5):704–11.
34. Parrino L, Milioli G, De Paolis F, Grassi A, Terzano MG. Paradoxical insomnia: the role of CAP and arousals in sleep misperception. Sleep Med. 2009;10(10):1139–45.
35. Luyster FS, Buysse DJ, Strollo Jr PJ. Comorbid insomnia and obstructive sleep apnea: challenges for clinical practice and research. J Clin Sleep Med. 2010;6(2):196–204.
36. Ong JC, Gress JL, San Pedro-Salcedo MG, Manber R. Frequency and predictors of obstructive sleep apnea among individuals with major depressive disorder and insomnia. J Psychosom Res. 2009;67(2):135–41.
37. Bianchi MT. Screening for obstructive sleep apnea: Bayes weighs in. Open Sleep J. 2009;2:56–9.
38. Mallon L, Broman JE, Hetta J. Relationship between insomnia, depression, and mortality: a 12-year follow-up of older adults in the community. Int Psychogeriatr. 2000;12(3):295–306.
39. Vollrath M, Wicki W, Angst J. The Zurich study. VIII. Insomnia: association with depression, anxiety, somatic syndromes, and course of insomnia. Eur Arch Psychiatry Neurol Sci. 1989;239(2):113–24.
40. Ford DE, Kamerow DB. Epidemiologic study of sleep disturbances and psychiatric disorders. An opportunity for prevention? JAMA. 1989;262(11):1479–84.
41. Mellinger GD, Balter MB, Uhlenhuth EH. Insomnia and its treatment. Prevalence and correlates. Arch Gen Psychiatry. 1985;42(3):225–32.
42. Weissman MM, Greenwald S, Nino-Murcia G, Dement WC. The morbidity of insomnia uncomplicated by psychiatric disorders. Gen Hosp Psychiatry. 1997;19(4):245–50.
43. Lustberg L, Reynolds CF. Depression and insomnia: questions of cause and effect. Sleep Med Rev. 2000;4(3):253–62.
44. Riemann D. Insomnia and comorbid psychiatric disorders. Sleep Med. 2007;8 Suppl 4:S15–20.
45. Benca RM, Peterson MJ. Insomnia and depression. Sleep Med. 2008;9 Suppl 1:S3–9.
46. Fava M. Daytime sleepiness and insomnia as correlates of depression. J Clin Psychiatry. 2004;65 Suppl 16:27–32.
47. Fava M, Asnis GM, Shrivastava RK, et al. Improved insomnia symptoms and sleep-related next-day functioning in patients with comorbid major depressive disorder and insomnia following concomitant zolpidem extended-release 12.5 mg and escitalopram treatment: a randomized controlled trial. J Clin Psychiatry. 2011;72(7):914–28.
48. Fava M, McCall WV, Krystal A, et al. Eszopiclone co-administered with fluoxetine in patients with insomnia coexisting with major depressive disorder. Biol Psychiatry. 2006;59(11):1052–60.
49. Cole MG, Dendukuri N. Risk factors for depression among elderly community subjects: a systematic

review and meta-analysis. Am J Psychiatry. 2003;160(6):1147–56.
50. Perlis ML, Smith LJ, Lyness JM, et al. Insomnia as a risk factor for onset of depression in the elderly. Behav Sleep Med. 2006;4(2):104–13.
51. Buysse DJ, Angst J, Gamma A, Ajdacic V, Eich D, Rossler W. Prevalence, course, and comorbidity of insomnia and depression in young adults. Sleep. 2008;31(4):473–80.
52. Neckelmann D, Mykletun A, Dahl AA. Chronic insomnia as a risk factor for developing anxiety and depression. Sleep. 2007;30(7):873–80.
53. Breslau N, Roth T, Rosenthal L, Andreski P. Sleep disturbance and psychiatric disorders: a longitudinal epidemiological study of young adults. Biol Psychiatry. 1996;39(6):411–8.
54. Yokoyama E, Kaneita Y, Saito Y, et al. Association between depression and insomnia subtypes: a longitudinal study on the elderly in Japan. Sleep. 2010;33(12):1693–702.
55. Vallieres A, Ivers H, Beaulieu-Bonneau S, Morin CM. Predictability of sleep in patients with insomnia. Sleep. 2011;34(5):609–17.
56. Vallieres A, Ivers H, Bastien CH, Beaulieu-Bonneau S, Morin CM. Variability and predictability in sleep patterns of chronic insomniacs. J Sleep Res. 2005;14(4):447–53.
57. Edinger JD, Fins AI, Goeke JM, et al. The empirical identification of insomnia subtypes: a cluster analytic approach. Sleep. 1996;19(5):398–411.
58. LeBlanc M, Merette C, Savard J, Ivers H, Baillargeon L, Morin CM. Incidence and risk factors of insomnia in a population-based sample. Sleep. 2009;32(8):1027–37.
59. Singareddy R, Vgontzas AN, Fernandez-Mendoza J, et al. Risk factors for incident chronic insomnia: a general population prospective study. Sleep Med. 2012;13(4):346–53.
60. Salo P, Sivertsen B, Oksanen T, et al. Insomnia symptoms as a predictor of incident treatment for depression: prospective cohort study of 40,791 men and women. Sleep Med. 2012;13(3):278–84.
61. Kripke DF. Greater incidence of depression with hypnotic use than with placebo. BMC Psychiatry. 2007;7:42.
62. Kim JM, Stewart R, Kim SW, Yang SJ, Shin IS, Yoon JS. Insomnia, depression, and physical disorders in late life: a 2-year longitudinal community study in Koreans. Sleep. 2009;32(9):1221–8.
63. Morphy H, Dunn KM, Lewis M, Boardman HF, Croft PR. Epidemiology of insomnia: a longitudinal study in a UK population. Sleep. 2007;30(3):274–80.
64. Perlis ML, Giles DE, Buysse DJ, Tu X, Kupfer DJ. Self-reported sleep disturbance as a prodromal symptom in recurrent depression. J Affect Disord. 1997;42(2–3):209–12.
65. Pigeon WR, Hegel M, Unutzer J, et al. Is insomnia a perpetuating factor for late-life depression in the IMPACT cohort? Sleep. 2008;31(4):481–8.
66. Iovieno N, van Nieuwenhuizen A, Clain A, Baer L, Nierenberg AA. Residual symptoms after remission of major depressive disorder with fluoxetine and risk of relapse. Depress Anxiety. 2011;28(2):137–44.
67. Fava M, Asnis GM, Shrivastava R, et al. Zolpidem extended-release improves sleep and next-day symptoms in comorbid insomnia and generalized anxiety disorder. J Clin Psychopharmacol. 2009;29(3): 222–30.
68. Krystal A, Fava M, Rubens R, et al. Evaluation of eszopiclone discontinuation after cotherapy with fluoxetine for insomnia with coexisting depression. J Clin Sleep Med. 2007;3(1):48–55.
69. Krystal AD, McCall WV, Fava M, et al. Eszopiclone treatment for insomnia: effect size comparisons in patients with primary insomnia and insomnia with medical and psychiatric comorbidity. Prim Care Companion CNS Disord. 2012;14(4): PCC.11m01296.
70. McCall WV, Blocker JN, D'Agostino Jr R, et al. Treatment of insomnia in depressed insomniacs: effects on health-related quality of life, objective and self-reported sleep, and depression. J Clin Sleep Med. 2010;6(4):322–9.
71. Manber R, Edinger JD, Gress JL, San Pedro-Salcedo MG, Kuo TF, Kalista T. Cognitive behavioral therapy for insomnia enhances depression outcome in patients with comorbid major depressive disorder and insomnia. Sleep. 2008;31(4):489–95.
72. Harris M, Glozier N, Ratnavadivel R, Grunstein RR. Obstructive sleep apnea and depression. Sleep Med Rev. 2009;13(6):437–44.
73. Eiseman NA, Westover MB, Mietus JE, Thomas RJ, Bianchi MT. Classification algorithms for predicting sleepiness and sleep apnea severity. J Sleep Res. 2012;21(1):101–12.
74. Sil A, Barr G. Assessment of predictive ability of Epworth scoring in screening of patients with sleep apnoea. J Laryngol Otol. 2012;126(4):372–9.
75. Ohayon MM. The effects of breathing-related sleep disorders on mood disturbances in the general population. J Clin Psychiatry. 2003;64(10):1195–200. quiz, 1274–1196.
76. Wheaton AG, Perry GS, Chapman DP, Croft JB. Sleep disordered breathing and depression among U.S. adults: National Health and Nutrition Examination Survey, 2005–2008. Sleep. 2012;35(4): 461–7.
77. Sharafkhaneh A, Giray N, Richardson P, Young T, Hirshkowitz M. Association of psychiatric disorders and sleep apnea in a large cohort. Sleep. 2005;28(11): 1405–11.
78. Peppard PE, Szklo-Coxe M, Hla KM, Young T. Longitudinal association of sleep-related breathing disorder and depression. Arch Intern Med. 2006;166(16):1709–15.
79. Giles TL, Lasserson TJ, Smith BH, White J, Wright J, Cates CJ. Continuous positive airways pressure for obstructive sleep apnoea in adults. Cochrane Database Syst Rev. 2006;(3):CD001106.

80. Yu BH, Ancoli-Israel S, Dimsdale JE. Effect of CPAP treatment on mood states in patients with sleep apnea. J Psychiatr Res. 1999;33(5):427–32.
81. Haensel A, Norman D, Natarajan L, Bardwell WA, Ancoli-Israel S, Dimsdale JE. Effect of a 2 week CPAP treatment on mood states in patients with obstructive sleep apnea: a double-blind trial. Sleep Breath. 2007;11(4):239–44.
82. Lee IS, Bardwell W, Ancoli-Israel S, Loredo JS, Dimsdale JE. Effect of three weeks of continuous positive airway pressure treatment on mood in patients with obstructive sleep apnoea: a randomized placebo-controlled study. Sleep Med. 2012;13(2):161–6.
83. Kjelsberg FN, Ruud EA, Stavem K. Predictors of symptoms of anxiety and depression in obstructive sleep apnea. Sleep Med. 2005;6(4):341–6.
84. Li Y, Mirzaei F, O'Reilly EJ, et al. Prospective study of restless legs syndrome and risk of depression in women. Am J Epidemiol. 2012;176(4):279–88.
85. Chervin RD. The multiple sleep latency test and Epworth sleepiness scale in the assessment of daytime sleepiness. J Sleep Res. 2000;9(4):399–401.
86. Chervin RD, Aldrich MS. The Epworth Sleepiness Scale may not reflect objective measures of sleepiness or sleep apnea. Neurology. 1999;52(1):125–31.
87. Plante DT, Winkelman JW. Sleep disturbance in bipolar disorder: therapeutic implications. Am J Psychiatry. 2008;165(7):830–43.
88. Jackson A, Cavanagh J, Scott J. A systematic review of manic and depressive prodromes. J Affect Disord. 2003;74(3):209–17.
89. Wu JC, Bunney WE. The biological basis of an antidepressant response to sleep deprivation and relapse: review and hypothesis. Am J Psychiatry. 1990;147(1): 14–21.
90. Wu JC, Kelsoe JR, Schachat C, et al. Rapid and sustained antidepressant response with sleep deprivation and chronotherapy in bipolar disorder. Biol Psychiatry. 2009;66(3):298–301.
91. Soreca I, Levenson J, Lotz M, Frank E, Kupfer DJ. Sleep apnea risk and clinical correlates in patients with bipolar disorder. Bipolar Disord. 2012; 14(6):672–6.
92. Strakowski SM, Hudson JI, Keck Jr PE, et al. Four cases of obstructive sleep apnea associated with treatment-resistant mania. J Clin Psychiatry. 1991; 52(4):156–8.
93. Calhoun PS, Wiley M, Dennis MF, Means MK, Edinger JD, Beckham JC. Objective evidence of sleep disturbance in women with posttraumatic stress disorder. J Trauma Stress. 2007;20(6):1009–18.
94. Habukawa M, Uchimura N, Maeda M, Kotorii N, Maeda H. Sleep findings in young adult patients with posttraumatic stress disorder. Biol Psychiatry. 2007;62(10):1179–82.
95. Capaldi 2nd VF, Guerrero ML, Killgore WD. Sleep disruptions among returning combat veterans from Iraq and Afghanistan. Mil Med. 2011;176(8):879–88.
96. Yetkin S, Aydin H, Ozgen F. Polysomnography in patients with post-traumatic stress disorder. Psychiatry Clin Neurosci. 2010;64(3):309–17.
97. Kobayashi I, Boarts JM, Delahanty DL. Polysomnographically measured sleep abnormalities in PTSD: a meta-analytic review. Psychophysiology. 2007;44(4):660–9.
98. Kobayashi I, Huntley E, Lavela J, Mellman TA. Subjectively and objectively measured sleep with and without posttraumatic stress disorder and trauma exposure. Sleep. 2012;35(7):957–65.
99. Yesavage JA, Kinoshita LM, Kimball T, et al. Sleep-disordered breathing in Vietnam veterans with post-traumatic stress disorder. Am J Geriatr Psychiatry. 2012;20(3):199–204.
100. van Liempt S, Vermetten E, Lentjes E, Arends J, Westenberg H. Decreased nocturnal growth hormone secretion and sleep fragmentation in combat-related posttraumatic stress disorder; potential predictors of impaired memory consolidation. Psychoneuroendocrinology. 2011;36(9):1361–9.
101. Woodward SH, Arsenault NJ, Voelker K, et al. Autonomic activation during sleep in posttraumatic stress disorder and panic: a mattress actigraphic study. Biol Psychiatry. 2009;66(1):41–6.
102. Ulmer CS, Calhoun PS, Edinger JD, Wagner HR, Beckham JC. Sleep disturbance and baroreceptor sensitivity in women with posttraumatic stress disorder. J Trauma Stress. 2009;22(6):643–7.
103. Cohrs S. Sleep disturbances in patients with schizophrenia: impact and effect of antipsychotics. CNS Drugs. 2008;22(11):939–62.
104. Auslander LA, Jeste DV. Perceptions of problems and needs for service among middle-aged and elderly outpatients with schizophrenia and related psychotic disorders. Community Ment Health J. 2002;38(5):391–402.
105. Manoach DS, Stickgold R. Does abnormal sleep impair memory consolidation in schizophrenia? Front Hum Neurosci. 2009;3:21.
106. Monti JM, Monti D. Sleep disturbance in schizophrenia. Int Rev Psychiatry. 2005;17(4):247–53.
107. Pritchett D, Wulff K, Oliver PL, et al. Evaluating the links between schizophrenia and sleep and circadian rhythm disruption. J Neural Transm. 2012;119(10): 1061–75.
108. Norra C, Richter N, Juckel G. Sleep disturbances and suicidality: a common association to look for in clinical practise and preventive care. EPMA J. 2011;2(3):295–307.
109. Hall RC, Platt DE, Hall RC. Suicide risk assessment: a review of risk factors for suicide in 100 patients who made severe suicide attempts. Evaluation of suicide risk in a time of managed care. Psychosomatics. 1999;40(1):18–27.
110. Sjostrom N, Waern M, Hetta J. Nightmares and sleep disturbances in relation to suicidality in suicide attempters. Sleep. 2007;30(1):91–5.

111. Wojnar M, Ilgen MA, Wojnar J, McCammon RJ, Valenstein M, Brower KJ. Sleep problems and suicidality in the National Comorbidity Survey Replication. J Psychiatr Res. 2009;43(5):526–31.
112. Chin YR, Lee HY, So ES. Suicidal ideation and associated factors by sex in Korean adults: a population-based cross-sectional survey. Int J Public Health. 2011;56(4):429–39.
113. Yang AC, Yang CH, Hong CJ, et al. Sleep state instabilities in major depressive disorder: detection and quantification with electrocardiogram-based cardiopulmonary coupling analysis. Psychophysiology. 2010. [Epub ahead of print]

Sleep Deprivation as a Therapy in Psychiatry

7

Sara Dallaspezia and Francesco Benedetti

Introduction

The antidepressant effect of sleep deprivation (SD) was first described in 1959 in Germany, where Schulte suggested a therapeutic use of SD for depressed subjects basing on anecdotal reports of depressed patients that accidentally stayed awake all night [1]. His collaborators Pflug and Tölle carried out systematic investigations thereof, starting an important research field in psychiatry [2]. Until recently, the observation that the clinical efficacy of SD alone seemed to be hampered by early relapse after subsequent recovery sleep [3] restricted the application of the chronobiological treatment in the context of experimental settings aimed at increasing knowledge about the pathophysiology of mood disorders and discouraged its use in common clinical practice. In recent years, however, different methods for increasing and sustaining the efficacy of sleep deprivation via combinatorial strategies have been studied and the chronobiological intervention could be considered the most rapid antidepressant therapy available today [4]. Little research has been conducted about the use of SD as a therapy for psychiatric disorders other than mood disorders.

S. Dallaspezia, M.D. (✉) • F. Benedetti, M.D.
Department of Clinical Neurosciences,
Ospedale San Raffaele, Milan, Italy
e-mail: dallaspezia.sara@hsr.it; benedetti.francesco@hsr.it

Indication and Contraindication

The principal indication of therapeutic SD is the presence of depression, where an extraordinarily broad response to the chronobiological treatment has been described, irrespective of the syndromal classification. Indeed, an antidepressant effect of SD has been described in endogenous unipolar, bipolar, and schizoaffective depression, reactive depression, depression associated with pregnancy, postpartum and premenstrual dysphoric disorder, depression in the elderly, depression secondary to Parkinson's disease, or schizophrenia [5]. When comparing clinical conditions, the antidepressant efficacy of the chronobiological treatment is higher in endogenous primary depression compared to reactive and/or secondary types (75 % vs. 48 %) [6], and bipolar depressed patients were shown to respond more often than recurrent unipolar ones [7, 8], with the antidepressant effect seeming to be proportional to the patient susceptibility to develop mania. Moreover, the clinical benefit of SD was shown even in drug-resistant depression [9, 10]. Men and women respond equally well. Neither age, number of hospitalizations, earlier treatments, duration of the episode or severity of depression appears consistently related to responsiveness to SD [11].

The influence of SD on mood strictly depends on diagnosis of mood disorder. Indeed, healthy subjects experience either no changes or indeed a worsening of mood after SD [12]. There is little experience regarding its use in other psychiatric disorders. When administered to patients affected

M.T. Bianchi (ed.), *Sleep Deprivation and Disease: Effects on the Body, Brain and Behavior*,
DOI 10.1007/978-1-4614-9087-6_7, © Springer Science+Business Media New York 2014

by obsessive-compulsive [13] or panic [14] disorder the chronobiological treatment led to both improvements or worsening of the symptomatology. While a proven efficacy was showed in schizophrenic patients affected by secondary depression [15], in nondepressed chronic schizophrenic patients treated by 100 h of SD an exacerbation of psychotic symptoms was detected [16]. A recent study by a Japanese group evaluated the effect of SD in subjects affected by posttraumatic stress disorder. The authors suggested that sleep deprivation extinguishes the fear-magnifying effects of memory during sleep, and that insomnia as an acute stress response might provide prophylactic benefits in reducing the development of the disorder [17].

When considering therapeutic SD, a medical examination is suggested before the beginning of the treatment. Indeed, staying awake all night is associated with a nonspecific stress which, although generally well tolerated by healthy people, could unexpectedly precipitate unsuspected medical conditions, e.g., undetected severe cardiovascular diseases [18, 19].

The only known contraindication to SD is the presence of epilepsy, because of the increased risk of seizure induction linked to sleep reduction [20].

Since sleep loss is associated with a marked increase in dopaminergic neurotransmission, caution should be used in administering antidepressant SD to patients affected by Parkinson's disease in which contrasting results have been reported. Indeed, while improvement in motor scores associated with a more prolonged amelioration of depressive symptoms [21] was shown in patients affected by Parkinson's disease after both total [22] and partial [23] SD, in other studies a worsening has been reported after the treatment [24].

For the same reason, the presence of psychotic symptoms should be carefully evaluated, even if no controlled trial has been already done. Indeed, anecdotal reports in literature showed that a worsening of overall symptomatology including an increased extension and pressure of delusions was found after the treatment when SD was administered in delusional depression [25]. Moreover, patients affected by delusional depression showed a larger negative response after recovery sleep even if they had a better response than nonpsychotic depressives to total SD combined with clomipramine [26].

Sleep Deprivation: How Many Hours?

The standard treatment is called "total" SD (TSD) because wake is prolonged throughout the night of treatment. It begins with the extension of daytime wake into the night and lasts about 36 h until the evening of the day after. During this period any napping should be avoided. This is made easier by a nocturnal activity program which however does not seem to have any influence to the therapeutic effect [27]. Indeed, SD has a specific effect which is independent and greater than that of physical exercise [28]. It is still debated if a short nap can block the powerful antidepressant effects of SD, because controversial results have been found. Indeed, while a mood worsening has been shown not only after napping [29] but also even after subjectively unrecognized microsleeps [30], some researchers reported no changes in mood or even a mood amelioration after napping [31]. Moreover, a circadian variation of propensity to relapse into depression as a function of nap timing was suggested (better in the afternoon, but with longer naps in the morning paradoxically less detrimental than shorter ones) [32].

Actually, it is still unclear how many hours of SD are needed to achieve its full antidepressant effect and the minimum amount of sleep restriction needed to obtain any antidepressant effects has not been determined. Over recent years, variants of TSD, such as REM sleep deprivation and partial sleep deprivation (PSD), have been developed.

Selective REM sleep deprivation was suggested to have an antidepressant effect, basing on the observation of REM sleep suppression associated with almost all antidepressants. In 1975 Vogel and colleagues found that depressed patients treated with 3 weeks of REM sleep deprivation by selective awakenings without pharmacological intervention showed a response comparable to that of imipramine, while a control group of patients deprived of non-REM sleep by selective awakenings did not show any clinical improvement [33]. This finding has not been replicated by the only other study focusing on this topic with a methodologically improved design [34]. The authors compared selective REM sleep deprivation with the same amount of well-balanced awakenings leading to non-REM sleep deprivation in depressed subjects. Even though REM deprivation induced an antidepressant effect in this second study too, the non-REM deprivation group, however, exhibited an even stronger antidepressant response, showing that the antidepressant effects of REM sleep disrupting awakenings was similar to that of nonspecific stage II or slow wave sleep disruption. The use of REM sleep deprivation has always been restricted in the context of experimental settings and it has never been incorporated in clinical practice.

In PSD sleep is allowed during one-half of the night and is called late (LPSD) or early (EPSD) according to the part of the night chosen to be sleep deprived. Schilgen and Tölle [35] deliberately chose the second half of the night for partial SD, introducing LPSD in which patients are woken up at 1:30 a.m. and remain awake till the next evening. They considered it to be decisive to deprive the patients of sleep in the early morning hours because at this time the circadian course of several bodily functions changes direction. Initially, L-PSD was considered as effective as TSD and more effective than EPSD [36], consisting in staying awake until 1:30 then sleeping until 7:00. Thus, it was proposed as the SD method of choice [11]. Regarding the issue of timing for partial SD, subsequent trials specifically addressing the issue of comparative efficacy showed either a better efficacy of late partial SD [37] or similar efficacy of both treatments [38]. According to present knowledge, it seems to be irrelevant whether partial SD takes place during the first or the second half of the night, provided the remaining sleep is equal in duration. Moreover, despite overall response rates being similar, studies directly comparing total and partial SD found indeed TSD to be more effective than partial SD [39].

Response Rates

Cross-sectional data on many hundreds of depressed patients of all diagnostic subcategories show substantial positive responses the day following a TSD [40]. The reported response rates to TSD range from 50 to 80 % of patients, with a mean response rate of 60 % of treated patients across all diagnostic subgroups [40]. Thus, response rates to SD are similar to those observed with antidepressant drugs, but, response to SD becomes clinically relevant in a matter of hours after the beginning of treatment with an improvement which can last for weeks, while antidepressant drugs show longer response latencies. The time course of a positive response to SD usually begins in the second half of the sleep deprived night, but approximately 10–15 % of all patients undergoing SD only react to SD after nocturnal recovery sleep (day-2 responders) [38]. The term "non-response" ranges from lack of any change to extremely negative response [41]. Moreover, lack of antidepressant response to the first SD does not mean that the patient will not respond to further SDs, with about 27 % of not responding to the first night showing positive responses to further SD [40].

Predictors of Response

From a clinical point of view, some patient characteristics seem to be of major importance for the responsiveness to SD. It is one of the most reliable findings in therapeutic SD research that patients with a marked variability of symptoms respond better to SD than those with more stable signs and symptoms. Patients' diurnal variation of mood appears to predict antidepressant response: subjects having the typical diurnal mood fluctuation with an evening mood improvement tend to respond more favorably than those showing a symptomatology worsening in the evening [42]. It was found that average tiredness on the day prior to SD was related to the SD response with patients reporting a relatively low degree of tiredness on the day preceding SD improving more [43], independently from the severity of depression. Other clinical variables, such as sex, age, age at first onset of illness, duration, or severity of the acute episode have not consistently been related to responsiveness [11].

When patients' sleep characteristics before SD were considered as a predictor of response to the chronobiological treatment, contradictory results were found. In some investigations, patients characterized by short sleep time, low sleep efficiency, and little slow wave sleep showed better response to SD, but other researchers found the opposite or no relationship [44]. Similarly, considering REM-latency and REM-density [44] both positive and negative correlations with response to SD were found. One study concerning spectral analysis of NREM sleep EEG found a correlation between delta sleep and antidepressant effect of SD with a high delta sleep ratio being a positive predictor for response to treatment [45].

Studies on the possible biological predictors of the SD response have yielded disparate results. Response to SD seems to be favored by low peripheral sympathetic activity and high central noradrenergic activity, as indicated by levels of transmitter metabolites in urine and cerebrospinal fluid [11]. An abnormal dexamethasone suppression test (DST) result was found to be a positive predictor of response. Patients who show a trend for normalization of the DST after the treatment have a better antidepressant response [46]. Basal thyroid function was related to the SD antidepressant efficacy with a higher function predicting a better response [47]. Moreover, neuroinflammatory marker production is known to be enhanced in patients affected by a major depressive episode and to affect response to antidepressant drugs [48, 49]. In particular, the response to SD was found to be influenced by interleukine-6 levels: patients characterized by lower baseline levels showed a better response [50]. Indeed, SD influences the nocturnal production of cytokines in depressed patients [51], thus possibly normalizing the disrupted pattern of cytokine production associated with depression [52].

Since the clinical effects of SD are paralleled by specific effects on the brain, a group of brain imaging studies with different techniques considered cerebral cortex activation in specific areas as predictors of response. Responders to SD showed higher relative metabolic rates in the ventral anterior cingulate, medial prefrontal cortex, and posterior subcallosal cortex at baseline than either normal volunteers or depressed patients who did not respond to SD [53], with higher baseline levels being linked with better antidepressant effects.

Finally, the same genetic polymorphisms shown to influence antidepressant response to drugs were found to influence the antidepressant efficacy of SD [54]. In particular, significant associations have been observed with gene variants affecting the promoter of the serotonin transporter [55], the serotonin receptor 2A [56], the catechol-*O*-methyltransferase [57], and the glycogen synthase kinase-3b promoter [58], with a recent research showing a gene–gene interaction between serotonin transporter and glycogen synthase kinase-3b [59].

Short-Term Relapses and Augmentation Therapies

The efficacy of one night of SD as antidepressant treatment was hampered by early relapse after subsequent recovery sleep [3]. Indeed, up to the 80 % of SD-responders relapse, even if incompletely, after the first night of recovery sleep [44] and in the following days patients generally show a trend of progressive worsening with the severity of depression returning to the same levels observed at baseline.

During recent years, many strategies have been developed to sustain the effects of SD over time, preventing the short-term relapses. Serial repetition of TSD was initially studied and was reported to produce more sustained antidepressant effects during treatment but with a delayed (1 month) relapse after treatment in 63 % of responders [60]. Moreover, anecdotal reports of tolerance to treatment in bipolar patients have also been noted [61].

Several studies showed better and maintained clinical responses with the combination of sleep deprivation and antidepressant drugs [3]. In particular, positive interactions were reported with fluoxetine, paroxetine, sertraline, nortryptiline, clomipramine, desipramine, and amitriptyline. The effect is synergistic: SD hastens the antidepressant action of drugs, or, conversely, drugs sustain over time the transient antidepressant effects of SD [61]. However, negative interactions were observed with trimipramine and amineptine [62, 63]. Lithium salts, the mainstay for the treatment of bipolar disorder, as well have been found to sustain over time the antidepressant effect of SD. This augmentation effect was found not only when lithium was used as a long-term treatment but different studies showed that starting lithium in previously untreated patients prolonged the effect of sleep deprivation for at least 30 days [64]. Lithium salts not only sustain response to SD, but it enhances it as well, probably by overcoming the effect of unfavorable genetic predispositions which affect the functioning of the serotonergic system [65].

Finally, antidepressant sleep SD has been successfully combined with other chronobiological treatment such as bright light therapy (BLT) or sleep phase advance (SPA). Early studies on SD combined with BLT showed that the effectiveness of SD became more significant when BLT was conducted in the morning [66]. Moreover, not only the exposure to BLT during and after wake therapy (TSD) was shown to stabilize the antidepressant effect of both partial [67] and TSD [68, 69], but also a more prolonged improvement of responders seem to be linked to the use of BLT during SD [70].

Early studies on SPA employed a 1-week schedule: after SD, bedtime started at 5 p.m. on the first recovery night and was shifted (delayed) daily by 1 h until reaching a more conventional bedtime of 11 p.m. [71–73]. Recent studies focused on a 3-day schedule in which the bedtime was delayed daily by 2 h until the conventional bedtime. This 3-day schedule was found to successfully prevent relapse as well as the 1-week schedule [74, 75].

In summary, Wirz-Justice et al. [4] concluded that relapse after SD can be prevented by concomitant medication, BLT, and/or SPA following SD, and combinations of these interventions can also prolong response duration. Combined (SD + SPA + BLT) chronobiological interventions have been demonstrated to have a good efficacy when added to ongoing antidepressant drug in depressed patients. Indeed, Wu and colleagues showed that the antidepressant efficacy of the three established circadian-related treatments as adjunctive treatment to lithium and antidepressants was more rapid and robust than the one of the drug treatments [74]. Recently, the combination of SD, SPA, and BLT as adjunctive treatment were shown to be effective also in drug-resistant depressed patients [10].

Our group has developed a treatment schedule which has been shown to prevent short-term relapses. It combines repeated SD with BLT and lithium salts [68]. It consists of three cycles of 36 h SD separated by 1 night of recovery sleep. Inpatients stay awake from 7 a.m. until 7 p.m. the following day, during the first, third, and fifth day. Then, they are allowed to sleep during the night of the second, fourth, and sixth day. The alternation of 3 nights of undisturbed sleep means that the period of sleep–wake cycle is enlarged from the usual 24 h length to 48 h. Moreover, patients are administered BLT during the SD night at 3 a.m. and in the morning after recovery sleep between 8 and 9 a.m. Lithium salts administration, if not already ongoing, is started at the beginning of the chronotherapeutic procedure. This combination treatment was found to have an antidepressant efficacy even in drug-resistant bipolar depression [9], with an acute antidepressant response in the 44 % of patients who did not show a response to antidepressant drug.

Safety

Several studies have confirmed the safety of SD which has very few side effects. However, worsening of depressive symptoms occurs in 2–7 % of therapeutic SDs. We note that a paradoxical acute worsening of suicidal ideation and/or attempts, and of completed suicide, is possible with all antidepressant treatments and every clinical psychiatrist knows that antidepressant treatments may transiently increase these risks before leading to the remission of the depressive syndrome and of the depressive cognitive distortions (hopelessness/helplessness) linked with suicidal ideation. Current knowledge about antidepressants and suicidality suggests a transient increase in children, adolescents, and young adults under age 25; no transient suicidality effect in adults aged 25–64 and a protective effect in over 65-year-old people [76]. Even if there is no reason to think that SD should be an exception to this rule, no report associated therapeutic SD with a worsening of suicidality [5]. Moreover, two studies described rapid amelioration of depressive cognitive distortions after SD alone [77] or combined with SPA [5].

Independent of depression, SD can provoke epileptic seizures in predisposed persons. Other side effects are headaches and gastrointestinal complaints [44]. The most common and obvious adverse effect is daytime sleepiness with a degree of sleepiness showing a high individual variability.

In bipolar patients undergoing SD, there have been occasional reports of switches into hypomania or mania with approximate 5 % switch rate into mania and 6 % into hypomania. The switch rate is influenced by a concomitant use of drugs: it is reduced by mood stabilizers and increased to 10–15 % by antidepressant drugs. When treating rapid cycling bipolar depressed patients, a high rate of manic switches is expected after SD, as well as after any antidepressant medication [78]. In conclusion, in bipolar depressed patients treated by SD, the mania switch rate is similar to those observed with SSRIs and placebo, and lower than those reported with tricyclic antidepressants [79] used as antidepressant treatments, and much lower than those reported (10–29 %) in bipolar patients receiving antidepressant drugs as maintenance treatment [80]. It should be noted that the severity of mania induced by TSD is mild or moderate in the majority of patients. Indeed, one third of switched patients return to euthymia after a good night of recovery sleep (facilitated by benzodiazepines), without the need of any further treatment during the next days, and less than half of the patients need to combine antipsychotic medication with mood stabilizers to get out of mania [81].

Bipolar patients can be affected also by mixed states which are characterized by the simultaneous presence of depressive and manic symptoms pertaining to both depression and mania are simultaneous. Current guidelines on diagnosis and treatment compare mixed states to bipolar mania, and suggest to avoid antidepressants because they may worsen intraepisodic mood lability [82]. In cases of a mixed episode with prevalent depressive symptoms, the administration of antidepressant SD may precipitate mania.

When Panic Attacks disorder is comorbid with Mood Disorder, the anxiety disorder will be expected to worsen during the night of sleep deprivation without any negative influence on the antidepressant effect. Patients should be informed about this condition [81].

Mechanism of Action

SD is a complex intervention and it should be considered multi-target in nature. Thus, the mechanisms explaining its antidepressant effect can be looked for on many levels. Sleep deprivation differentially affects neurotransmitter systems, including serotoninergic, cholinergic, noradrenergic, and dopaminergic function [83–85]. Biological factors affecting the activity of these pathways, such as genotypic variants [53, 55, 56, 86], basal neurotransmitter levels [87], or the extent of receptor occupancy [88], affect the clinical response thus confirming a critical role for changes in monoaminergic neurotransmission in the clinical effect of SD. One of the most consistent findings comes from data showing that SD enhances serotonergic function, similar to many antidepressant medications [89] both in humans [90] and animals [91, 92]. Moreover, a functional polymorphism within the promoter of the serotonin transport gene, serotonin transporter-linked polymorphic region, may influence antidepressant response to SD [55].

SD increases the levels of thyroid hormones [93, 94], and interacts with emerging specific targets for the treatment of mood disorders such as glycogen synthase kinase 3-β [58] and glutamate [95]. Indeed, SD was found to alter glutamate metabolism with a reduction in cortical glutamate concentrations paralleling clinical response to the treatment [95]. Remarkably, the effects were detected in the same cerebral area, such as the dorsal anterior cingulate cortex, where changes in 5-HT function were found to influence neural responses to depressive cognitive stimuli [53]. According to this finding, glutamate neurotransmission and its interaction with monoamines could have a role in the rapid antidepressant effects of SD. Research in animal models showed that SD promoted a synaptic potentiation increasing the inhibitory phosphorylation of GSK3-β [96] which is an essential element of the Wnt/beta-catenin pathway and plays major roles in neurodevelopment and in regulation of neuronal plasticity and cell survival [97]. Moreover, GSK3-β is supposed to be involved in the mechanism of action of lithium and serotonergic antidepressants and its Drosophila orthologue SHAGGY was found to be implicated in the regulation of the molecular clock located in the suprachiasmatic nucleus of the hypothalamus [98]. A promoter single nucleotide functional (greater activity of the T allele) polymorphism of GSK3-β (−50 T/C; rs334558) was found to influence the response to SD. Indeed, bipolar depressed homozygote carriers of the C allele showed a better mood amelioration after SD and a relapse similar to the other subjects after recovery sleep [58]. Moreover, recently a gene–gene interaction between rs334558 and serotonin transporter gene in influencing antidepressant response to SD was found [59].

SD can influence the activity of the suprachiasmatic nucleus of the hypothalamus by modifying vigilance state transitions and sleep states [99]. Changes in sleep homeostasis have been hypothesized to play a major role in the mechanism of action of sleep deprivation [40]. According to the recent "synaptic homeostasis hypothesis" of sleep [100], the antidepressant action of SD could be related to the marked changes in neuronal connectivity leading to major changes in brain metabolism and function caused by the chronobiological treatment. Moreover, recently SD was found to influence the expression of some genes of the biological clock which are known to contribute to the homeostatic aspect of sleep regulation [101]. Since it is hypothesized that a subset of patients with severe depression who experience circadian rhythm abnormalities, including mood, sleep, hormonal, and/or temperature regulation, have a state-related defect in clock gene machinery, SD could be supposed to have an antidepressant effect by stabilizing clock gene machinery [102].

References

1. Schulte W. Zum Priblem der provokation und kupierung von Melancholischen Phasen. Schweiz Arch Neurol Neurochir Psychiatr. 1971;109:427–35.
2. Pflug B, Tolle R. Therapy of endogenous depressions using sleep deprivation. Practical and theoretical consequences. Nervenarzt. 1971;42:117–24.
3. Leibenluft E, Wehr TA. Is sleep deprivation useful in the treatment of depression? Am J Psychiatry. 1992;149:159–68.
4. Wirz-Justice A, Benedetti F, Berger M, Lam RW, Martiny K, Terman M, Wu JC. Chronotherapeutics (light and wake therapy) in affective disorders. Psychol Med. 2005;35:939–44.
5. Benedetti F, Barbini B, Colombo C, Smeraldi E. Chronotherapeutics in a psychiatric ward. Sleep Med Rev. 2007;11:509–22.
6. Wu JC, Bunney WE. The biological basis of an antidepressant response to sleep deprivation and relapse: review and hypothesis. Am J Psychiatry. 1990; 147:14–21.
7. Szuba MP, Baxter Jr LR, Fairbanks LA, Guze BH, Schwartz JM. Effects of partial sleep deprivation on the diurnal variation of mood and motor activity in major depression. Biol Psychiatry. 1991;30:817–29.
8. Barbini B, Colombo C, Benedetti F, Campori E, Bellodi L, Smeraldi E. The unipolar-bipolar dichotomy and the response to sleep deprivation. Psychiatry Res. 1998;79:43–50.
9. Benedetti F, Barbini B, Fulgosi MC, Colombo C, Dallaspezia S, Pontiggia A, Smeraldi E. Combined total sleep deprivation and light therapy in the treatment of drug-resistant bipolar depression: acute response and long-term remission rates. J Clin Psychiatry. 2005;66:1535–40.
10. Echizenya M, Suda H, Takeshima M, Inomata Y, Shimizu T. Total sleep deprivation followed by sleep phase advance and bright light therapy in drug-resistant mood disorders. J Affect Disord. 2012; 144(1–2):28–33.
11. Kuhs H, Tolle R. Sleep deprivation therapy. Biol Psychiatry. 1991;29:1129–48.
12. Babson KA, Trainor CD, Feldner MT, Blumenthal H. A test of the effects of acute sleep deprivation on

general and specific self-reported anxiety and depressive symptoms: an experimental extension. J Behav Ther Exp Psychiatry. 2010;41:297–303.
13. Joffe RT, Swinson RP. Total sleep deprivation in patients with obsessive-compulsive disorder. Acta Psychiatr Scand. 1988;77:483–7.
14. Roy-Byrne PP, Uhde TW, Post RM. Effects of one night's sleep deprivation on mood and behavior in panic disorder. Patients with panic disorder compared with depressed patients and normal controls. Arch Gen Psychiatry. 1986;43:895–9.
15. Fahndrich E. Effects of sleep deprivation on depressed patients of different nosological groups. Psychiatry Res. 1981;5:277–85.
16. Koranyi EK, Lehmann HE. Experimental sleep deprivation in schizophrenic patients. AMA Arch Gen Psychiatry. 1960;2:534–44.
17. Kuriyama K. Sleep medicine for the prevention of prolonged stress and posttraumatic stress disorder. Seishin Shinkeigaku Zasshi. 2012;114:136–43.
18. Delva NJ, Woo M, Southmayd SE, Hawken ER. Myocardial infarction during sleep deprivation in a patient with dextrocardia—a case report. Angiology. 2001;52:83–6.
19. Suh SY, Kim JW, Choi CU, Kim EJ, Rha SW, Park CG, Seo HS, Oh DJ. Spontaneous coronary dissection associated with sleep deprivation presenting with acute myocardial infarction. Int J Cardiol. 2007;115:e78–9.
20. Nakken KO, Solaas MH, Kjeldsen MJ, Friis ML, Pellock JM, Corey LA. Which seizure-precipitating factors do patients with epilepsy most frequently report? Epilepsy Behav. 2005;6:85–9.
21. Bertolucci PH, Andrade LA, Lima JG, Carlini EA. Total sleep deprivation and Parkinson disease. Arq Neuropsiquiatr. 1987;45:224–30.
22. Demet EM, Chicz-Demet A, Fallon JH, Sokolski KN. Sleep deprivation therapy in depressive illness and Parkinson's disease. Prog Neuropsychopharmacol Biol Psychiatry. 1999;23:753–84.
23. Hogl B, Peralta C, Wetter TC, Gershanik O, Trenkwalder C. Effect of sleep deprivation on motor performance in patients with Parkinson's disease. Mov Disord. 2001;16:616–21.
24. Lauterbach EC. Sleep benefit and sleep deprivation in subgroups of depressed patients with Parkinson's disease. Am J Psychiatry. 1994;151:782–3.
25. Benedetti F, Zanardi R, Colombo C, Smeraldi E. Worsening of delusional depression after sleep deprivation: case reports. J Psychiatr Res. 1999; 33:69–72.
26. Elsenga S, Beersma D, Van den Hoofdakker RH. Total and partial sleep deprivation in clomipramine-treated endogenous depressives. J Psychiatr Res. 1990;24:111–9.
27. Fischer H, Tolle R, Telger K. Sleep deprivation: temporal aspects of partial sleep deprivation in the treatment of depression. Schweiz Arch Neurol Psychiatr. 1990;141:351–9.
28. Martiny K, Refsgaard E, Lund V, Lunde M, Sorensen L, Thougaard B, Lindberg L, Bech P. A 9-week randomized trial comparing a chronotherapeutic intervention (wake and light therapy) to exercise in major depressive disorder patients treated with duloxetine. J Clin Psychiatry. 2012;73:1234–42.
29. Riemann D, Wiegand M, Lauer CJ, Berger M. Naps after total sleep deprivation in depressed patients: are they depressiogenic? Psychiatry Res. 1993;49:109–20.
30. Hemmeter U, Bischof R, Hatzinger M, Seifritz E, Holsboer-Trachsler E. Microsleep during partial sleep deprivation in depression. Biol Psychiatry. 1998;43:829–39.
31. Gillin JC, Kripke DF, Janowsky DS, Risch SC. Effects of brief naps on mood and sleep in sleep-deprived depressed patients. Psychiatry Res. 1989;27:253–65.
32. Wiegand M, Riemann D, Schreiber W, Lauer CJ, Berger M. Effect of morning and afternoon naps on mood after total sleep deprivation in patients with major depression. Biol Psychiatry. 1993;33:467–76.
33. Vogel GW, Vogel F, McAbee RS, Thurmond AJ. Improvement of depression by REM sleep deprivation. New findings and a theory. Arch Gen Psychiatry. 1980;37:247–53.
34. Grozinger M, Kogel P, Roschke J. Effects of REM sleep awakenings and related wakening paradigms on the ultradian sleep cycle and the symptoms in depression. J Psychiatr Res. 2002;36:299–308.
35. Schilgen B, Tolle R. Partial sleep deprivation as therapy for depression. Arch Gen Psychiatry. 1980; 37:267–71.
36. Goetze U, Tolle R. Antidepressive effect of partial sleep deprivation during the 1st half of the night. Psychiatr Clin (Basel). 1981;14:129–49.
37. Sack DA, Duncan W, Rosenthal NE, Mendelson WE, Wehr TA. The timing and duration of sleep in partial sleep deprivation therapy of depression. Acta Psychiatr Scand. 1988;77:219–24.
38. Giedke H, Geilenkirchen R, Hauser M. The timing of partial sleep deprivation in depression. J Affect Disord. 1992;25:117–28.
39. Giedke H, Wormstall H, Haffner HT. Therapeutic sleep deprivation in depressives, restricted to the two nocturnal hours between 3:00 and 5:00. Prog Neuropsychopharmacol Biol Psychiatry. 1990; 14:37–47.
40. Wirz-Justice A, Van den Hoofdakker RH. Sleep deprivation in depression: what do we know, where do we go? Biol Psychiatry. 1999;46:445–53.
41. Van den Hoofdakker RH, Beersma DG. On the contribution of sleep wake physiology to the explanation and the treatment of depression. Acta Psychiatr Scand Suppl. 1988;341:53–71.
42. Reinink E, Bouhuys AL, Gordijn MC, Van Den Hoofdakker RH. Prediction of the antidepressant response to total sleep deprivation of depressed patients: longitudinal versus single day assessment

of diurnal mood variation. Biol Psychiatry. 1993;34:471–81.
43. Bouhuys AL, van den Burg W, van den Hoofdakker RH. The relationship between tiredness prior to sleep deprivation and the antidepressant response to sleep deprivation in depression. Biol Psychiatry. 1995;37:457–61.
44. Giedke H, Schwarzler F. Therapeutic use of sleep deprivation in depression. Sleep Med Rev. 2002;6:361–77.
45. Nissen C, Feige B, Konig A, Voderholzer U, Berger M, Riemann D. Delta sleep ratio as a predictor of sleep deprivation response in major depression. J Psychiatr Res. 2001;35:155–63.
46. Kasper S, Moises HW, Beckmann H. Dexamethasone suppression test combined with total sleep deprivation in depressed patients. Psychiatr Clin (Basel). 1983;16:17–25.
47. Baumgartner A, Riemann D, Berger M. Neuroendocrinological investigations during sleep deprivation in depression. II. Longitudinal measurement of thyrotropin, TH, cortisol, prolactin, GH, and LH during sleep and sleep deprivation. Biol Psychiatry. 1990;28:569–87.
48. Lanquillon S, Krieg JC, Bening-Abu-Shach U, Vedder H. Cytokine production and treatment response in major depressive disorder. Neuropsychopharmacology. 2000;22:370–9.
49. Sluzewska A, Sobieska M, Rybakowski JK. Changes in acute-phase proteins during lithium potentiation of antidepressants in refractory depression. Neuropsychobiology. 1997;35:123–7.
50. Benedetti F, Lucca A, Brambilla F, Colombo C, Smeraldi E. Interleukine-6 serum levels correlate with response to antidepressant sleep deprivation and sleep phase advance. Prog Neuropsychopharmacol Biol Psychiatry. 2002;26:1167–70.
51. Voderholzer U, Fiebich BL, Dersch R, Feige B, Piosczyk H, Kopasz M, Riemann D, Lieb K. Effects of sleep deprivation on nocturnal cytokine concentrations in depressed patients and healthy control subjects. J Neuropsychiatry Clin Neurosci. 2012; 24:354–66.
52. Alesci S, Martinez PE, Kelkar S, Ilias I, Ronsaville DS, Listwak SJ, Ayala AR, Licinio J, Gold HK, Kling MA, Chrousos GP, Gold PW. Major depression is associated with significant diurnal elevations in plasma interleukin-6 levels, a shift of its circadian rhythm, and loss of physiological complexity in its secretion: clinical implications. J Clin Endocrinol Metab. 2005;90:2522–30.
53. Benedetti F, Bernasconi A, Blasi V, Cadioli M, Colombo C, Falini A, Lorenzi C, Radaelli D, Scotti G, Smeraldi E. Neural and genetic correlates of antidepressant response to sleep deprivation: a functional magnetic resonance imaging study of moral valence decision in bipolar depression. Arch Gen Psychiatry. 2007;64:179–87.
54. Benedetti F, Smeraldi E. Neuroimaging and genetics of antidepressant response to sleep deprivation: implications for drug development. Curr Pharm Des. 2009;15:2637–49.
55. Benedetti F, Serretti A, Colombo C, Campori E, Barbini B, di Bella D, Smeraldi E. Influence of a functional polymorphism within the promoter of the serotonin transporter gene on the effects of total sleep deprivation in bipolar depression. Am J Psychiatry. 1999;156:1450–2.
56. Benedetti F, Barbini B, Bernasconi A, Fulgosi MC, Colombo C, Dallaspezia S, Gavinelli C, Marino E, Pirovano A, Radaelli D, Smeraldi E. Serotonin 5-HT2A receptor gene variants influence antidepressant response to repeated total sleep deprivation in bipolar depression. Prog Neuropsychopharmacol Biol Psychiatry. 2008;32:1863–6.
57. Benedetti F, Barbini B, Bernasconi A, Fulgosi MC, Dallaspezia S, Gavinelli C, Locatelli C, Lorenzi C, Pirovano A, Radaelli D, Smeraldi E, Colombo C. Acute antidepressant response to sleep deprivation combined with light therapy is influenced by the catechol-O-methyltransferase Val(108/158)Met polymorphism. J Affect Disord. 2010;121:68–72.
58. Benedetti F, Serretti A, Colombo C, Lorenzi C, Tubazio V, Smeraldi E. A glycogen synthase kinase 3-beta promoter gene single nucleotide polymorphism is associated with age at onset and response to total sleep deprivation in bipolar depression. Neurosci Lett. 2004;368:123–6.
59. Benedetti F, Dallaspezia S, Lorenzi C, Pirovano A, Radaelli D, Locatelli C, Poletti S, Colombo C, Smeraldi E. Gene-gene interaction of glycogen synthase kinase 3-beta and serotonin transporter on human antidepressant response to sleep deprivation. J Affect Disord. 2011;136:514–9.
60. Kvist J, Kirkegaard C. Effect of repeated sleep deprivation on clinical symptoms and the TRH test in endogenous depression. Acta Psychiatr Scand. 1980; 62:494–502.
61. Benedetti F, Colombo C. Sleep deprivation in mood disorders. Neuropsychobiology. 2011;64:141–51.
62. Holsboer-Trachsler E, Hemmeter U, Hatzinger M, Seifritz E, Gerhard U, Hobi V. Sleep deprivation and bright light as potential augmenters of antidepressant drug treatment–neurobiological and psychometric assessment of course. J Psychiatr Res. 1994; 28:381–99.
63. Benedetti F, Barbini B, Campori E, Colombo C, Smeraldi E. Dopamine agonist amineptine prevents the antidepressant effect of sleep deprivation. Psychiatry Res. 1996;65:179–84.
64. Szuba MP, Baxter Jr LR, Altshuler LL, Allen EM, Guze BH, Schwartz JM, Liston EH. Lithium sustains the acute antidepressant effects of sleep deprivation: preliminary findings from a controlled study. Psychiatry Res. 1994;51:283–95.
65. Benedetti F, Barbini B, Bernasconi A, Fulgosi MC, Campori E, Colombo C, Dallaspezia S, Lorenzi C, Pontiggia A, Radaelli D, Smeraldi E. Lithium overcomes the influence of 5-HTTLPR gene polymorphism on antidepressant response to sleep

deprivation. J Clin Psychopharmacol. 2008; 28:249–51.
66. Wehr TA, Rosenthal NE, Sack DA, Gillin JC. Antidepressant effects of sleep deprivation in bright and dim light. Acta Psychiatr Scand. 1985; 72:161–5.
67. Neumeister A, Goessler R, Lucht M, Kapitany T, Bamas C, Kasper S. Bright light therapy stabilizes the antidepressant effect of partial sleep deprivation. Biol Psychiatry. 1996;39:16–21.
68. Colombo C, Lucca A, Benedetti F, Barbini B, Campori E, Smeraldi E. Total sleep deprivation combined with lithium and light therapy in the treatment of bipolar depression: replication of main effects and interaction. Psychiatry Res. 2000;95:43–53.
69. Loving RT, Kripke DF, Shuchter SR. Bright light augments antidepressant effects of medication and wake therapy. Depress Anxiety. 2002;16:1–3.
70. van den Burg W, Bouhuys AL, van den Hoofdakker RH, Beersma DG. Sleep deprivation in bright and dim light: antidepressant effects on major depressive disorder. J Affect Disord. 1990;19:109–17.
71. Albert R, Merz A, Schubert J, Ebert D. Sleep deprivation and subsequent sleep phase advance stabilizes the positive effect of sleep deprivation in depressive episodes. Nervenarzt. 1998;69:66–9.
72. Berger M, Vollmann J, Hohagen F, Konig A, Lohner H, Voderholzer U, Riemann D. Sleep deprivation combined with consecutive sleep phase advance as a fast-acting therapy in depression: an open pilot trial in medicated and unmedicated patients. Am J Psychiatry. 1997;154:870–2.
73. Riemann D, Konig A, Hohagen F, Kiemen A, Voderholzer U, Backhaus J, Bunz J, Wesiack B, Hermle L, Berger M. How to preserve the antidepressive effect of sleep deprivation: a comparison of sleep phase advance and sleep phase delay. Eur Arch Psychiatry Clin Neurosci. 1999;249:231–7.
74. Wu JC, Kelsoe JR, Schachat C, Bunney BG, DeModena A, Golshan S, Gillin JC, Potkin SG, Bunney WE. Rapid and sustained antidepressant response with sleep deprivation and chronotherapy in bipolar disorder. Biol Psychiatry. 2009;66:298–301.
75. Benedetti F, Barbini B, Campori E, Fulgosi MC, Pontiggia A, Colombo C. Sleep phase advance and lithium to sustain the antidepressant effect of total sleep deprivation in bipolar depression: new findings supporting the internal coincidence model? J Psychiatr Res. 2001;35:323–9.
76. Stone M, Laughren T, Jones ML, Levenson M, Holland PC, Hughes A, Hammad TA, Temple R, Rochester G. Risk of suicidality in clinical trials of antidepressants in adults: analysis of proprietary data submitted to US Food and Drug Administration. BMJ. 2009;339:b2880.
77. Baving L, Maes H, Bohus M, Lis S, Krieger S, Olbrich H, Berger M. Can negative self-schemes in depressives be altered through sleep deprivation? J Affect Disord. 1997;42:93–101.
78. Wehr TA, Goodwin FK, Wirz-Justice A, Breitmaier J, Craig C. 48-hour sleep-wake cycles in manic-depressive illness: naturalistic observations and sleep deprivation experiments. Arch Gen Psychiatry. 1982;39:559–65.
79. Peet M. Induction of mania with selective serotonin re-uptake inhibitors and tricyclic antidepressants. Br J Psychiatry. 1994;164:549–50.
80. Frye MA, Helleman G, McElroy SL, Altshuler LL, Black DO, Keck Jr PE, Nolen WA, Kupka R, Leverich GS, Grunze H, Mintz J, Post RM, Suppes T. Correlates of treatment-emergent mania associated with antidepressant treatment in bipolar depression. Am J Psychiatry. 2009;166:164–72.
81. Wirz-Justice A, Benedetti F, Terman M. Chronotherapeutics for affective disorders A clinician's manual for light and wake therapy. Basel: Karger; 2009.
82. Kruger S, Trevor Young L, Braunig P. Pharmacotherapy of bipolar mixed states. Bipolar Disord. 2005;7:205–15.
83. Basheer R, Bauer A, Elmenhorst D, Ramesh V, McCarley RW. Sleep deprivation upregulates A1 adenosine receptors in the rat basal forebrain. Neuroreport. 2007;18:1895–9.
84. Conti B, Maier R, Barr AM, Morale MC, Lu X, Sanna PP, Bilbe G, Hoyer D, Bartfai T. Region-specific transcriptional changes following the three antidepressant treatments electro convulsive therapy, sleep deprivation and fluoxetine. Mol Psychiatry. 2007;12:167–89.
85. Wirz-Justice A, Tobler I, Kafka MS, Naber D, Marangos PJ, Borbely AA, Wehr TA. Sleep deprivation: effects on circadian rhythms of rat brain neurotransmitter receptors. Psychiatry Res. 1981;5:67–76.
86. Benedetti F, Colombo C, Serretti A, Lorenzi C, Pontiggia A, Barbini B, Smeraldi E. Antidepressant effects of light therapy combined with sleep deprivation are influenced by a functional polymorphism within the promoter of the serotonin transporter gene. Biol Psychiatry. 2003;54:687–92.
87. Gerner RH, Post RM, Gillin JC, Bunney Jr WE. Biological and behavioral effects of one night's sleep deprivation in depressed patients and normals. J Psychiatr Res. 1979;15:21–40.
88. Ebert D, Feistel H, Kaschka W, Barocka A, Pirner A. Single photon emission computerized tomography assessment of cerebral dopamine D2 receptor blockade in depression before and after sleep deprivation–preliminary results. Biol Psychiatry. 1994;35:880–5.
89. Ressler KJ, Nemeroff CB. Role of serotonergic and noradrenergic systems in the pathophysiology of depression and anxiety disorders. Depress Anxiety. 2000;12 Suppl 1:2–19.
90. Salomon RM, Delgado PL, Licinio J, Krystal JH, Heninger GR, Charney DS. Effects of sleep deprivation on serotonin function in depression. Biol Psychiatry. 1994;36:840–6.

91. Grossman GH, Mistlberger RE, Antle MC, Ehlen JC, Glass JD. Sleep deprivation stimulates serotonin release in the suprachiasmatic nucleus. Neuroreport. 2000;11:1929–32.
92. Zant JC, Leenaars CH, Kostin A, Van Someren EJ, Porkka-Heiskanen T. Increases in extracellular serotonin and dopamine metabolite levels in the basal forebrain during sleep deprivation. Brain Res. 2011;1399:40–8.
93. Parekh PI, Ketter TA, Altshuler L, Frye MA, Callahan A, Marangell L, Post RM. Relationships between thyroid hormone and antidepressant responses to total sleep deprivation in mood disorder patients. Biol Psychiatry. 1998;43:392–4.
94. Szuba MP, Altshuler LL, Baxter Jr LR. Thyroid function and partial sleep deprivation response. Arch Gen Psychiatry. 1992;49:581–2.
95. Benedetti F, Calabrese G, Bernasconi A, Cadioli M, Colombo C, Dallaspezia S, Falini A, Radaelli D, Scotti G, Smeraldi E. Spectroscopic correlate of antidepressant response to sleep deprivation and light therapy: a 3.0 T study of bipolar depression. Psychiatry Res. 2009;173(3):238–42.
96. Vyazovskiy VV, Cirelli C, Pfister-Genskow M, Faraguna U, Tononi G. Molecular and electrophysiological evidence for net synaptic potentiation in wake and depression in sleep. Nat Neurosci. 2008;11:200–8.
97. Grimes CA, Jope RS. The multifaceted roles of glycogen synthase kinase 3beta in cellular signaling. Prog Neurobiol. 2001;65:391–426.
98. Martinek S, Inonog S, Manoukian AS, Young MW. A role for the segment polarity gene shaggy/GSK-3 in the drosophila circadian clock. Cell. 2001;105:769–79.
99. Deboer T, Vansteensel MJ, Detari L, Meijer JH. Sleep states alter activity of suprachiasmatic nucleus neurons. Nat Neurosci. 2003;6:1086–90.
100. Tononi G, Cirelli C. Sleep and synaptic homeostasis: a hypothesis. Brain Res Bull. 2003;62:143–50.
101. Mongrain V, La Spada F, Curie T, Franken P. Sleep loss reduces the DNA-binding of BMAL1, CLOCK, and NPAS2 to specific clock genes in the mouse cerebral cortex. PLoS One. 2011;6:e26622.
102. Bunney BG, Bunney WE. Mechanisms of rapid antidepressant effects of sleep deprivation therapy: clock genes and circadian rhythms. Biol Psychiatry. 2012;73(12):1164–71.

Part IV

Sleep and Medical Topics

Sleep Deprivation and Human Development

8

Nishi Bhopal and Umakanth Khatwa

Normal Sleep and Development

Sleep is defined as a behavioral state characterized by a period of reduced motor activity, associated with specific postures such as lying down with eyes closed, decreased interaction with the environment, reduced responsiveness to external stimuli, and easy reversibility.

Sleep patterns and requirements change with age (see Table 8.1). Sleep onset in the first year of life is usually through rapid eye movement (REM) sleep, also referred to as "active sleep" in infants [1]. In the normal adult, sleep is entered through non-REM (NREM), while REM sleep occurs after about 80 min [1]. The characteristic electroencephalogram (EEG) patterns of NREM sleep are not developed until the ages of 2–6 months. The slow wave EEG patterns of NREM stages 3 and 4 begin to emerge as the brain continues to develop in infancy. Slow wave sleep is prominent in young children and is more intense in quality than in adults, as children are "virtually" non-arousable from slow wave sleep during the first sleep cycle. Slow wave sleep declines markedly by mid-adolescence and sleep patterns begin to resemble those of young adults (see Fig. 8.1). By the age of 60, slow wave sleep may be absent altogether, especially in men [1].

Sleep cycles between NREM and REM, which averages 50–60 min in infants and 90 min in adults. In full term infants, REM sleep accounts for approximately 50 % of total sleep time. The proportion of REM sleep declines with age, decreasing to 30–35 % of sleep time by age 2 years down to 25 % by age 10 years, then remaining stable through adulthood until approximately age 65 when the percentage of REM sleep begins to decline further. REM sleep declines markedly in the cases of organic brain disorders [1, 2] and the absolute amount of REM sleep has been shown to correlate with cognitive functioning [1].

The optimal amount of sleep and the capacity to tolerate to sleep deprivation varies between individuals. There is great variability in the amount of sleep required, as there are short sleepers and long sleepers, "morning larks" and "night owls," and those that are more sensitive to sleep restriction and fragmentation than others. Sleep deprivation refers to a reduction in the optimal amount of sleep for an individual at a given age, associated with medical, behavioral, psychiatric, and neurocognitive morbidity. Sleep deprivation affects overall well-being and may exacerbate underlying medical conditions.

N. Bhopal, M.D. (✉)
Department of Sleep Medicine, Beth Israel Deaconess Medical Center, Boston, MA, USA
e-mail: nkbhopal1@gmail.com

U. Khatwa, M.D.
Sleep Laboratory, Division of Respiratory, Department of Medicine, Boston Children's Hospital, Boston, MA, USA

M.T. Bianchi (ed.), *Sleep Deprivation and Disease: Effects on the Body, Brain and Behavior*,
DOI 10.1007/978-1-4614-9087-6_8, © Springer Science+Business Media New York 2014

Sleep, Learning, and Memory: An Overview

Memories must be consolidated before they are rendered available for delayed retrieval [3]. Sleep is an integral part of the necessary processes of encoding, consolidating, retrieving, and integrating memories [3]. This may have a greater impact on neuropsychiatric development and functioning, as proper encoding and consolidation of memories may be important for the development of cognitive function and behavioral regulation. Functional magnetic resonance imaging (fMRI) studies have shown decreased hippocampal activity after sleep deprivation [4]. Although early studies focused primarily on the role of REM sleep in learning, studies of adult human subjects have suggested that NREM and REM sleep are both implicated in memory consolidation. Tasks learned during wakefulness are transferred from the cortex and encoded in the hippocampus, a process that is facilitated by cholinergic activity. Cholinergic pathways are active during both wake and REM sleep and are reduced during slow wave sleep. This reduction of cholinergic activity in slow wave sleep is thought to suppress the direction of encoding from the cortex to the hippocampus and to promote memory consolidation by reactivating the hippocampal memory and its transfer to cortical structures [4]. Slow wave sleep is thought to be important in the formation of declarative memory while REM is postulated to be involved primarily in non-declarative memory, although in actuality the pathways are likely far more complex.

Table 8.1 Average sleep requirements by age

Age	Hours of sleep per 24 h
Newborns (0–2 months)	10–19
Infants (2–12 months)	12–13
Toddlers (1–3 years)	11–13
Ages 3–5 years	9–10
Adolescents (12–18 years)	9–9¼
Adults	7.5–8.5

Source: data from Mindell et al. [6]

Consequence of Sleep Deprivation on Human Development: Causes of Sleep Deprivation

Sleep deprivation can be caused by sleep restriction (behavioral, intentional, or medical causes of decreased sleep opportunity) or by sleep fragmentation. The common causes vary with age (see Table 8.2).

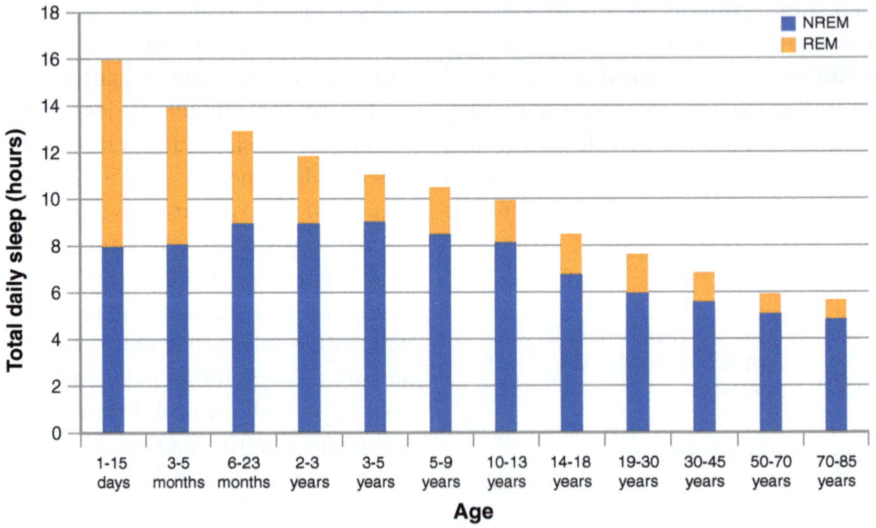

Fig. 8.1 The changes in total daily sleep, REM sleep, and NREM sleep with age. Notice the large amount of REM sleep in the neonate and infant (Based on data from Roffwarg et al. [42])

Table 8.2 Common causes of sleep disturbances

Infancy	Behavioral insomnia of childhood
	Medical problems
	Sleep disordered breathing
Early childhood	Behavioral insomnia of childhood
	Poor sleep hygiene
	Medical problems
	Sleep disordered breathing
	Periodic limb movements of sleep
Adolescence	Circadian rhythm disorders
	Medical and psychiatric disorders
	Psychophysiologic insomnia
	Sleep disordered breathing
	Periodic limb movements of sleep
Adulthood	Sleep disordered breathing
	Periodic limb movements of sleep
	Circadian rhythm disorders
	Medical and psychiatric disorders
	Psychophysiologic insomnia

Neurocognitive Effects of Sleep Deprivation in Infancy

Sleep is the primary activity of the brain during infancy. By the age of 2 years, the average child has spent nearly 14 months asleep and only 10 months awake [5]. Most newborns (aged 0–2 months) require 10–19 h of sleep per 24-h period [6]. Premature babies may have higher sleep requirements. In the first few weeks of life, sleep is polyphasic without clear nocturnal or diurnal patterns, as sleep occurs throughout the day and night. Sleep begins to consolidate around 3 months of age with emerging diurnal patterns of nighttime sleep and daytime wakefulness. Infants (aged 2–12 months) require an average of 9–10 h of sleep at night with naps averaging 3–4 h, resulting in an average of 12–13 h of sleep across the 24-h period.

Extensive research has been done on the implications of inadequate sleep on cognition and behavior in children and adolescents, but there is a paucity of literature on the same in infants. A study by Montgomery-Downs and Gozal [7] found that healthy 8-month-old infants who snored, without any polysomnogram (PSG) evidence of other sleep disorders, scored lower on assessments of cognitive function. Infants were assessed after PSG using the Bayley Scales of Infant Development II (BSID-II), which includes the Mental Development Index (MDI) and the Motor Scale. The MDI assesses sensory/perceptual acuities, discriminations, and response; acquisition of object constancy; memory learning and problem solving; vocalization and beginning of verbal communication. It was found that infants with higher snoring-arousal indices had lower scores on the BSID-II.

Bernier et al. [8] investigated the contribution of sleep disturbances to the development of executive function and impulse control. Sleep regulation was assessed at the ages of 12 and 18 months with a parent sleep diary. Executive functioning was assessed at age 18 and 26 months. Higher total sleep times at 12 months were related to executive function and impulse control at 26 months. Total sleep times at 18 months were related to concurrent working memory and later impulse control. Furthermore, it was found that children who obtained a higher percentage of their total sleep time at night were more advanced in their development of executive functioning. Thus, not only are total sleep times important for neurocognitive development, but the ratio of daytime to nighttime sleep is an important indicator of development and sleep consolidation.

Furthermore, Dionne et al. [9] examined the association between sleep consolidation in infancy and language development in early childhood. Sleep consolidation was measured by parental reports of day and night sleep durations in twins at the ages of 6, 18, and 30 months. Language skills were assessed at the ages of 18 and 30 months with the MacArthur Communicative Development Inventory and at the age of 60 months with the Peabody Picture Vocabulary Test. It was found that children who exhibited language delays at the age of 60 months had less mature sleep consolidation at 6 and 18 months than children without language delays or with only transient early delays. Genetic and environmental influences were also shown to play a role. The authors concluded that poor sleep consolidation within the first 2 years of life may be a risk factor for impaired development of language skills and that good sleep consolidation may enhance language development.

Neurocognitive Effects of Sleep Deprivation in Childhood

Sleep requirements and patterns continue to change throughout childhood. Toddlers require an average of 9.5–10.5 h of sleep at night with 2–3 h of naptime during the day, for an overall sleep requirement of 11–13 h per 24-h period. Around the age of 18 months, the number of naps decreases from two to one nap per day. By the age of 3 years, only about half of children take a nap. Children aged 3–5 years require an average of 9–10 h of nighttime sleep. About 25 % of 4 year olds and 15 % of 5 year olds take a nap. By the school years, children aged 6–12 years require an average of 9–10 h of sleep over 24 h. A circadian sleep phase preference may begin to emerge during the school years. Children with circadian phase delay may be at high risk for sleep deprivation as sleep onset difficulties associated with phase delay are often compounded by early school start times.

Sleep disturbances in children are common, as 25–40 % of children experience some kind of sleep problem during childhood, ranging from transient issues with insomnia and nighttime wakings to primary sleep disorders such as obstructive sleep apnea [10, 11].

Sleep disruption leads to impairments in neurocognitive and behavioral functioning regardless of the underlying cause (sleep restriction, sleep-related breathing disorders, etc.) [12]. It has been well established that sleep disruption in children can cause ADHD-like symptoms including hyperactivity, poor concentration, inattention, impulsivity, irritability, and poor academic performance. It is estimated that 25–50 % of children and adolescents with a diagnosis of ADHD have reported problems with sleep during clinical visits [13]. Furthermore, comorbid psychiatric conditions including mood disorders, learning disorders, and externalizing behaviors such as conduct disorder and oppositional defiant disorder are common in children and adolescents with ADHD. Such comorbidities have also been implicated in sleep disruption [14].

The relationship between sleep, behavior, mood, and cognition is bidirectional. Mood disorders and behavioral problems often result in sleep disturbance. In turn, sleep deprivation frequently causes problems with mood, cognitive impairment, behavioral disturbances, and inattention.

Reduced sleep duration is shown to be associated with high emotional lability scores [15, 16]. Holly et al. [17] found that reduced sleep duration, measured in absolute minutes by actigraphy, may be a risk factor for childhood conduct problems. Furthermore, their research suggested that an absolute reduction in the number of minutes of sleep is correlated with an increase in conduct problem scores, and that a 60-min reduction in sleep duration may in itself be a risk factor for conduct problems. As stated above, the relationship between sleep and behavior is bidirectional. Thus, it remains unclear to what extent conduct problems cause sleep disruption and vice versa.

Whereas conduct disorders, which fall under the spectrum of externalizing behaviors, are linked with sleep disruption, internalizing behaviors may also develop in association with sleep disorders. The spectrum of internalizing behaviors includes emotional withdrawal, somatization, depression, and anxiety, and these are thought to affect up to 40 % of youth [18]. Again, the interaction between sleep and mood is bidirectional—sleep problems may be a symptom of anxiety and depression, while feelings of anxiety and depression may develop as a consequence of chronic sleep problems. The risk of developing internalizing problems, particularly anxiety, in the setting of chronic sleep issues is increased across all ages, from toddlers to adults [19, 20].

It has been shown that sleep problems can result in long lasting issues with emotional internalizing [18]. Touchette et al. [18] studied a sample of over 1,500 French subjects over the course of 18 years. They found that children with sleep problems were 4.5 times more likely to experience persistently high levels of internalizing symptoms into young adulthood than those without sleep problems, after accounting for important covariates such as sex, age, childhood temperament, externalizing problems, stressful life events, socioeconomic status, and parental depression. These findings were equal in males and females.

The underlying mechanisms of sleep problems leading to internalizing remain unclear. Several physiologic mechanisms have been postulated, including alterations in monoaminergic and glutaminergic pathways, changes in the hypothalamic–pituitary–adrenal axis from chronic stress caused by sleep problems, and decreased daytime vigilance resulting in emotional dysregulation. Environmental factors may include parental behaviors and childhood temperament. Further investigation is needed into these mechanisms and into whether treating sleep disorders early in life can reduce the likelihood of later development of internalizing disorders [18].

Neurocognitive Effects of Sleep Deprivation in Adolescence

Adolescents (age 12–18 years) require on average 9–9¼ h of sleep per night, ranging from 10 h for 12 year olds down to 8.5 h for 18 year olds [21]. Most teenagers, however, report only 7 h of sleep at night [22] and thus are chronically sleep deprived. Sleep times on non-school nights average 9 h, so even attempts to catch up on missed sleep during the school week are inadequate [6]. Average bedtimes become progressively later, ranging from 9:30 p.m. for 6th graders to 11:00 p.m. for 12th graders on school nights and 10:30 p.m. for 6th graders and 12:45 a.m. for 12th graders on non-school nights (see Fig. 8.2) [6]. These patterns are similar across cultures and countries, including those in North America, Europe, Asia, and South America [23]. Many parents are unaware of their teens' sleeping requirements and habits [23] which may exacerbate the problem. A 2006 poll by the National Sleep Foundation [24] found that 90 % of caregivers believed their adolescent was getting enough sleep at least a few nights a week on school nights, whereas the same poll found that only 20 % of adolescents received the optimal 9 h of sleep per night. Given the significant physical, cognitive, and psychological development that occur during adolescence, teenagers may be particularly vulnerable to the effects of sleep deprivation [23].

Adolescents undergo a significant change in their circadian phase, usually delayed phase, around the onset of puberty. Along with changes in hormone secretion, there is a shift in the

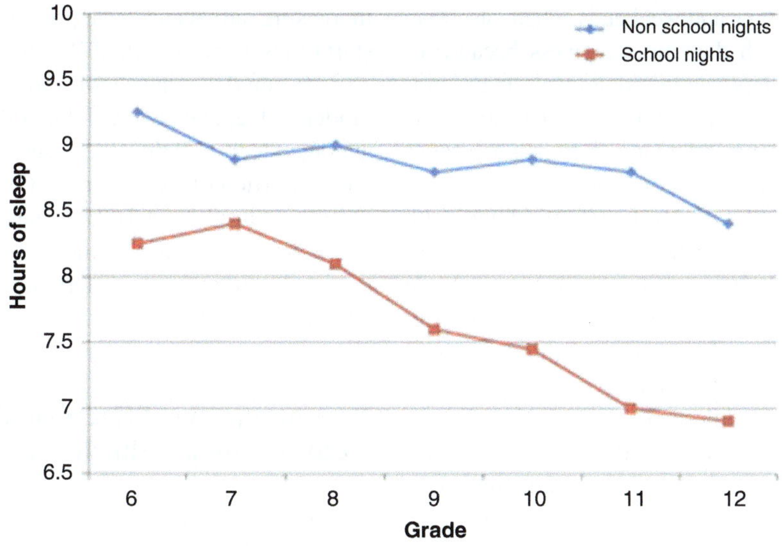

Fig. 8.2 Sleep duration in children (Reprinted with permission from the National Sleep Foundation [24])

secretion of melatonin that results in a 2-h phase delay relative to middle childhood [25]; this hormonal and circadian shift is correlated with Tanner stage rather than chronological age [6]. The circadian phase delay manifests as later sleep onset and later wake times, which tends to conflict with the early start times of most high schools. As a result, many adolescents are at school during their "biological night" [26]. The fundamental biological sleep requirements are not met because of social constraints, resulting in chronic sleep deprivation.

Delayed sleep phase syndrome (DSPS) is common amongst adolescents but may also affect younger children. It is estimated that 7–16 % of adolescents are affected by DSPS [6]. As there is a mismatch between environmental light and dark cues and sleep onset, adolescents often complain of sleep onset insomnia when attempting to initiate sleep sooner than their preferred bedtime. However, when bedtimes are delayed to their preferred time, sleep onset is usually quick, sleep maintenance is good, and the quality of sleep is normal. Children with DSPS experience significant difficulties waking up at required times for school and weekend extracurricular activities and have decreased levels of alertness in the morning. On weekends and vacations, they often extend their sleep times until the late morning or early afternoon hours. Hence these children are in a state of constant jet lag between weekdays and weekends. There also may be problems with daytime sleepiness because of chronic sleep deprivation; adolescents may complain of feeling sleepy or dozing off in the afternoons and they may take long afternoon naps after school to make up for chronic sleep loss.

DSPS can cause significant problems with daytime sleepiness, school performance, behavior, and mood. It has been shown in multiple studies that inadequate sleep is associated with lower academic achievement in middle school through college [22]. Excessive daytime sleepiness also puts adolescents at risk for drowsy driving-related accidents, reduced physical activity which can contribute to obesity and metabolic issues, and the use of stimulants such as caffeine and prescription medications [27].

DSPS has been associated with mood disorders. Thorpy et al. [28] found that more than half of adolescent patients with DSPS had symptoms of depression, measured objectively by the Beck Depression Inventory, Minnesota Multiphasic Personality Inventory (MMPI), or formal psychological evaluation. Furthermore, Lee et al. [29] have suggested that DSPS is partially comorbid with seasonal affective disorder (SAD), as there may be a shared circadian physiology causing delayed sleep phase.

Sleep problems in adolescents, whether related to DSPS, sleep restriction, or other sleep disturbances, can be a risk factor for impulsivity and other behavioral problems. A study by Moore et al. [30] showed that sleep problems in adolescents are associated with increased measures of negative affectivity and poorer effortful control, corresponding with increased impulsivity. A meta-analysis by Pigeon et al. [31] found an increased relative risk for suicidality, including suicidal ideation, suicide attempts, and completed suicide in adolescents with sleep problems. Furthermore, Fitzgerald et al. [32] found that extremes in total sleep time, whether short or long sleep times, are associated with suicidal ideation and behavior after controlling for age, sex, levels of sadness, and substance abuse. They postulated that extremes in sleep times may contribute to suicidality by influencing mood instability and impulsivity.

As the appreciation and understanding of the impact of sleep restriction in adolescents is increasing, advocates have proposed later school start times. Owens et al. [27] examined the effects of a 30-min delay in school start times on 9–12th graders' sleep, behavior, and mood. Adolescents' average sleep duration increased by 45 min and the proportion of students reporting at least 8 h of sleep increased from 16 % to nearly 55 %. This had a positive impact on motivation, class attendance, daytime alertness, fatigue, mood, and satisfaction with sleep.

Neurocognitive Effects of Sleep Deprivation in Adulthood

The average healthy adult requires between 7.5 and 8.5 h sleep per night in the absence of sleep debt. However, many adults do not get enough sleep. Data from the National Health Interview

Survey [33] conducted from 2005 to 2007 showed that nearly 30 % of the US adults reported getting 6 or less hours of sleep per day. A survey of 1,000 adults [34] found that adults who slept less than 6 h on work nights were significantly more likely to be obese than adults who slept at least 8 h (41 % vs. 28 %). Ongoing sleep issues in adulthood may have detrimental effects on overall health, exacerbating underlying medical issues such cardiovascular and metabolic disorders, psychiatric disorders such as depression and anxiety, and causing impairment in overall well-being and neurocognitive functioning.

Acute and chronic sleep deprivation result in important and serious deficits in cognition and performance on everyday tasks such as driving. It is estimated by the National Department of Transportation [35] that drowsy driving is responsible for 1,550 fatalities and 40,000 nonfatal injuries annually in the United States. A 2008 poll by the National Sleep Foundation [34] found that 32 % of adults working full-time had driven drowsy at least once a month in the past year, and this number was as high as 48 % in shift workers.

Although we live in a society in which chronic partial sleep restriction is rampant and becoming an increasingly important public health issue, the vast majority of studies have looked at the effects of total sleep deprivation rather than chronic sleep restriction. There are several studies, however, examining the effects of chronic partial sleep restriction. All forms of sleep deprivation, including total sleep deprivation, partial sleep deprivation, and chronic partial sleep restriction, are associated with negative affectivity including irritability, depression, anxiety, confusion, sleepiness, and fatigue [36]. Cognitive performance, including executive function and working memory, are negatively affected by total sleep deprivation. Studies have shown that chronic sleep restriction over several days is associated with a degree of impairment in cognitive performance similar to that seen in acute severe total sleep deprivation [36]. There is significant interindividual variability, however, as some individuals seem to be more sensitive to the effects of sleep loss than others. The underlying neurobiological mechanisms of this variability remain unclear, although it has been postulated that differences between individuals may be based on genes that regulate sleep homeostasis and circadian rhythms [37]. Interestingly, as most individuals become increasingly cognitively impaired as a result of sleep loss, they tend to underestimate the degree of impairment and report only moderate levels of sleepiness [38].

Sleep disruption, whether secondary to medical conditions or environmental disturbances, is also an important contributor to neurocognitive and behavioral problems but is the least studied form of sleep loss [38]. Studies of sleep disruption have shown impaired performance on the psychomotor vigilance test (PVT), reduced speed of cognitive processing, and impairments in working memory [39]. This can have an important impact on functioning in the workplace. Up to 40 % of adults report becoming impatient with others at work at least a few days a month [34] while nearly 30 % report problems with concentration. About 20 % of workers have reported issues with reduced productivity at least a few days a month [34].

Primary sleep disorders that contribute to sleep disruption and fragmentation, such as obstructive sleep apnea, restless legs syndrome, and periodic limb movement disorder, may also contribute to sleep deprivation and problems with neurocognitive impairment.

Electronic Media and Sleep Hygiene

Electronic media are ubiquitous and have become an important contributor to poor sleep habits and sleep deprivation across all ages. In a survey by the National Sleep Foundation, 95 % of respondents reported using some form of electronic device within the hour before bedtime, including televisions, video games, computers, and cell phones. Exposure to artificial light affects the production of melatonin and enhances alertness, which may cause difficulties with sleep onset and alterations in the circadian system [40]. Furthermore, engaging with interactive devices such as cell phones, computers, and video games is thought to be more disruptive to sleep than using passive media such as televisions [40]. About 40 % of Americans use their cell phones when trying to go to sleep [41], with a higher prevalence of use amongst adolescents and young adults (72 % of 13–18 year olds and 67 % of 19–29 year olds). Texting at bedtime is common in adolescents and young adults and has been shown to result in subjectively less restful sleep, waking up unrefreshed, scoring "sleepy" on the Epworth Sleepiness Scale, and a higher likelihood of drowsy driving [41]. Cell phones can be a further sleep disturbance during the night if not turned off or set to silent when going to bed. Up to 60 % of adults and over 70 % of teens and young adults use their computers or laptops in their bedrooms during the hour before bedtime; this has similar results to cell phone use on subjective sleep quality and levels of daytime alertness.

Informing patients about good sleep hygiene is important in minimizing sleep deprivation. Avoiding light exposure and use of electronic media before bedtime, having a relaxing presleep ritual, keeping the bedroom cool and comfortable, and avoiding strenuous exercise, caffeine, alcohol, and large meals before bedtime are conducive to good quality sleep. Adequate sleep duration and good quality sleep are important for overall health, well-being, and development.

Summary

Sleep deprivation can be caused by sleep restriction or sleep fragmentation, with similar effects on overall neurocognitive development regardless of the cause.

Sleep is vital for neurocognitive development and sleep deprivation can have detrimental effects on cognition and functioning across the lifespan. Infants who are sleep deprived show deficits in language development, executive function, and impulse control in early childhood. Sleep disorders in childhood are common and often manifest in ADHD-like symptoms, including poor school performance, inattention, hyperactivity, and behavioral issues. Children with sleep disorders may develop problems with emotional internalizing, such as anxiety and depression, in young adulthood. As children enter adolescence, there is a shift in circadian biology resulting in a phase delay which is often worsened by the use of electronic media. This, compounded with early school start times, social demands such extracurricular activities, and lack of parental understanding of adolescents' sleep needs, leads to chronic sleep restriction and deprivation. Sleep deprivation puts adolescents at risk for poor school performance, drowsy driving, impulsivity, mood dysregulation, and suicidality. Later school start times have been shown to have a positive impact on adolescent cognition, mood, and behavior. As we live in a 24-h society, many adults are chronically sleep deprived. More studies need to be done on chronic partial sleep restriction. However, chronic sleep restriction is associated with poor psychomotor vigilance, cognitive impairment, and mood disorders. Good sleep hygiene and early recognition of sleep problems are important for overall health, development, and functioning. A detailed sleep evaluation should be a part of the well-child visit and the annual health check-up for adults. Screening for subtle sleep disorders should be routine and attention toward good sleep hygiene is recommended to help minimize the adverse effects of sleep deprivation.

References

1. Carskadon MA, Dement WC. Normal human sleep: an overview. Principles and practice of sleep medicine. 5th ed. Elsevier Saunders: St. Louis; 2011.
2. Lovell K, Liszewski C. Normal sleep patterns and sleep disorders. http://learn.chm.msu.edu/neuroed/neurobiology_disease/content/otheresources/sleepdisorders.pdf. Accessed Jan 2012.
3. Kopasz M, Loessl B, Hornyak M, et al. Sleep and memory in healthy children and adolescents—a critical review. Sleep Med Rev. 2010;14(3):167–77.
4. Hill C, Hogan A, Karmiloff-Smith A. To sleep, perchance to enrich learning? Arch Dis Child. 2007;92(7):637–43.
5. Dahl R. The impact of inadequate sleep on children's daytime cognitive function. Semin Pediatr Neurol. 1996;3(1):44–50.
6. Mindell J, Owens J. A clinical guide to pediatric sleep: diagnosis and management of sleep problems. 2nd ed. Philadelphia: Lippincott Williams & Wilkins; 2010.
7. Montgomery-Downs HE, Gozal D. Snore-associated sleep fragmentation in infancy: mental development effects and contribution of secondhand cigarette smoke exposure. Pediatrics. 2006;117(3):e496–502.

8. Bernier A, Carlson SM, Bordeleau S, Carrier J. Relations between physiological and cognitive regulatory systems: infant sleep regulation and subsequent executive functioning. Child Dev. 2010;81(6): 1739–52.
9. Dionne G, Touchette E, Forget-Dubois N, et al. Associations between sleep-wake consolidation and language development in early childhood: a longitudinal twin study. Sleep. 2011;34(8):987–95.
10. Owens J. Classification and epidemiology of childhood sleep disorders. Prim Care. 2008;35(3): 533–46.
11. Owens J. Epidemiology of sleep disorders during childhood. In: Sheldon S, Ferber R, Kryger MH, editors. Principles and practice of pediatric sleep medicine. Philadelphia: Elsevier Saunders; 2005.
12. O'Brien LM. The neurocognitive effects of sleep disruption in children and adolescents. Child Adolesc Psychiatr Clin N Am. 2009;18(4):813–23.
13. Owens J. The ADHD and sleep conundrum: a review. J Dev Behav Pediatr. 2005;26(4):312–22.
14. Gruber R. Sleep characteristics of children and adolescents with attention deficit hyperactivity disorder. Child Adolesc Psychiatr Clin N Am. 2009; 18(4): 863–76.
15. Nixon GM, Thompson JM, Han DY, et al. Short sleep duration in middle childhood: risk factors and consequences. Sleep. 2008;31(1):71–8.
16. Rosen CL, Storfer-Isser A, Taylor HG, Kirchner HL, Emancipator JL, Redline S. Increased behavioral morbidity in school-aged children with sleep-disordered breathing. Pediatrics. 2004;114(6):1640–8.
17. Holley S, Hill CM, Stevenson J. An hour less sleep is a risk factor for childhood conduct problems. Child Care Health Dev. 2011;37(4):563–70.
18. Touchette E, Chollet A, Galera C, et al. Prior sleep problems predict internalising problems later in life. J Affect Disord. 2012;143(1–3):166–71.
19. Jansen PW, Saridjan NS, Hofman A, Jaddoe VW, Verlhulst FC, Tiemeier H. Does disturbed sleeping precede symptoms of anxiety or depression in toddlers? The generation R study. Psychosom Med. 2011;73(3):242–9.
20. Gregory AM, O'Connor TG. Sleep problems in childhood: a longitudinal study of developmental change and association with behavioral problems. J Am Acad Child Adolesc Psychiatry. 2002;41(8):964–71.
21. National Institutes of Health, NIH Office of Science Education. Information about sleep. science.education.nih.gov. Accessed Jan 2013.
22. Wolfson AR, Carskadon MA. Understanding adolescents' sleep patterns and school performance: a critical appraisal. Sleep Med Rev. 2003;7(6):491–506.
23. Leger D, Beck F, Richard JB, Godeau E. Total sleep time severely drops during adolescence. PLoS One. 2012;7(10):e45204.
24. National Sleep Foundation. 2006 Teens and sleep. Sleep in America polls. 2006. http://www.sleepfoundation.org/article/sleep-america-polls/2006-teens-and-sleep. Accessed Jan 2013.
25. Carskadon MA, Acebo C. Regulation of sleepiness in adolescents: update, insights, and speculation. Sleep. 2002;25(6):606–14.
26. Meltzer LJ, Mindell JA. Sleep and sleep disorders in children and adolescents. Psychiatr Clin North Am. 2006;29(4):1059–76.
27. Owens JA, Belon K, Moss P. Impact of delaying school start time on adolescent sleep, mood, and behavior. Arch Pediatr Adolesc Med. 2010;164(7):608–14.
28. Thorpy MJ, Korman E, Spielman AJ, Glovinsky PB. Delayed sleep phase syndrome in adolescents. J Adolesc Health Care. 1988;9(1):22–7.
29. Lee HJ, Rex KM, Nievergelt CM, Kelsoe JR, Kripke DF. Delayed sleep phase syndrome is related to seasonal affective disorder. J Affect Disord. 2011; 133(3):573–9.
30. Moore M, Slane J, Mindell JA, Burt SA, Klump KL. Sleep problems and temperament in adolescents. Child Care Health Dev. 2011;37(4):559–62.
31. Pigeon WR, Pinquart M, Conner K. Meta-analysis of sleep disturbance and suicidal thoughts and behaviors. J Clin Psychiatry. 2012;73(9):e1160–7.
32. Fitzgerald CT, Messias E, Buysse DJ. Teen sleep and suicidality: results from the youth risk behavior surveys of 2007 and 2009. J Clin Sleep Med. 2011;7(4): 351–6.
33. Schoenborn CA, Adams PF. Health behaviors of adults: United States, 2005–2007. Vital Health Stat. 2010;245:1–132.
34. National Sleep Foundation. 2008 Sleep, performance and the workplace. 2008. http://www.sleepfoundation.org/article/sleep-america-polls/2008-sleep-performance-and-the-workplace. Accessed Jan 2013.
35. US Dept of Transportation. Drowsy driving and automobile crashes. National Center on Sleep Disorders Research. http://www.nhtsa.gov/people/injury/drowsy_driving1/Drowsy.html#NCSDR/NHTSA
36. Durmer JS, Dinges DF. Neurocognitive consequences of sleep deprivation. Semin Neurol. 2005; 25(1):117–29.
37. Goel N, Rao H, Durmer JS, Dinges DF. Neurocognitive consequences of sleep deprivation. Semin Neurol. 2009;29(4):320–39.
38. Reynolds AC, Banks S. Total sleep deprivation, chronic sleep restriction and sleep disruption. Prog Brain Res. 2010;185:91–103.
39. Bonnet MH, Arand DL. Clinical effects of sleep fragmentation versus sleep deprivation. Sleep Med Rev. 2003;7(4):297–310.
40. National Sleep Foundation. Sleepy connected Americans. 2011. http://www.sleepfoundation.org/article/press-release/annual-sleep-america-poll-exploring-connections-communications-technology-use. Accessed Jan 2013.
41. National Sleep Foundation. 2011 Sleep in America poll: communications technology in the bedroom. 2011. http://www.sleepfoundation.org/article/sleep-america-polls/2011-communications-technology-use-and-sleep.
42. Roffwarg HP, Muzio JN, Dement WC. Ontogenetic development of the human sleep-dream cycle. Science. 1966;152(3722):604–19.

Sleep Deprivation and Pregnancy

9

Mihaela H. Bazalakova, Matt T. Bianchi, and Aleksandar K. Stanic

Introduction

Pregnancy is anecdotally equated with sleep disturbance, most commonly resulting in sleep deprivation, with the possible exception of the first trimester when hypersomnia is frequently reported [1–4]. The relationship between gestational stage and maternal sleep is likely bidirectional. For example, the dynamic hormonal and physiological changes of pregnancy are known to impact a large variety of sleep parameters, including homeostatic sleep drive, sleep latency, sleep maintenance, duration of sleep, sleep fragmentation, perceived sleep quality, and objectively measured sleep stage cycling. Conversely, sleep disturbance of any kind, including decreased total sleep amount or increased fragmentation, with or without respiratory disturbance, negatively impacts pregnancy outcomes, including gestational hypertensive disease, labor type and duration, prematurity, and birth weight. Thus, while the relationship is undoubtedly complicated, pregnancy provides a natural "experiment" informing the role of reproductive hormones on sleep characteristics, while the interplay of sleep disturbance and pregnancy outcomes alerts to the physiological significance of sleep and its electrophysiological and subjective characteristics. In this chapter, we will review the various aspects of sleep disturbance that may lead to sleep deprivation during pregnancy and the existing evidence that sleep deprivation and disturbance affect pregnancy outcomes.

Characteristics of Sleep During Pregnancy

The growing volume of literature attempting to characterize sleep during pregnancy consists of both self-reported, frequently sleep diary-based, and objective, or actigraphy and polysomnography (PSG)-based data. Not surprisingly, given the involved nature of overnight laboratory PSG instrumentation, the paucity of validated home sleep testing devices and the length of gestation, there are few longitudinal prospective studies of sleep during pregnancy utilizing objective data recording. In addition, many studies are underpowered due to small sample sizes and pre-pregnancy baselines are

M.H. Bazalakova, M.D., Ph.D. (✉)
Division of Sleep Medicine, Department of Neurology, Massachusetts General Hospital, Harvard Medical School, Boston, MA, USA

Division of Sleep Medicine, Department of Medicine, Brigham and Women's Hospital, Harvard Medical School, Boston, MA, USA
e-mail: mbazalakova@partners.org

M.T. Bianchi, M.D., Ph.D., M.M.Sc.
Division of Sleep Medicine, Department of Neurology, Massachusetts General Hospital, Boston, MA, USA

A.K. Stanic, M.D., Ph.D.
Division of Reproductive Endocrinology and Infertility, Gynecology and Reproductive Biology, Vincent Department of Obstetrics and Gynecology, Harvard Medical School; Massachusetts General Hospital, Boston, MA, USA

M.T. Bianchi (ed.), *Sleep Deprivation and Disease: Effects on the Body, Brain and Behavior*, DOI 10.1007/978-1-4614-9087-6_9, © Springer Science+Business Media New York 2014

understandably difficult to obtain in order to serve as control data. Nonpregnant controls are also difficult to compare with women at various gestational points, as reproductive hormones, which are suspected to play a key role in sleep changes during pregnancy, vary during the menstrual cycle, albeit to a smaller degree than during gestation. Thus, objective data of the incidence and prevalence of sleep disturbance is scant. Nevertheless, some patterns have emerged, including in large epidemiological surveys.

Prevalence of Sleep Disturbance During Pregnancy

A national poll by the National Science Foundation (NSF) in 2007 of 1,003 women, 150 of whom were pregnant, revealed that 84 % of pregnant women experienced some sleep problem at least a few nights a week, compared to 67 % of women in general, and 40 % of pregnant women reported getting a good night's sleep only a few nights a month or less compared to 29 % of all women [5]. In a retrospective study of 100 women in their 38th week of pregnancy, 14 % recalled sleep disturbance in the first trimester citing as the primary reasons nausea and vomiting, back pain, and urinary frequency [6]. Dreams and heartburn emerged as additional sources of sleep disruption during the second trimester in the NSF sample [5], and leg cramps, shortness of breath, and fetal movement became increasingly disruptive during the third trimester [5], when sleep disturbance/insomnia has been reported in greater than 50 % of pregnant women [7, 8].

Evidence for Sleep Deprivation During Pregnancy

Given the prevalence of self-reported gestational sleep disturbance and declining quality of sleep, the question arises, does pregnancy lead to objective sleep deprivation and if so, which sleep parameters are affected and when during pregnancy do these changes occur.

Sleep Variables

Specific sleep variables, such as sleep onset latency (SOL), total sleep time (TST), wake after sleep onset (WASO), and number of awakenings, have been evaluated in pregnancy using subjective and objective means. Okun et al. report increasing number of awakenings and longer awake time at night starting early in the first trimester, based on sleep diary data from 19 pregnant women [9]. In a postal survey of 244 pregnant women, Hutchison et al. report a mean nighttime TST of 7.5 h during the last week of pregnancy, 35.8 min shorter than retrospectively recalled pre-pregnancy TST of 8.1 h, as well as increasing number of awakenings in the third trimester [10]. Self-reported mean TST also decreased from the first trimester, gestational weeks 13.8 ± 3.8 (7.4 h), to the third trimester, gestational weeks 30 ± 2.2 (7 h), in a serial questionnaire prospective study of 198 women by Facco et al. [8].

Daytime napping, although frequently not addressed in studies, appears to increase in frequency at higher gestational ages and complicates the evaluation of sleep deprivation in pregnancy [10, 11]. For example, shorter nighttime sleep duration may be compensated by more frequent and longer naps, resulting in unchanged overall sleep time per 24 h, as reported by Hutchison et al. (8.6 h pre-pregnancy versus 8.7 h in the last week of pregnancy) [10]. While they agree that nighttime TST objectively measured by PSG decreases between the beginning and end of pregnancy, Lee et al. and Hertz et al. report no change in TST between pre-pregnancy and the last trimester of pregnancy in their prospective and cross-sectional studies, respectively [12, 13]. However, they do not account for daytime naps, thus again raising the possibility that total sleep duration per 24 h may not differ significantly or may even be greater, albeit noncontinuous, at the end of pregnancy compared to the first trimester or the nonpregnant state. Whether napping can physiologically compensate for lost nighttime sleep, and how obstetrical outcomes may be affected, remain as unknowns.

Interestingly, mean TST was actually longer by 0.7 h during the first trimester compared to pre-pregnancy TST in a questionnaire study of 325 women [7], a phenomenon consistent with anecdotal increased daytime sleepiness and fatigue as an early marker of pregnancy and possibly due to the soporific effects of rising progesterone levels. This subjective finding has been replicated by objective PSG data, as reported by Lee et al. who used in-home PSG in a rare prospective study following 33 women from pre-pregnancy through the postpartum period, demonstrating an increase from 6.8 to 7.4 h in mean sleep duration from pre-pregnancy to gestational weeks 11–12 [12].

Of note, a recent study comparing overnight PSG with perceived SOL and TST by 16 women in the first trimester, 33 women in the third trimester of pregnancy, and ten nonpregnant controls, demonstrated that the first trimester and nonpregnant groups underestimated TST, while the third trimester group overestimated TST compared to objective PSG data, and all groups overestimated SOL, further highlighting the difficulty in integrating subjective and objective sleep data [14].

Sleep Stages

Changes in sleep stage architecture during pregnancy may result in sleep disturbance and/or deprivation by various mechanisms, including decreased sleep stability and higher number of awakenings as a result of more frequent stage changes, or heightened brain excitability as seen in rapid eye movement (REM) sleep [15]. There is a paucity of PSG studies allowing for quantification of sleep stages in pregnancy. Although often contradictory, the data appears to increasingly support a decrease in REM sleep in pregnancy [13, 16–18], possibly potentiated by rising progesterone and cortisol levels, and more frequent [13, 16, 19] or longer [17, 18, 20] awakenings with increasing gestational age. However conclusions on slow wave sleep (SWS) trends are difficult to arrive at, as studies report decreased SWS in the first trimester [12, 16], increased SWS during the second trimester [18], and decreased [16, 19, 20], increased [18] or unchanged [17] SWS in the third trimester. Increased stage N1 has also been reported in the third trimester of pregnancy [13, 16].

In summary, as discussed earlier, varying study designs and methodologies and limited sample sizes confound the interpretation of sometimes conflicting reports of sleep characteristics during pregnancy. Nevertheless, although not universally demonstrated, an overall pattern emerges of increased sleep duration during the first trimester compared to pre-pregnancy levels, followed by a decline in nocturnal TST with increasing gestational age, but possibly preserved to slightly increased TST per 24 h compared to pre-pregnancy states, due to increasing frequency and/or duration of daytime naps. In addition, REM sleep suppression and increasing wake time, the latter due to either more frequent or longer awakenings, are seen as pregnancy progresses, consistent with an insomnia pattern and sleep deprivation in relation to gestational age. As less intrusive recording technologies become available, larger longitudinal prospective studies, recording sleep on multiple nights at various gestational points, should conclusively determine sleep characteristics of pregnancy.

Suspected Hormonal, Physiological, and Physical Mechanisms of Sleep Disturbance During Pregnancy

Hormones and Sleep Disturbance in Pregnancy

Sex Hormones

Pregnancy is characterized by a steady rise in the reproductive steroid hormones progesterone and estrogen, peaking at term, followed by a rapid decline postpartum [21]. By the end of pregnancy, progesterone levels can be 1,000-fold higher than pre-pregnancy values in the follicular phase of the menstrual cycle [22]. Progesterone has soporific effects, thought to be exerted through the $GABA_A$ receptor agonist properties of progesterone's metabolites, 5-α-dihydroprogesterone (allopregnanolone), and 5-β-dihydroprogesterone (pregnanolone) [23], and is speculated to contribute to increased sleepiness and sleep duration during the first trimester. Indeed, exogenous administration of progesterone has been shown to increase drowsiness in both men and women [24]. However, progesterone also inhibits the urinary tract smooth muscle resulting in urinary frequency, a well-known factor of sleep disruption especially during the first and third trimesters [5].

Progesterone is also thermogenic, and studies in healthy, nonpregnant, menstruating women demonstrate increased 24-h mean core body temperature (CBT) post-ovulation and during the luteal phase, when progesterone and the progesterone/estrogen ratio rise [25]. The thermogenic effects of progesterone likely contribute to the REM suppression seen with increasing gestational age, as an inverse relationship between REM sleep and CBT has been reported [26].

Finally, exogenous administration of progesterone in men resulted in increased non-REM sleep [27]. However, spectral analysis of EEG frequency revealed decreases in the slow wave frequency (<4.3 Hz) range, potentially consistent with decreases in SWS reported by some, although not all, PSG studies, especially during the third trimester of pregnancy. In contrast, progesterone supplementation in hypogonadal women did not change sleep architecture when sleep disturbance was not present, but resulted in reduced WASO and increased SWS when sleep was disrupted artificially [28].

Estrogen supplementation in hypogonadal women has been associated with decreased sleep latency [29], less time spent awake and fewer awakenings, as well as increases in REM sleep [30]. Prolactin also increases during pregnancy [31], and has been hypothesized to contribute to increased SWS, as increased SWS has been described in lactating women [32, 33] and patients with prolactinomas [33].

Cortisol

Cortisol levels increase during pregnancy, particularly during the third trimester [34]. Exogenous nighttime pulsatile administration of cortisol, a catabolic hormone, in healthy young men resulted in significant reduction in REM sleep, increase in SWS, and higher plasma growth hormone (GH) concentrations [35]. This data provides evidence for cortisol-activated GH secretion and, perhaps more importantly, emphasizes the importance of SWS for GH secretion, a significant relationship established in studies as early as 1969 [36] leading to the "restorative" theory of sleep, and SWS in particular. Conversely, sleep deprivation in young men has been shown to increase cortisol secretion [37].

These findings are relevant to sleep during pregnancy, as sleep, SWS especially, as well as the first two trimesters of pregnancy are considered anabolic states, while the third trimester is considered a catabolic state [38]. If the restorative theory of SWS [39] is correct, then we may expect to see changes in SWS, possibly in a trimester-specific pattern, in relation to changing hormonal levels and metabolic demands, but also in response to sleep disturbance or deprivation during pregnancy. While SWS duration in pregnancy has been examined, with contradictory and inconclusive results, (see above), the hypothesis that SWS disturbance may affect pregnancy outcomes has yet to be explored to our knowledge.

In summary, we would expect a bidirectional relationship between changing hormonal levels and sleep characteristics in pregnancy. In one simplified model, increased SWS as percent of TST in the early to mid-pregnancy, possibly potentiated by rising progesterone and/or prolactin levels, may be necessary for higher GH secretion during what is considered to be an anabolic state. Conversely, sleep disturbance and deprivation may lead to SWS decrease or fragmentation in the late second-early third trimesters, in turn potentiating increased cortisol secretion and the catabolic portion of pregnancy. Further studies are needed to elucidate these complicated relationships and the relationship between sleep changes and pregnancy outcomes.

Physio-anatomical Changes and Primary Sleep Disorders in Pregnancy

Sleep Disordered Breathing

Sleep disordered breathing (SDB) refers to impaired airflow during sleep due to either obstructive (OSA) or central (CSA) sleep apnea, distinguished by the presence or absence of respiratory effort, respectively. Obstructive SDB represents a spectrum from partial to total closure of the airway, ranging from mild airway narrowing in primary snoring to complete airway collapse in OSA. SDB results in sleep disturbance and fragmentation secondary to recurrent microarousals in response to repeated oxygen desaturations and sympathetic surges.

Incidence of snoring appears to increase during pregnancy, with 14 % of pregnant versus 4 % of nonpregnant women reporting snoring in one prospective survey [40], and OSA (defined as apnea hypopnea index (AHI) >5) prevalence, although poorly studied, has been reported in up to 15 % of pregnant women [41]. Pregnancy is both protective and also presents risk factors for pregnancy-onset SDB. Protective features include REM sleep decrease, as OSA tends to be exacerbated by REM atonia, in women especially [42]; avoidance of the supine sleep position [43], also known to worsen OSA [44]; a possible estrogen-related reduction in AHI as seen in estrogen supplementation in postmenopausal women [45]; progesterone-induced phasic and tonic activity of pharyngeal dilator muscles [46], and higher propensity for increased minute ventilation secondary to progesterone-driven increased respiratory drive. Two caveats to consider include evidence that progesterone increases the sensitivity of the respiratory centers to CO_2 [47] and increased ventilatory drive may enhance respiratory instability, both of which may result in CSA [48], a possibility which has not been investigated in pregnant women.

Risk factors for pregnancy-onset SDB include estrogen-mediated nasopharyngeal edema, hyperemia, and vasomotor rhinitis, decreasing nasopharyngeal patency and increasing airflow resistance [49]; weight gain, commonly up to 20 % of body weight over the course of pregnancy [50], with a similar degree of weight gain translating in 70 % AHI exacerbation in nonpregnant subjects with gradual weight gain [51]; decreased functional residual capacity (FRC) secondary to upward displacement of the diaphragm, and decreased oxygen reserve secondary to increased oxygen consumption and decreased FRC [3].

Restless Legs Syndrome

Pregnancy is a well-known secondary cause of restless legs syndrome (RLS), with 20–25 % of pregnant women reporting pregnancy-onset symptoms, most prevalent in the third trimester. RLS can lead to sleep disturbance and deprivation secondary to shorter self-reported sleep duration [52] and longer SOL [53].

To summarize, pregnancy can predispose to or exacerbate new-onset or preexisting primary sleep disorders respectively. Both SDB and RLS can lead to sleep disturbance and deprivation via shortened TST, increased SOL, and increased sleep fragmentation, in the case of respiratory events with or without significant oxygen desaturations (mean oxygen nadir even in pregnant women with moderate to severe OSA/average AHI 22, was only 87 %, range 84–90 % [54]). We will discuss the reciprocal effect of sleep disturbance on pregnancy outcomes below.

Sleep Disturbance and Pregnancy Outcomes

Sleep disturbance, including short and long sleep duration and SDB, has been associated with increased mortality [55], hypertension [56, 57], cardiovascular disease [58], obesity [59], altered glucose metabolism [60] and diabetes mellitus [61], and impaired immune cell activity [62, 63] in nonpregnant populations. As early as 1990, a large questionnaire-based study described increased risk of preterm labor (11 % versus 6 %), preterm delivery (9.8 % versus 4.6 %), and preeclampsia (8.8 % versus 3.5 %) in a large registry of pregnant resident physicians compared to spouses of male colleagues [64]. Although sleep was not directly assessed, the difference in pregnancy outcomes was attributed to suspected sleep disturbance and deprivation, as the physician group worked significantly longer hours than the control group (as high as 73 hrs/week in the first trimester in the physician group compared to 38 hrs/week in the non-physician group). Since then, a growing body of literature has addressed the relationship between sleep disturbance and pregnancy outcomes as discussed below.

Pregnancy Complications

Gestational Hypertensive Spectrum

As has been described in nonpregnant populations, both short (<6 h) and long (>10 h) self-reported sleep durations were associated with 3.72 and 4.21 mmHg elevations in third trimester systolic blood pressures respectively, compared to systolic blood pressures in subjects with intermediate sleep durations (6-10 hrs/night), in a prospective cohort study of 1,272 pregnant women [65]. In a survey of 1,719 women in the third trimester of pregnancy, pregnancy-onset, but not chronic snoring was independently associated with gestational hypertension and preeclampsia but not gestational diabetes (GDM) [66], although frequent snoring was shown to be associated with GDM in other studies [67]. In a retrospective cross-sectional study, Franklin et al. asked 502 women on the day of delivery whether they snored prior to pregnancy (4 %) or during the last week of pregnancy (23 % of women reported snoring every night during the last week). Gestational hypertension and preeclampsia developed in 14 % and 10 % of snorers, compared with 6 % and 4 % of non-snorers [68].

In a retrospective cohort study, Louis et al. found an association between PSG-confirmed OSA in 57 women (median AHI 22, median oxygen saturation nadir 87 %, range 84–90 %) and incidence of preeclampsia (19 % in OSA patients versus 7 % in a control cohort of 115 women), as well as preterm birth (30 % versus 12). However their study was complicated by preexisting comorbid characteristics of the OSA cohort, including higher BMI and chronic hypertension, as well as iatrogenically-induced medically-indicated preterm delivery in the context of preeclampsia [54]. Chen et al. also found increased risk of preeclampsia and preterm birth, but not GDM, in 791 pregnant women with confirmed OSA [69]. Finally, a recent study has found an independent association between OSA and preeclampsia even when confounding comorbidities such as BMI, maternal age, and diabetes were controlled for [41].

Conversely, in a cross-sectional study, Reid et al. found higher prevalence of PSG-confirmed OSA (defined as RDI >5) in pregnant women with gestational hypertension (53 %) compared to healthy pregnancy controls (12 %) [70]. Importantly, early OSA treatment with continuous positive airway pressure (CPAP) during the first 8 weeks of pregnancy in women at risk for preeclampsia resulted in improved blood pressure control, lower antihypertensive medication requirements, and improved pregnancy outcomes [71, 72].

Gestational Diabetes

In contrast to the findings of O'Brien et al., frequent snoring (>3 nights/week) was independently associated with increased incidence of GDM in a prospective cohort study of 189 healthy nulliparous women, and so was self-reported short sleep duration (<7 h) [67]. Qui et al. also describe an association between GDM and self-reported snoring and short sleep (<4 h). However their findings also implicate long (>10 h) sleep duration, as well as elevated BMI (>25 kg/m^2) with increased incidence of GDM [73].

Labor Complications

Lee and Gay used 48 hour actigraphy and sleep questionnaires in a prospective study of 131 women in the third trimester of pregnancy, and reported increased duration of labor and a 5.2 higher likelihood of cesarean delivery in women with actigraphy-derived WASO>15 % compared to WASO<10 %, as well as longer labors and 4.5 times greater likelihood of cesarean delivery in women reporting <6 h of sleep compared to at least 7 h of sleep. Higher rates of cesarean delivery were also associated with self-reported poor sleep quality occurring more frequently than 3 days per week [74]. Higher cesarean rates have also been reported in association with PSG-confirmed OSA during pregnancy, 65 % versus 4 % in the non-OSA pregnant controls, although higher BMI and incidence of chronic hypertension in the OSA compared to the control groups were significant confounders [41].

Perinatal Complications

In addition to an association between pregnancy-onset snoring and gestational hypertension, Franklin et al. reported snoring as a risk factor for growth retardation of the fetus, with 7.1 % of small for gestational age (SGA) infants born to snoring mothers versus 2.6 % in non-snorers. APGAR scores were also <7 at 1 and 5 min, respectively, in 12 % and 3.5 % of babies born to snorers, compared with 3.6 % and 0.3 % of babies born to non-snorers [68]. SGA and low Apgar scores at 5 min, as well as low gestational weight (LGW) have also been reported in babies of moms with confirmed OSA [69]. Finally, Louis et al. describe higher rates of neonatal intensive care unit (NICU) admissions of infants born to mothers with confirmed OSA [41].

In summary, sleep disturbance has been described as a risk factor for adverse pregnancy outcomes, including increased incidence of gestational hypertension/diabetes, cesarean delivery, and longer labor in self-reported short sleep during pregnancy, as well as increased risk of gestational hypertension/diabetes, preeclampsia, higher cesarean rates, LGW, lower APGAR scores, and higher rates of NICU admissions in pregnancies complicated by SDB, especially in the OSA end of the SDB spectrum. Activation of inflammatory pathways [75], including up-regulation of cytokine secretion [76, 77], may represent the pathophysiological link between sleep disruption and adverse pregnancy outcomes. For example, Okun et al. report increased circulating and stimulated interleukin (IL)-6 levels in association with self-reported poor sleep quality (PSQI) and short sleep duration in mid- and late pregnancy [78], while IL-6 levels are elevated in preeclampsia [79].

Finally, despite the importance of sleep characterization in this population, there are no published studies definitively linking objective sleep measures (i.e. sleep stage as percent of TST, or arousal index) with maternal and neonatal outcomes. For example, although altered sleep architecture by PSG has been reported in preeclampsia [80], there are no prospective data on sleep disturbance as a cause rather than effect of preeclampsia.

In conclusion, a growing research effort is underway to build upon and further refine the existing body of work describing sleep disruption during pregnancy and the complicated relationship between sleep parameters and pregnancy outcomes. As methodologies for objective sleep evaluation and proteogenomic characterization become more sophisticated and widely available, longitudinal prospective studies with large numbers of participants will undoubtedly shed light on these important and fascinating topics http://www.sleepfoundation.org/article/sleep-america-polls/2007-women-and-sleep.

References

1. Pien GW, Schwab RJ. Sleep disorders during pregnancy. Sleep. 2004;27(7):1405–17.
2. Lee KA. Alterations in sleep during pregnancy and postpartum: a review of 30 years of research. Sleep Med Rev. 1998;2(4):231–42.
3. Sahota PK, Jain SS, Dhand R. Sleep disorders in pregnancy. Curr Opin Pulm Med. 2003;9(6):477–83.
4. Chang JJ, Pien GW, Duntley SP, Macones GA. Sleep deprivation during pregnancy and aternal and fetal outcomes: is there a relationship? Sleep Med Rev. 2010;14(2):107–14.
5. Foundation NS. Sleep in America Poll. 2007. http://www.sleepfoundation.org/article/sleep-america-polls/2007-women-and-slee.
6. Schweiger MS. Sleep disturbance in pregnancy. A subjective survey. Am J Obstet Gynecol. 1972;114(7):879–82.
7. Hedman C, Pohjasvaara T, Tolonen U, Suhonen-Malm AS, Myllyla VV. Effects of pregnancy on mothers' sleep. Sleep Med. 2002;3(1):37–42.
8. Facco FL, Kramer J, Ho KH, Zee PC, Grobman WA. Sleep disturbances in pregnancy. Obstet Gynecol. 2010;115(1):77–83.
9. Okun ML, Coussons-Read ME. Sleep disruption during pregnancy: how does it influence serum cytokines? J Reprod Immunol. 2007;73(2):158–65.
10. Hutchison BL, Stone PR, McCowan LM, Stewart AW, Thompson JM, Mitchell EA. A postal survey of maternal sleep in late pregnancy. BMC Pregnancy Childbirth. 2012;12:144.
11. Mindell JA, Jacobson BJ. Sleep disturbances during pregnancy. J Obstet Gynecol Neonatal Nurs. 2000;29(6):590–7.
12. Lee KA, Zaffke ME, McEnany G. Parity and sleep patterns during and after pregnancy. Obstet Gynecol. 2000;95(1):14–8.
13. Hertz G, Fast A, Feinsilver SH, Albertario CL, Schulman H, Fein AM. Sleep in normal late pregnancy. Sleep. 1992;15(3):246–51.
14. Wilson DL, Fung A, Walker SP, Barnes M. Subjective reports versus objective measurement of sleep latency and sleep duration in pregnancy. Behav Sleep Med. 2013;11(3):207–21.
15. Mallick BN, Singh A. REM sleep loss increases brain excitability: role of noradrenaline and its mechanism of action. Sleep Med Rev. 2011;15(3):165–78.

16. Wilson DL, Barnes M, Ellett L, Permezel M, Jackson M, Crowe SF. Decreased sleep efficiency, increased wake after sleep onset and increased cortical arousals in late pregnancy. Aust N Z J Obstet Gynaecol. 2011;51(1):38–46.
17. Brunner DP, Munch M, Biedermann K, Huch R, Huch A, Borbely AA. Changes in sleep and sleep electroencephalogram during pregnancy. Sleep. 1994;17(7): 576–82.
18. Driver HS, Shapiro CM. A longitudinal study of sleep stages in young women during pregnancy and postpartum. Sleep. 1992;15(5):449–53.
19. Karacan I, Heine W, Agnew HW, Williams RL, Webb WB, Ross JJ. Characteristics of sleep patterns during late pregnancy and postpartum periods. Am J Obstet Gynecol. 1968;101(5):579–86.
20. Hoppenbrouwers T, Hodgman JE, Arakawa K, et al. Sleep apnea as part of a sequence of events: a comparison of three months old infants at low and increased risk for sudden infant death syndrome (SIDS). Neuropadiatrie. 1978;9(4):320–37.
21. Speroff L, Fritz MA. Clinical gynecologic endocrinology and infertility. 7th ed. Philadelphia: Lippincott Williams & Wilkins; 2005.
22. Lee KA, McEnany G, Zaffke ME. REM sleep and mood state in childbearing women: sleepy or weepy? Sleep. 2000;23(7):877–85.
23. Lancel M, Faulhaber J, Holsboer F, Rupprecht R. Progesterone induces changes in sleep comparable to those of agonistic GABAA receptor modulators. Am J Physiol. 1996;271(4 Pt 1):E763–72.
24. Soderpalm AH, Lindsey S, Purdy RH, Hauger R, de Wit H. Administration of progesterone produces mild sedative-like effects in men and women. Psychoneuroendocrinology. 2004;29(3):339–54.
25. Cagnacci A, Volpe A, Paoletti AM, Melis GB. Regulation of the 24-hour rhythm of body temperature in menstrual cycles with spontaneous and gonadotropin-induced ovulation. Fertil Steril. 1997; 68(3):421–5.
26. Baker FC, Driver HS, Rogers GG, Paiker J, Mitchell D. High nocturnal body temperatures and disturbed sleep in women with primary dysmenorrhea. Am J Physiol. 1999;277(6 Pt 1):E1013–21.
27. Friess E, Tagaya H, Trachsel L, Holsboer F, Rupprecht R. Progesterone-induced changes in sleep in male subjects. Am J Physiol. 1997;272(5 Pt 1):E885–91.
28. Caufriez A, Leproult R, L'Hermite-Baleriaux M, Kerkhofs M, Copinschi G. Progesterone prevents sleep disturbances and modulates GH, TSH, and melatonin secretion in postmenopausal women. J Clin Endocrinol Metab. 2011;96(4):E614–23.
29. Regestein QR, Schiff I, Tulchinsky D, Ryan KJ. Relationship among estrogen-induced psychophysiological changes in hypogonadal women. Psychosom Med. 1981;43(2):147–55.
30. Thomson J, Oswald I. Effect of oestrogen on the sleep, mood, and anxiety of menopausal women. Br Med J. 1977;2(6098):1317–9.
31. Rigg LA, Lein A, Yen SS. Pattern of increase in circulating prolactin levels during human gestation. Am J Obstet Gynecol. 1977;129(4):454–6.
32. Blyton DM, Sullivan CE, Edwards N. Lactation is associated with an increase in slow-wave sleep in women. J Sleep Res. 2002;11(4):297–303.
33. Frieboes RM, Murck H, Stalla GK, Antonijevic IA, Steiger A. Enhanced slow wave sleep in patients with prolactinoma. J Clin Endocrinol Metab. 1998;83(8):2706–10.
34. Allolio B, Hoffmann J, Linton EA, Winkelmann W, Kusche M, Schulte HM. Diurnal salivary cortisol patterns during pregnancy and after delivery: relationship to plasma corticotrophin-releasing-hormone. Clin Endocrinol (Oxf). 1990;33(2):279–89.
35. Friess E, V Bardeleben U, Wiedemann K, Lauer CJ, Holsboer F. Effects of pulsatile cortisol infusion on sleep-EEG and nocturnal growth hormone release in healthy men. J Sleep Res. 1994;3(2):73–9.
36. Sassin JF, Parker DC, Mace JW, Gotlin RW, Johnson LC, Rossman LG. Human growth hormone release: relation to slow-wave sleep and sleep-walking cycles. Science. 1969;165(3892):513–5.
37. Leproult R, Copinschi G, Buxton O, Van Cauter E. Sleep loss results in an elevation of cortisol levels the next evening. Sleep. 1997;20(10):865–70.
38. Lain KY, Catalano PM. Metabolic changes in pregnancy. Clin Obstet Gynecol. 2007;50(4):938–48.
39. Adam K, Oswald I. Protein synthesis, bodily renewal and the sleep-wake cycle. Clin Sci (Lond). 1983; 65(6):561–7.
40. Loube DI, Poceta JS, Morales MC, Peacock MD, Mitler MM. Self-reported snoring in pregnancy. Association with fetal outcome. Chest. 1996; 109(4):885–9.
41. Louis J, Auckley D, Miladinovic B, et al. Perinatal outcomes associated with obstructive sleep apnea in obese pregnant women. Obstet Gynecol. 2012;120(5):1085–92.
42. O'Connor C, Thornley KS, Hanly PJ. Gender differences in the polysomnographic features of obstructive sleep apnea. Am J Respir Crit Care Med. 2000;161(5):1465–72.
43. Mills GH, Chaffe AG. Sleeping positions adopted by pregnant women of more than 30 weeks gestation. Anaesthesia. 1994;49(3):249–50.
44. Itasaka Y, Miyazaki S, Ishikawa K, Togawa K. The influence of sleep position and obesity on sleep apnea. Psychiatry Clin Neurosci. 2000;54(3):340–1.
45. Manber R, Kuo TF, Cataldo N, Colrain IM. The effects of hormone replacement therapy on sleep-disordered breathing in postmenopausal women: a pilot study. Sleep. 2003;26(2):163–8.
46. Popovic RM, White DP. Upper airway muscle activity in normal women: influence of hormonal status. J Appl Physiol. 1998;84(3):1055–62.
47. Zwillich CW, Natalino MR, Sutton FD, Weil JV. Effects of progesterone on chemosensitivity in normal men. J Lab Clin Med. 1978;92(2):262–9.
48. Bradley TD, McNicholas WT, Rutherford R, Popkin J, Zamel N, Phillipson EA. Clinical and physiologic heterogeneity of the central sleep apnea syndrome. Am Rev Respir Dis. 1986;134(2):217–21.
49. Elkus R, Popovich Jr J. Respiratory physiology in pregnancy. Clin Chest Med. 1992;13(4):555–65.

50. Gunderson EP, Abrams B. Epidemiology of gestational weight gain and body weight changes after pregnancy. Epidemiol Rev. 1999;21(2):261–75.
51. Peppard PE, Young T, Palta M, Dempsey J, Skatrud J. Longitudinal study of moderate weight change and sleep-disordered breathing. JAMA. 2000;284(23):3015–21.
52. Suzuki K, Ohida T, Sone T, et al. The prevalence of restless legs syndrome among pregnant women in japan and the relationship between restless legs syndrome and sleep problems. Sleep. 2003;26(6):673–7.
53. Lee KA, Zaffke ME, Baratte-Beebe K. Restless legs syndrome and sleep disturbance during pregnancy: the role of folate and iron. J Womens Health Gend Based Med. 2001;10(4):335–41.
54. Louis JM, Auckley D, Sokol RJ, Mercer BM. Maternal and neonatal morbidities associated with obstructive sleep apnea complicating pregnancy. Am J Obstet Gynecol. 2010;202(3):261. e1-5.
55. Hublin C, Partinen M, Koskenvuo M, Kaprio J. Sleep and mortality: a population-based 22-year follow-up study. Sleep. 2007;30(10):1245–53.
56. Peppard PE, Young T, Palta M, Skatrud J. Prospective study of the association between sleep-disordered breathing and hypertension. N Engl J Med. 2000;342(19):1378–84.
57. Gottlieb DJ, Redline S, Nieto FJ, et al. Association of usual sleep duration with hypertension: the sleep heart health study. Sleep. 2006;29(8):1009–14.
58. Meisinger C, Heier M, Lowel H, Schneider A, Doring A. Sleep duration and sleep complaints and risk of myocardial infarction in middle-aged men and women from the general population: the MONICA/KORA Augsburg cohort study. Sleep. 2007;30(9):1121–7.
59. Bjorvatn B, Sagen IM, Oyane N, et al. The association between sleep duration, body mass index and metabolic measures in the Hordaland Health Study. J Sleep Res. 2007;16(1):66–76.
60. Spiegel K, Leproult R, Van Cauter E. Impact of sleep debt on metabolic and endocrine function. Lancet. 1999;354(9188):1435–9.
61. Gottlieb DJ, Punjabi NM, Newman AB, et al. Association of sleep time with diabetes mellitus and impaired glucose tolerance. Arch Intern Med. 2005;165(8):863–7.
62. Irwin M, McClintick J, Costlow C, Fortner M, White J, Gillin JC. Partial night sleep deprivation reduces natural killer and cellular immune responses in humans. FASEB J. 1996;10(5):643–53.
63. Bollinger T, Bollinger A, Naujoks J, Lange T, Solbach W. The influence of regulatory T cells and diurnal hormone rhythms on T helper cell activity. Immunology. 2010;131(4):488–500.
64. Klebanoff MA, Shiono PH, Rhoads GG. Outcomes of pregnancy in a national sample of resident physicians. N Engl J Med. 1990;323(15):1040–5.
65. Williams MA, Miller RS, Qiu C, Cripe SM, Gelaye B, Enquobahrie D. Associations of early pregnancy sleep duration with trimester-specific blood pressures and hypertensive disorders in pregnancy. Sleep. 2010;33(10):1363–71.
66. O'Brien LM, Bullough AS, Owusu JT, et al. Pregnancy-onset habitual snoring, gestational hypertension, and preeclampsia: prospective cohort study. Am J Obstet Gynecol. 2012;207(6):487. e1-9.
67. Facco FL, Grobman WA, Kramer J, Ho KH, Zee PC. Self-reported short sleep duration and frequent snoring in pregnancy: impact on glucose metabolism. Am J Obstet Gynecol. 2010;203(2):142. e1-5.
68. Franklin KA, Holmgren PA, Jonsson F, Poromaa N, Stenlund H, Svanborg E. Snoring, pregnancy-induced hypertension, and growth retardation of the fetus. Chest. 2000;117(1):137–41.
69. Chen YH, Kang JH, Lin CC, Wang IT, Keller JJ, Lin HC. Obstructive sleep apnea and the risk of adverse pregnancy outcomes. Am J Obstet Gynecol. 2012;206(2):136. e1-5.
70. Reid J, Skomro R, Cotton D, et al. Pregnant women with gestational hypertension may have a high frequency of sleep disordered breathing. Sleep. 2011;34(8):1033–8.
71. Poyares D, Guilleminault C, Hachul H, et al. Pre-eclampsia and nasal CPAP: part 2. Hypertension during pregnancy, chronic snoring, and early nasal CPAP intervention. Sleep Med. 2007;9(1):15–21.
72. Guilleminault C, Palombini L, Poyares D, Takaoka S, Huynh NT, El-Sayed Y. Pre-eclampsia and nasal CPAP: part 1. Early intervention with nasal CPAP in pregnant women with risk-factors for pre-eclampsia: preliminary findings. Sleep Med. 2007;9(1):9–14.
73. Retnakaran R, Qi Y, Connelly PW, Sermer M, Hanley AJ, Zinman B. Risk of early progression to prediabetes or diabetes in women with recent gestational dysglycaemia but normal glucose tolerance at 3-month postpartum. Clin Endocrinol (Oxf). 2010;73(4):476–83.
74. Lee KA, Gay CL. Sleep in late pregnancy predicts length of labor and type of delivery. Am J Obstet Gynecol. 2004;191(6):2041–6.
75. Okun ML, Roberts JM, Marsland AL, Hall M. How disturbed sleep may be a risk factor for adverse pregnancy outcomes. Obstet Gynecol Surv. 2009;64(4):273–80.
76. Gozal D, Serpero LD, Kheirandish-Gozal L, Capdevila OS, Khalyfa A, Tauman R. Sleep measures and morning plasma TNF-alpha levels in children with sleep-disordered breathing. Sleep. 2010;33(3):319–25.
77. Irwin MR, Wang M, Campomayor CO, Collado-Hidalgo A, Cole S. Sleep deprivation and activation of morning levels of cellular and genomic markers of inflammation. Arch Intern Med. 2006;166(16):1756–62.
78. Okun ML, Hall M, Coussons-Read ME. Sleep disturbances increase interleukin-6 production during pregnancy: implications for pregnancy complications. Reprod Sci. 2007;14(6):560–7.
79. Prins JR, Gomez-Lopez N, Robertson SA. Interleukin-6 in pregnancy and gestational disorders. J Reprod Immunol. 2012;95(1–2):1–14.
80. Edwards N, Blyton CM, Kesby GJ, Wilcox I, Sullivan CE. Pre-eclampsia is associated with marked alterations in sleep architecture. Sleep. 2000;23(5):619–25.

Sleep Deprivation and Metabolism

10

Erin C. Hanlon and Kristen L. Knutson

Introduction

The prevalence of overweight and obesity has steadily increased worldwide since approximately 1980 [1], but the acceleration in the United States has been particularly alarming [2]. According to data collected by the Center for Disease Control's (CDC) Behavioral Risk Factor Surveillance System (BRFSS), in 1985 no participating states had obesity rates greater than 15 %, but by 2009 only one state had obesity rates lower than 20 %, while 9 states reported a prevalence of obesity equal to or greater than 30 % of the state's population. As of 2011, 27.8 % of the American population could be categorized as obese (body mass index (BMI) greater than 30 kg/m^2), while 35.8 % of population was overweight (BMI 25–29.9 kg/m^2). Disorders commonly associated with obesity, such as cardiovascular disease and type II diabetes, have concurrently increased [3, 4]. Due to their close association with one another, these disorders, obesity, diabetes, and cardiovascular diseases, are collectively termed "cardiometabolic diseases." Considering that cardiometabolic diseases can lead to significant healthcare costs and adverse health outcomes, including reduced quality of life and life expectancy, elucidating potential contributing factors to the increased incidence of obesity will have important implications for public health. Generally speaking, obesity is the result of energy intake exceeding energy expenditure. Thus, traditional causes for the increase in the prevalence of overweight and obesity include, but are not limited to, increased portion size, increased availability of high-calorie/high fat foods, and decreased physical activity. In recent years, other putative causal mechanisms have begun to emerge, including chronic partial sleep loss [5]. The present chapter will focus on the association between sleep deficiency and increased risk of diabetes and cardiovascular disease (i.e., cardiometabolic disease).

Epidemiological Evidence

Sleep deficiency would include insufficient sleep durations and/or reduced sleep quality. As the incidence of obesity has increased, average sleep times appear to have decreased. Polls conducted by the CDC, National Sleep Foundation (NSF), as well as large scale epidemiological studies have indicated that many Americans experience chronic partial sleep restriction because of voluntary bedtime curtailment [6–8]. In1960, a study conducted by the American Cancer Society

E.C. Hanlon, Ph.D. (✉)
Section of Endocrinology, Diabetes, and Metabolism, Department of Medicine, Sleep, Metabolism, and Health Center, University of Chicago, Chicago, IL, USA
e-mail: ehanlon@medicine.bsd.uchicago.edu

K.L. Knutson, Ph.D.
Section of Pulmonary and Critical Care, Department of Medicine, Sleep, Metabolism, and Health Center, University of Chicago, Chicago, IL, USA

M.T. Bianchi (ed.), *Sleep Deprivation and Disease: Effects on the Body, Brain and Behavior*, DOI 10.1007/978-1-4614-9087-6_10, © Springer Science+Business Media New York 2014

found that the majority of respondents reported sleeping 8–8.9 h/night [9]. However, simultaneously, some studies were already reporting reductions in average self-reported sleep times to 7–8 h/night [10–12]. As evidenced by the 2009 NSF poll, average self-reported sleep times have continued to decline in adults to 6 h and 40 min on weeknights and 7 h and 7 min on the weekend [8]. The 2010 NSF poll detailed average self-reported sleep times across racial/ethnic groups where all groups combined reported sleep times less than 7 h/week night with Whites reporting on average 6 h and 52 min, African-Americans 6 h and 14 min, Asians 6 h and 48 min and, Hispanics 6 h and 34 min [13]. Interestingly, many studies have reported that African-Americans, a group at increased risk of cardiometabolic diseases, have shorter sleep durations and poorer sleep quality than Whites [14–17]. Although self-reported sleep duration may be underestimated (e.g., in patients with insomnia), it is also important to recognize that actual sleep times may be lower than what is estimated with self-reports. Sleep can be reliably estimated with wrist actigraphy; a watch-like device worn on the wrist that utilizes movement (or lack thereof) to distinguish sleep versus wake states. Using wrist actigraphy, a study conducted between 1990 and 1994 found that participants 40–64 years of age slept on average 6.2 h/ night [16]. Recently, in the Coronary Artery Risk Development in Young Adults (CARDIA) Sleep Study (2000–2006), sleep duration ascertained from several days of wrist actigraphy among a sample of 35–50 year olds revealed average sleep times of 6.1 h/night [18] while self-reported sleep averaged 6.7 h/ weeknight and 7.3 h/weekend night [17]. As evidenced by the 2011 and 2012 NSF polls, declines in sleep time can be attributed, in part, to extended work schedules including shift work, long commuting times, stressful lifestyles, modern conveniences such as 24-h television and computer/internet usage, and social and leisure activities [19, 20].

There is a growing body of observational evidence suggesting a link between insufficient sleep duration and increased risk of obesity and type II diabetes. Many studies reveal an association between short sleep duration and increased prevalence of obesity or higher BMI and have been previously reviewed [21–23]. The majority of both cross-sectional and prospective studies, whether in children or adults, found significant associations between short sleep and increased obesity risk after controlling for multiple confounders. Importantly, the strength of the association between obesity and insufficient sleep may be greater in children than adults [22]. Nonetheless, the relationship between short sleep and elevated BMI persists in both older men and women as demonstrated in a large study that used actigraphy to assess sleep duration in more than 6,000 adults aged 67–99 years [24]. Interestingly, a recent longitudinal observational study of self-reported sleep durations showed that short sleepers (<6 h) who were found subsequently to have extended their sleep to 7–8 h per night had less fat mass and lower increases in BMI than those that maintained the short sleep schedule over a 6-year period [25]. To that end, two population-based studies have also reported associations between short sleep duration and alterations in circulating peptides known to modulate feeding behavior (leptin, a signal of energy deficiency, and the orexigenic hormone ghrelin; described in detail below) consistent with an upregulation of appetite [26, 27]. Moreover, these associations were independent of BMI and other possible confounding factors. Intriguingly, Taheri and colleagues reported a U-shape relationship between self-reported average nightly sleep and BMI after adjustment for age and sex, such that those with greater than 9 h/night of average nightly sleep also had higher BMI [26]. Similarly, Chaput and colleagues revealed that when compared to those that reported sleeping 7–8 h/night, long sleepers (9–10 h/night) had increased adjusted odds ratio for overweight/obesity (1.38) [27]. To that end, although the main focus of this chapter is the effect of *sleep restriction* on metabolism, the findings that long sleep may also be associated with adverse outcomes is discussed below.

There is also strong epidemiologic evidence for a link between self-reported sleep duration and an increased risk of type II diabetes and cardiovascular disease. The majority of prospective studies (which provide some indication regarding direction of causality) revealed a significantly elevated risk of diabetes in short sleepers [28]. A recent meta-analysis combining data from 90,623 individuals concluded that for short sleep duration (≤5–6 h/night), the relative risk of developing diabetes was 1.28 compared to those sleeping 7–8 h/night after controlling for multiple factors [29]. Interestingly, long sleep (>8 h/night) was also associated with an increased relative risk (1.48) of type II diabetes in this study. Not included in this meta-analysis is the largest study to date [30], which included 174,542 adults and observed that individuals who reported sleeping <5 h per night, relative to those reporting 7–8 h per night, had a 46 % higher risk of developing type II diabetes, after controlling for multiple confounders, including adiposity. In regard to cardiovascular disease, a meta-analysis revealed that in 474,684 male and female participants, short sleep duration was associated with a greater risk of developing or dying from coronary heart disease [31]. This analysis also revealed that long sleep (8–9 h/night) was associated with increased relative risk for coronary heart disease (1.38) and cardiovascular disease (1.41) [31]. Moreover, the CARDIA study revealed that short sleep duration and lower sleep maintenance, a component of sleep quality, predicted significantly higher blood pressure and greater increases in blood pressure over 5 years. Furthermore, in this study, short sleep duration was associated with increased odds of developing hypertension over 5 years [32]. Thus, there is a well-established link between sleep deficiency and increased risk for obesity, diabetes, and cardiovascular disease. A few controlled laboratory studies have been conducted that further strengthen this association and are discussed below.

Laboratory Studies

Although laboratory studies in human volunteers involve relatively small sample sizes (10–20 participants), there is the advantage of measuring various components of energy balance and glucose metabolism while stringently imposing different sleep conditions; normal bedtimes, restricted bedtimes, and extended bedtimes [33]. Further, polysomnography (PSG) can be obtained allowing for information on sleep architecture. Participants are typically young healthy lean volunteers that report habitual sleep schedules of approximately 8 h per night. Throughout the course of the laboratory study, caloric intake is rigorously controlled and sedentary conditions are enforced to control for activity levels. Each sleep condition involves 2–15 days with stringently controlled bedtimes and light-dark cycles.

In our laboratory, the center of the bedtime period is kept constant and light exposure is reduced in the evening and morning to avoid a shift of circadian phase. Since each participant is exposed to all bedtime conditions, within subject comparisons can be made between conditions, therefore any alterations observed are most likely due to the experimental intervention instead of other confounding factors. During the course of the study, participants complete questionnaires about mood, subjective sleepiness, alertness, hunger, and appetite multiple times per day. Each sleep condition involves at least one 24-h period when blood is frequently sampled which allows for 24-h profiles of blood constituents including glucose, insulin, and C-peptide (a marker of insulin secretion), cortisol, growth hormone, and the appetite-regulating hormones leptin and ghrelin. Intravenous glucose tolerance tests (ivGTT) are also conducted to examine glucose tolerance (Kg; rate of decrease of glucose levels following glucose injection), glucose effectiveness (Sg, a marker of non-insulin-dependent glucose utilization and therefore an indirect measure of brain glucose metabolism), insulin sensitivity (SI, which quantifies the amount of insulin needed to metabolize a given amount of glucose), acute insulin response to glucose (AIRg: the acute insulin response to glucose in the first 20 min following glucose injection), and the disposition index (a validated marker of diabetes risk; $DI = SI \times AIRg$). The response to oral glucose, which involves the gastro-intestinal tract and the so-called incretin effect, may also be tested on a separate day.

Laboratory studies of sleep restriction do have limitations in that they are generally constrained in duration and may not precisely mimic alterations in glucose metabolism, energy balance, or appetite and hunger produced by more chronic partial sleep loss. Thus, translating these results to real-life conditions is not straightforward. We acknowledge that the stress of sleep loss under the demands of normal life conditions, including professional and social demands, is also not replicated by laboratory conditions. Furthermore, although cross-sectional and prospective studies have reported associations between insufficient sleep duration and increased weight irrespective of sex differences, the vast majority of laboratory studies in both humans and animals have only been conducted on males. Thus, further examination of potential sex differences in regard to this relationship is necessary.

There have only been a few carefully controlled laboratory studies that have meticulously examined the effect of sleep deficiency on glucose metabolism, endocrine function, and feeding behavior or appetite regulation. The first controlled study examined 11 healthy young men for 16 consecutive nights in the laboratory with varying sleep allotments; 8 h in bed for 3 nights (baseline), restricted to 4 h in bed for the next 6 nights (sleep-debt), followed by 12 h in bed for 7 nights (sleep recovery) [34]. The protocol for this "sleep debt" study is shown in Fig. 10.1a. During the last 2 days of sleep debt and sleep-recovery conditions, while subjected to bed rest, participants were given identical carbohydrate-rich meals and an intravenous glucose tolerance test (ivGTT) was conducted followed by a 24-h period of frequent blood sampling. This seminal study of recurring partial sleep loss was successful in producing repeated sleep restriction in the laboratory; mean total sleep time during the baseline period was 7 h and 14 min and during sleep debt it was 3 h and 49 min in comparison to the 9 h and 3 min attained during the period of sleep recovery. The proportion of slow-wave sleep (stage III of non-REM sleep, also termed "deep sleep") was higher during the sleep-debt condition in comparison to baseline and sleep recovery, revealing an increased pressure for slow-wave sleep. The period of sleep debt was primarily characterized by a loss of REM sleep which was reduced from approximately 90 min at baseline to 40 min during the last 2 short nights. Following the period of sleep restriction, glucose and insulin responses to breakfast and the ivGTT were consistent with an impairment of carbohydrate tolerance consistent with a prediabetic state. In contrast, the glucose and insulin responses subsequent to the sleep-recovery period were in the normal range. As illustrated in Fig. 10.2, the ivGTT revealed 40 % lower glucose clearance, a 25–30 % reduction in both glucose effectiveness and insulin sensitivity, and a disposition index 40 % lower in the sleep-restricted than the sleep-extension condition [34, 35]. The 24-h assessments revealed that the post-breakfast Homeostatic Model Assessment (HOMA) values (a marker of insulin resistance) increased 56 % in the sleep-debt condition compared to sleep recovery, due to elevated glucose levels in response to breakfast despite the fact that insulin levels tended to be also higher. Interestingly, neither the glucose nor insulin response differed between the sleep-debt and sleep-recovery conditions in response to lunch or dinner. In contrast, evening cortisol (total cortisol measured from plasma and free cortisol from saliva) and sympathetic nervous system activation were increased; both are risk factors for the development of insulin resistance and obesity. The 24-h profile of blood constituents revealed that levels of the satiety signal leptin are particularly sensitive to sleep duration [36], confirming an early study that reported significantly decreased leptin levels following sleep restriction to 4 h/night for 7 nights [37]. Mean leptin levels were 19 % lower in the sleep-debt vs. sleep-recovery condition and were intermediate with 8-h bedtimes (shown in the upper panel of Fig. 10.3). Further, both the nocturnal acrophase and amplitude of the diurnal variation of leptin were decreased (26 % and 20 %, respectively). Interestingly, these changes occurred without fluctuations in BMI and despite similar caloric intake and activity levels [36]. These observed decreases in leptin concentrations are somewhat larger than those observed in young adults after 3 days of dietary restriction by ~900 kcal/day [38]. Thus, not only does sleep debt alter metabolic systems promoting diabetes

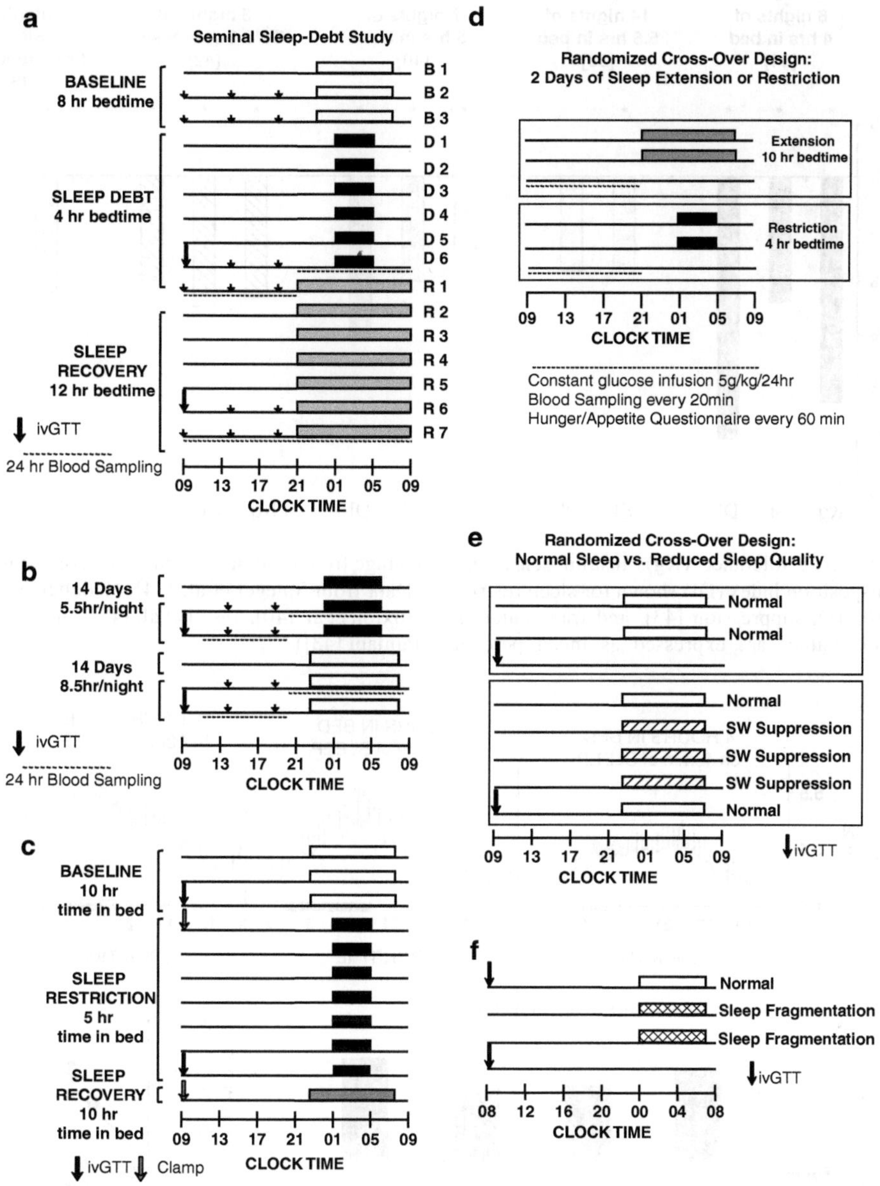

Fig. 10.1 (**a**) Experimental protocol included three baseline nights of 8 h in bed (white bars), followed by 6 night of sleep restriction (4 h in bed—*black bars*), ending with a 7 night period of sleep extension (12 h in bed—*light grey bars*). The last 2 days of the sleep debt and sleep-extension periods included identical meals for breakfast, lunch, and dinner (denoted by *small arrows*), an ivGTT to assess glucose metabolism (indicated by a large *arrow*), and 24 h blood sampling to examine circulating hormonal profiles (*dashed lines*). (**b**) A randomized cross-over design that included two 14-day in-laboratory sessions, with either 5.5 or 8.5 h/night in bed. The last 48 h of each session included 24-h blood sampling (*dashed lines*) and an ivGTT (indicated by a *large arrow*). During this period, identical carbohydrate-rich meals were served at 14:00 and 19:00 (denoted by *small arrows*). (**c**) Experimental protocol included three baseline nights of 10 h in bed (*white bars*), followed by 7 nights of sleep restriction (5 h in bed—*black bars*), ending with one night of sleep recovery (10 h in bed—*grey bar*). To assess glucose metabolism an ivGTT was conducted following 2 nights of baseline and 6 nights of sleep restriction (indicated with *black arrow*), and the euglycemic-hyperinsulinemic clamp procedure was done after 3 baseline nights and 7 nights of sleep restriction (indicated with *grey arrow*). (**d**) In a randomized cross-over design, two nights of either bedtime extension (10 h in bed—*dark grey bars*) or sleep restriction (4 h in bed—*black bars*) were followed by 12 h of blood sampling, coupled with a constant glucose infusion and hourly questionnaires regarding hunger/appetite, mood, and sleepiness. (**e**) In a randomized cross-over design, 2 nights of normal sleep (8 h in bed—*white bars*) or three nights of slow-wave sleep suppression (*hatched bars*) were followed by an ivGTT (denoted with an *arrow*) to assess glucose metabolism. (**f**) Study protocol included one night of uninterrupted sleep followed by 2 nights of sleep fragmentation. Glucose metabolism was assessed with ivGTT the morning prior to normal sleep and following 2 nights of sleep fragmentation (denoted with *black arrow*). (Adapted from Hanlon [33])

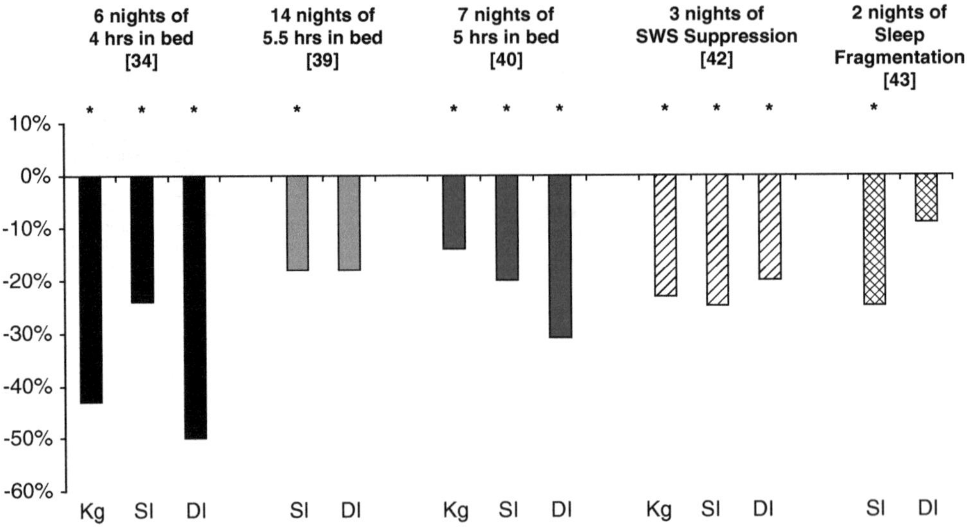

Fig. 10.2 Glucose tolerance (Kg), insulin sensitivity (SI), and disposition index (DI) shown for sleep restriction [35, 40, 41], suppression [43], and fragmentation [44] studies. Values are expressed as mean percent change from baseline/normal sleep condition. *$p < 0.05$. (Data from Spiegel et al. [34], Nedeltcheva et al. [39], Buxton et al. [40], Tasali et al. [42], and Stamatakis and Punjabi [43])

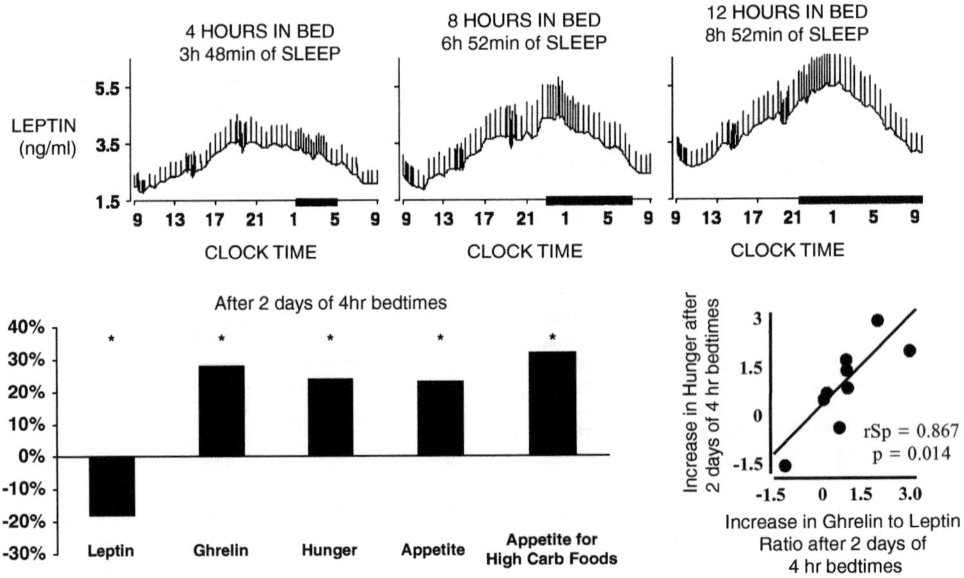

Fig. 10.3 *Upper panel*; mean (±SEM) 24 h plasma leptin profiles obtained from nine healthy lean men. Participants ate three identical carbohydrate-rich meals following 6 days of 4, 8, and 12 h in bed. The *dark bars* denote sleep periods. Comparisons of variables obtained during 8-, 4-, and 12-h bedtime conditions were performed using ANOVA for repeated measures. Time spent asleep in each condition was as follows; 3 h and 48 min in 4 h bedtime condition, 6 h and 52 min in 8 h bed condition, and 8 h and 52 min in the 12 h condition. Note that the characteristics of the 24-h leptin profile (amplitude, nocturnal maximum, and overall mean) increased from the 4 h to the 12 h bedtime condition. Lower panel, mean plasma leptin and ghrelin, as well as subjective hunger and appetite ratings observed in 12 healthy lean subjects after 2 days of 4 h bedtimes compared to 2 days with 10 h bedtimes. Comparisons between the two sleep conditions were performed using the Wilcoxon test for matched pairs; data shown as percent difference from 10 h bedtimes. Caloric intake was exclusively administered via a constant glucose infusion. Correlation of the change in hunger ratings and the ghrelin-to-leptin ratio were calculated using the Spearman rank test. Values were calculated using data from 4 h in bed minus the value obtained following 10 h in bed. The calculated value was negative when the variable measured after 10 h in bed was higher than that measured after 4 h in bed. *$p < 0.05$. (Data from Hanlon and Van Cauter [33] and Spiegel et al. [36])

risk, but leptin seems to be signaling a state of energy insufficiency/caloric deficit during the period of sleep debt, potentially leading to a reactive or compensatory hyperphagia.

Findings of decreased insulin sensitivity without adequate compensation by increased insulin release have been replicated in other studies of sleep restriction [39, 40]. In one study, the experimental design required the 11 lean, healthy participants (five males and six females) to complete two 14-day in laboratory study periods, in which they were either allotted 5.5 or 8.5 h/night in bed [39] (Fig. 10.1b). During this time, the participants were sedentary and had *ad libitum* access to food which resulted in positive energy balance and similar weight gain regardless of sleep condition. However, following the sleep restriction paradigm, oral glucose tolerance was reduced by 10 %, insulin sensitivity reduced by 18 %, and the disposition index by 18 % (although not statistically significant), without changes to the acute insulin response to glucose, suggesting that sleep restriction may interfere with β-cell compensation. Another study successfully recruited 20 healthy lean men to participate in a laboratory session in which activity and caloric intake was controlled [40]. After at least 5 days of 10 h/night in bed at home (validated with sleep diaries and wrist actigraphy), participants were required to spend 12 days in the laboratory;10 h/night for 3 nights (baseline), followed by 5 h/night for 7 nights (sleep restriction), and 10 h for the final night (recovery) (Fig. 10.1c). When assessed with an ivGTT and also with euglycemic-hyperinsulinemic clamp, insulin sensitivity was significantly lower in the sleep restriction condition than during baseline; 20 % and 11 % reductions, respectively. Again, this was observed without increases in acute insulin response to intravenous glucose. Glucose tolerance and disposition index were also significantly reduced following sleep restriction. Thus, 5.5 h or 5 h/night was sufficient to reduce insulin sensitivity in healthy lean young individuals in a manner expected to elevate diabetes risk if chronic.

Subsequent to the original laboratory sleep-debt experiment, a randomized cross-over study (Fig. 10.1d) was developed, in part to control for putative order effects in the "sleep debt" study, and examined metabolic parameters following 2 nights of either 4 or 10 h in bed [41]. Hormonal findings pertinent to appetite regulation are illustrated in the panels of Fig. 10.3. Leptin, a satiety signal released from adipose tissue, and ghrelin, an appetite stimulant produced in the stomach, were measured in this study. Consistent with the seminal study, sleep restriction was associated with decreased leptin concentration, even though meals were replaced by constant glucose infusion. Furthermore, this study revealed a concomitant increase in the orexigenic factor ghrelin (28 %), along with increased subjective hunger and appetite ratings (24 % and 23 %, respectively) in the short sleep condition compared to the well-rested condition [41]. Interestingly, appetite ratings tended to be greatest for carbohydrate-rich calorie-dense foods; foods likely to have high hedonic values (Fig. 10.3; and see below, *Mechanistic Pathways*). The change in the ghrelin-to-leptin ratio between the two experimental conditions was significantly and positively correlated with changes in hunger ratings, suggesting that sleep restriction-induced alterations in these hormones may, in part, be driving observed increases in hunger ratings. These results are consistent with the observational studies described above [26, 27]. Thus, sleep restriction or partial chronic sleep loss produces modifications in the profile of appetite-regulating hormones, favoring hyperphagia.

Interestingly, a few studies involving experimental manipulation of sleep quality without change in sleep duration have reported similar findings to those that only alter sleep duration [42, 43]. In a recent study of the metabolic impact of experimental reductions of sleep quality, 9 healthy lean participants (five men and four women) were tested under two conditions in randomized order: undisturbed baseline condition with 2 nights of 8.5 h in bed and 3 nights of 8.5 h with slow-wave sleep suppression [42]. Suppression of slow-wave sleep (SWS; non-REM stage III) was achieved with acoustic stimulation; as soon as slow-waves were identified on the EEG recording, a sound was sent to amplifiers on both sides of the subject's bed to elicit a microarousal and subsequent suppression of slow-wave activity (Fig. 10.1e). The acoustic stimulation administered during SWS suppression resulted in an increase in the lighter sleep stages, stages I and II, without changing total sleep time or the amount of REM sleep. As summarized in Fig. 10.2, metabolic alterations qualitatively similar to those observed following reductions in sleep duration emerged [42]. Following 3 nights of acoustic stimulation during SWS only, an ivGTT revealed that insulin sensitivity was decreased by 25 %, glucose tolerance by 23 %, and the disposition index decreased by 20 % compared to baseline. These values are typical of individuals who have impaired glucose tolerance and are at risk of developing diabetes. Interestingly, the magnitude of the changes for both insulin sensitivity and acute insulin response to glucose were correlated with the decreases in slow-wave sleep [42]. Similar to the previous studies of sleep restriction, elevated cardiac sympathetic nervous activity was apparent after 3 days of acoustic stimulation during SWS. Acoustic stimulation during SWS thus produces clear reductions in glucose tolerance and increases in markers of diabetes risk.

Consistent with this notion, an independent study of sleep fragmentation achieved via auditory and mechanical stimulation across all sleep stages (which however led to a greater decrease of slow-wave sleep than of other sleep stages) obtained similar findings as in the study of acoustic stimulation during SWS only [43]. Eleven young lean healthy individuals (9 men and 2 women) spent 3 nights in the laboratory. The first night was undisturbed and the following 2 nights had sleep fragmentation (Fig. 10.1f). An ivGTT to assess glucose metabolism was performed before the baseline night and after the second night of fragmentation. Total sleep time remained constant across all 3 nights, stage I significantly increased, while SWS and REM sleep were significantly reduced [43]. In congruence with previous studies, sleep fragmentation was associated with a decrease in insulin sensitivity by 25 % and glucose effectiveness by 21 % (Fig. 10.2). Further, an increase in sympathetic nervous system activity was observed following sleep fragmentation. Thus, it appears that not only the duration of sleep, but also the quality of sleep, is important for metabolic function. Considering that there are marked age-related changes in sleep quality, particularly reductions in slow-wave sleep, it is possible that the sleep disturbances of normal aging may also play a role in the increased diabetes risk in older populations. In contrast, a current ongoing clinical trial at NIH may offer interesting insight into the association between sleep duration and BMI. These investigators are examining whether extending sleep duration may reduce body weight in overweight individuals and improve other health markers, although findings have yet to be reported [44]. The potential mechanisms underlying the association between sleep deficiency and these outcomes are discussed below.

Mechanistic Pathways

The complexity of mechanisms within the periphery and central nervous system (CNS) that manage energy expenditure and feeding is intricate and involves redundant systems. However, dysfunction within only one of the nodes of the system can create alterations in feeding behavior and/or energy expenditure [45]. Here we focus on a few molecular signals found in the periphery and CNS that modulate feeding and energy expenditure.

Sleep loss may disturb appetite regulation and metabolism via alterations in activity of nuclei within the hypothalamus, as well as within hypothalamic communication with peripheral systems and/or other circuitry within the CNS. Stimulation and lesion experiments have revealed the role that hypothalamic nuclei play in energy homeostasis via feeding regulation; lesions of ventromedial, paraventricular, and dorsomedial nuclei or stimulation of the lateral hypothalamus (LH) produce hyperphagia [46, 47] while lesions of the LH inhibit feeding [48]. Peripheral circulating satiety signals, known to cross the blood brain barrier [49, 50], secreted from the stomach, fat tissue, and pancreas easily interact with the arcuate nucleus (Arc) of the hypothalamus, as it lies close to the third ventricle. A subset of neurons within the Arc produce and respond to neuropeptide Y (NPY) and agouti-related protein (AgRP), while another subset contain pro-opiomelanocortin (POMC) and cocaine- and amphetamine-regulated transcript (CART) [51–54]. Direct stimulation of NPY/AgRP neurons increases food intake and decreases energy expenditure/promote energy storage [55–58]. In contrast, excitation of POMC/CART neurons inhibits food intake and increases energy expenditure [53, 59]. Cells within the Arc directly project to the lateral hypothalamus which, in turn, projects to thalamo-cortical systems, central autonomic effectors, and motor pattern generators that influence regulation of feeding [60]. Thus, neurochemicals within the Arc influence feeding behavior via connections with the lateral hypothalamus.

Metabolic regulation and energy homeostasis is modulated by various peptides and hormones released from peripheral tissues including fat (such as leptin and adiponectin) and the gut (such as ghrelin, peptide YY, pancreatic polypeptide, and cholecystokinin). Receptors for these circulating peptides also lie within the CNS. Leptin and ghrelin are the two most studied peptides when considering the impact of sleep deficiency on energy balance, and thus this chapter focuses on these two pivotal players. Leptin, discovered in 1994 [61], is a peptide hormone encoded by the obesity gene (ob) that is secreted by white adipose tissue into the circulatory system [62]. Leptin is thought to be a signal of nutritional plenty; drops in leptin levels may be a key signal to the CNS that there is an imbalance in metabolism indicating a fasted state [63]. This signal would then promote increases in appetite and decreases in energy expenditure to regain energy homeostasis. Leptin acts most robustly on receptors located in the arcuate, ventromedial, and dorsomedial nuclei of the hypothalamus [64–69]. Leptin is also known to act on extrahypothalamic sites as well as peripheral tissues, although less is known about the mechanism of action in these areas [68–71]. Within the hypothalamus, both subsets of neurons containing NPY/AgRP and POMC/CART are responsive to leptin. In vitro, leptin directly activates, via depolarization, hypothalamic POMC/CART neurons; increases in both c-Fos and cytokine signaling 3 (SOC-3) expression, markers of neuronal activation and STAT-3 activation, respectively, in POMC neurons, suggest that leptin directly activates these neurons [72]. In contrast, leptin inhibits (hyperpolarizes) NPY/AgRP hypothalamic neurons [73, 74]. Additionally, NPY/AgRP neurons only express STAT-3 following leptin administration, suggesting that these cells are inhibited by leptin [75]. Thus, one mechanism by which leptin mediates energy homeostasis is via orexigenic NPY/AgRP and anorexigenic POMC/CART neurons within the hypothalamus. In regard to appetite regulation, individuals lacking leptin or the leptin receptor become obese [76] and in some individuals leptin replacement therapy has shown to improve obesity [77]. In normal weight individuals, plasma leptin levels increase consequent to food intake and decrease in response to food deprivation [78–81]. Interestingly, recent data have suggested a role for leptin in modulating glucose metabolism, independent of its effects on energy balance [45]. As an example, during controlled food intake paradigms, leptin administration to leptin-deficient humans and mice improves hyperinsulinemia and hyperglycemia [65, 81, 82].

A peripheral signal for satiety, ghrelin, a hormone produced by endocrine cells within the stomach, is thought to be a marker of energy insufficiency [83] and plays a role in stimulating the appetite, as well as promoting effective storage of consumed food [84]. Ghrelin, identified in 1999, was found to be primarily produced by the stomach [85, 86], although small amounts of this peptide are made in the hypothalamus [85] and various peripheral organs [87–89]. One mechanism by which ghrelin exerts its effects on feeding and energy homeostasis is via pathways that partly overlap leptin-sensitive pathways; ghrelin receptors are also located within the ventromedial and Arc nuclei of the hypothalamus [90]. NPY/AgRP cells within the Arc express ghrelin receptors [91] and ghrelin activates these neurons, evidenced by c-Fos expression [92, 93]. Further, ghrelin simultaneously increases inhibitory input to POMC/CART neurons [94]. With respect to appetite regulation, in humans there is a premeal rise in plasma ghrelin, suggesting a role for ghrelin in meal initiation [95]. Rodent studies have revealed that food deprivation increases ghrelin levels while food intake inhibits ghrelin expression [96]. It is apparent that ghrelin is involved in mediating energy homeostasis via feeding regulation; however, the exact mechanism of ghrelin action is still unclear.

Energy homeostasis and appetite regulation are also under the control of insulin. Insulin receptors are also present in the CNS [97]. Similar to leptin, insulin receptors are expressed in the Arc of the hypothalamus and may also inhibit NPY/AgRP neurons [98]. Intraventricular infusions of insulin decrease NPY mRNA in the Arc and insulin-deficient rats show elevated hypothalamic NPY mRNA expression [99–101]. Moreover, recent studies have shown that within discrete subpopulations within the Arc, insulin and leptin both exert effects on POMC neurons [83]. In regard to food intake, intraventricular infusions of insulin reduce food intake and body weight [83, 102, 103].

The energy balance regulating system of the hypothalamus is also intricately connected to the limbic system that encompasses circuitry involved in reward and motivation; the nucleus accumbens (Acb) has direct connections to the lateral hypothalamus (LH) and connects to the Arc, indirectly, through the LH [60]. Thus, regulation of food intake may also be manipulated by alterations in activation within the limbic system. The classic incentive-motivation theory posits that behavior is coordinated by motivational state; in regard to feeding behavior, energy deficit and incentive properties of food would drive feeding. The nucleus accumbens and other areas of the limbic system are involved in modulating reward value and/or incentive salience of food reward [60, 104]. In regard to human studies, a recent fMRI study revealed that obese individuals show elevated activation in reward systems when presented with pictures of high-calorie foods. Specifically, increased activation was observed within the medial and lateral orbitofrontal cortex, amygdala, nucleus accumbens/ventral striatum, medial prefrontal cortex, insula, anterior cingulate cortex (ACC), ventral pallidum, caudate, putamen, and hippocampus [105]. A more recent fMRI study found the ACC within the limbic system, which plays a role in determining the "pleasantness" and reward value of food [106], and the medial prefrontal cortex to be more highly activated in obese versus normal weight subjects when anticipating food [107]. An earlier PET study reported that the availability of striatal dopamine D2 receptors was significantly lower in obese versus control subjects [108]. Further, the decrement in availability was proportional to BMI; lower D2 receptors for higher BMI. In this study, the subjects examined had a BMI greater than 40 kg/m [2]. Thus, the reduction in D2 receptors may reflect a downregulation of receptors due to extended increased activation within the reward system from chronic/prolonged overeating. In all, these data suggest that alterations in systems involved in reward and motivation may indeed impact feeding behavior via altered activation in limbic system structures and other cortical areas involved in mediating the value of food as a reward. Along those lines, it should be noted that one study suggests that disinhibition eating behavior trait (the tendency to overeat and eat opportunistically) may explain weight gain in short sleepers; short sleepers with high disinhibition eating behavior trait were more likely to gain weight than short sleepers with low scores [109].

A few recent studies have begun to examine the effects of sleep restriction on these systems and brain areas. When assessed with fMRI in adolescents, short sleep duration and diminished subjective sleep quality were associated with less reactivity of the striatum [110], suggesting that more exciting rewards (higher hedonic value for food) are required to achieve a "normal" level of activity within the striatum during a period of sleep restriction. In adults assessed with fMRI, one night of total sleep deprivation increased activation of the right anterior cingulate cortex in response to food cues. Furthermore, activation was positively correlated with appetite ratings [111]. Another study conducted on adults reported that in response to food cues, multiple nights of partial sleep restriction (4 h/night for 6 nights) resulted in increased activity in prefrontal cortex, putamen, nucleus accumbens, thalamus, and insula [112].

PET studies have the ability to reveal alterations in neurotransmitter and receptor levels following sleep restriction. When assessed with PET, binding of a dopamine D2/D3 receptor radioligand, [11C]raclopride, in the striatum and thalamus was reduced after one night of total sleep deprivation compared to one rested night in 15 healthy male participants [113]. The magnitude of the reduction in binding was correlated with increases in fatigue and with deterioration in performance on cognitive tasks. At the time, these data were interpreted as increased dopamine levels within the striatum and thalamus following sleep deprivation but the authors acknowledged that these data could also reflect decreased receptor levels or affinity. In fact, a subsequent study by the same group revealed that one night of total sleep deprivation facilitates a down-regulation of D2/D3 receptors in the ventral striatum [114]. Interestingly, a down-regulation of D2/D3 receptors has been previously implicated in mediating attention, risk-taking, and with a greater risk for compulsive drug consumption [115–117]. Thus, sleep deficiency may be affecting reward systems and ultimately hunger, appetite, and feeding behavior via alterations in striatal dopamine. Furthermore, there is evidence showing that peripherally circulating hormones that regulate feeding behavior (i.e., leptin and ghrelin) modulate activity of brain regions involved in reward behavior [118, 119]. It has been reported that leptin therapy in patients with congenital leptin deficiency modulated striatal activation [118]. Activation in neural circuitry involved in moderating feeding behavior was also observed following intravenous ghrelin administration to healthy volunteers during functional magnetic resonance imaging when food cues were shown; increased activation was observed in regions involved in relating the incentive value of the food including the amygdala, orbitofrontal cortex, anterior insula, and striatum [119]. Sleep restriction is known to alter circulating levels leptin and ghrelin, in favor of increased feeding, thus revealing a potential mechanism by which sleep restriction may affect brain reward systems and modulate feeding behavior.

Sleep deprivation affects glucose metabolism through multiple pathways. The brain uses as much as 50 % of total glucose utilization in the fasting state (20 % in the fed state) which is ten times more than predicted on a mass basis. Imaging studies have shown that the sleep-deprived brain uses 7–8 % less glucose than the well-rested brain. A limitation of these imaging studies is that they have been conducted under conditions of total sleep deprivation. Thus, the impact of recurrent partial sleep restriction, a much more common condition, on brain glucose metabolism remains to be elucidated.

The autonomic nervous system is another major pathway linking sleep loss and peripheral function. Alterations of cardiac sympathovagal balance, indicating higher sympathetic nervous activity and lower vagal tone, have been documented in a number of studies of human sleep loss, including studies of partial sleep restriction [36]. Whether similar alterations of autonomic nervous system control in conditions of sleep loss occur at multiple organ levels is not known. A few studies have shown that norepinephrine levels are elevated during sleep deprivation [120] and in individuals suffering from obstructive sleep apnea [121], a sleep disorder resulting in disrupted sleep and sleep loss. The liver, pancreas, adipose tissue, and the gastro-intestinal tract are peripheral organs that play a major role in glucose regulation and are strongly affected by sympathetic nervous activity. Counter-regulatory hormones are also altered by sleep loss in a manner consistent with the promotion of hyperglycemia and/or insulin resistance. Indeed, elevations of evening cortisol levels [34, 121–123], increased release of growth hormone and ghrelin during daytime hours [124–126], and elevated daytime levels of epinephrine [41] have all been observed under sleep debt conditions.

A molecular link between sleep-wake behavior and the neuroendocrine control of appetite might be the orexin system [127]. Orexins A and B (also known as hypocretins) are produced by a small population of neurons located within the lateral hypothalamus and the orexin system activates the appetite promoting NPY neurons in the Arc [128]. In rodent studies, intracerebroventricular infusions of hypocretin increase food intake [129, 130] and hypocretin-deficient animals exhibit reduced food intake [130]. Orexinergic activity is influenced by both central and peripheral signals, with glucose and leptin exerting inhibitory effects while ghrelin promotes further activation. A role for the orexin system in reward processing and addiction has also been demonstrated, suggesting that orexins not only stimulate homeostatic food intake but also hedonic food intake [131, 132]. Relevant to the interactive regulation of arousal and feeding are findings that orexin neurons in the lateral hypothalamus are involved in reward processing for food [127], consistent with the fact that orexin neurons have dense projections to the dopaminergic ventrotegmental area (VTA) and nucleus accumbens (Acb); critical nodes in regard to the hedonic control of food intake. Feeding requires the maintenance of wakefulness and the orexin system appears to play a central role in this interaction between feeding and arousal [133]. There is evidence that orexins may stimulate food intake, particularly in the early part of the usual sleep period, which is when voluntary sleep deprivation most often occurs in humans [134, 135]. Orexin-containing neurons are active during waking and quiescent during sleep. Deficiencies in the orexin system are associated with sleep disorders that involve chronic excessive daytime sleepiness, including narcolepsy and obstructive sleep apnea. In contrast, when sleep deprivation is enforced behaviorally, the orexin system is overactive, most likely to maintain wakefulness against the increased sleep pressure [128, 136, 137]. A profound impact of sleep loss on appetite regulation should therefore be expected when considering the associations of these systems. While peripheral levels of circulating orexin may not be representative of central orexinergic activity, they would nonetheless be an interesting exploratory outcome measure in studies involving manipulations of sleep behavior. Of note, in a 2005 study from Japan, plasma orexin levels were found to decrease with the severity of obstructive sleep apnea and to increase following treatment with continuous positive airway pressure [138], in parallel with improvements in the arousal index (AI) and in Epworth Scale in those that had AI values of 60 events/h, suggesting that peripheral orexin levels may be related to obstructive sleep apnea-mediated sleep disturbance and/or daytime alertness.

A recent paper has revealed that sleep restriction may be acting directly on peripheral tissues, specifically adipocytes [139]. In a randomized cross-over design, subcutaneous fat biopsy samples were collected from seven healthy lean participants (6 men, 1 woman) following either 4 days of 4.5 h/night or 8 h/night of sleep in the laboratory. Again, physical activity and caloric intake were similar under both sleep conditions. Once collected, the isolated adipocytes were treated with incremental concentrations of insulin and levels of phosphorylated Akt (pAkt), a crucial step in the insulin-signaling pathway, were measured. Adipocytes collected from subcutaneous fat following 4 nights of sleep deficiency exhibited a 30 % reduction in insulin sensitivity than those collected following 4 nights of normal sleep [139]. Simply put, following 4 nights of sleep restriction, higher concentrations of insulin were necessary to elicit the same pAkt response as seen at lower concentrations in the tissue collected after normal sleep. The 30 % reduction in insulin sensitivity observed in this study is similar to that seen in obese individuals when compared to lean [140] and in diabetics compared to nondiabetics [141]. Thus, sleep deficiency may be directly acting on peripheral adipose tissue and affecting energy metabolism via alterations to insulin sensitivity within subcutaneous adipocytes.

A common argument to explain the association between sleep loss and increased food intake or appetite is that wakefulness requires greater energy expenditure than sleeping. A recent study quantified the caloric requirement of staying awake versus sleeping in healthy young adults and found that the energy cost of an entire night of total sleep deprivation under recumbent conditions averaged a modest 134 kcal (i.e., 17 kcal/h) [142]. Thus, in humans, the stimulation of appetite and subsequent food intake appears to be excessive in relation to the energy demands of extended wakefulness under comfortable sedentary conditions. In contrast, extreme sleep deprivation in rodent models results in weight loss despite increased caloric intake but experimental sleep deprivation invariably involves a substantial increase in energy expenditure. The large body of epidemiologic evidence linking short sleep duration and obesity suggests that in humans, the increase in energy intake resulting from sleep restriction exceeds the modest increase in energy needed to sustain extended wakefulness.

Some of the epidemiological studies report a U-shaped association between self-reported sleep duration and BMI, overweight/obesity risk, or diabetes risk. However, the mechanisms underlying the association between long self-reported sleep durations and mortality risk have not yet been identified. The laboratory experimental studies described above were in essence comparing short sleep durations (4–5.5 h) to long sleep durations (10–12 h) and observed that the long sleep condition was associated with more favorable metabolic outcomes [34, 40, 41]. These laboratory studies are short-term, however, and in two of these studies long sleep followed the short sleep condition and would therefore constitute recovery sleep. Whether objectively measured habitually long sleep durations are associated with increased obesity and diabetes risk remains to be determined. One study that explored the association between self-reported long sleep and mortality indicated that the presence of depression and low socioeconomic status were the most likely explanations for this association [143]. Furthermore, since these studies relied on self-reported sleep duration, it is not clear if long sleepers are actually obtaining more physiologic sleep or if they are just spending more time in bed. A study that recruited individuals who reported sleeping 9 or more hours per night suggests that many long sleepers may indeed be spending more time in bed not sleeping. They found that these self-reported long sleepers only obtained an average of 7–7.5 h of sleep per night based on wrist actigraphy [144]. The reason for the discrepancy between self-reported and objectively measured sleep duration remains to be identified, but could represent the presence of either a sleep disorder or other pathological condition. Given the large number of studies that have found an association between long sleep duration and morbidity and mortality risk, it is important that more research into possible mechanisms be conducted.

Conclusions

As rates of overweight and obesity continue to increase, chronic partial sleep loss and poor sleep quality (resulting in sleep deficiency) have also become endemic conditions. A growing body of epidemiologic and laboratory evidence suggests that the behavior of bedtime curtailment may be contributing to the epidemics of obesity and type II diabetes. While epidemiologic studies have revealed an association between short sleep times and increased BMI and increased diabetes risk, controlled laboratory studies are able to demonstrate a causal relationship between bedtime restriction and metabolic alterations. Sleep deficiency causes disturbances in glucose regulation potentially leading to increased risk for developing type II diabetes. Alterations in sympathovagal balance are also associated with sleep deficiency and further suggest an association with cardiovascular disease. Similarly, experimental reduction of sleep quality without change of sleep duration has also shown to be associated with impairment of glucose tolerance and sympathovagal balance. Moreover, sleep restriction leads to increases in hunger and appetite ratings along with modifications in hormonal profiles, lower leptin and higher ghrelin levels, that favor hyperphagia.

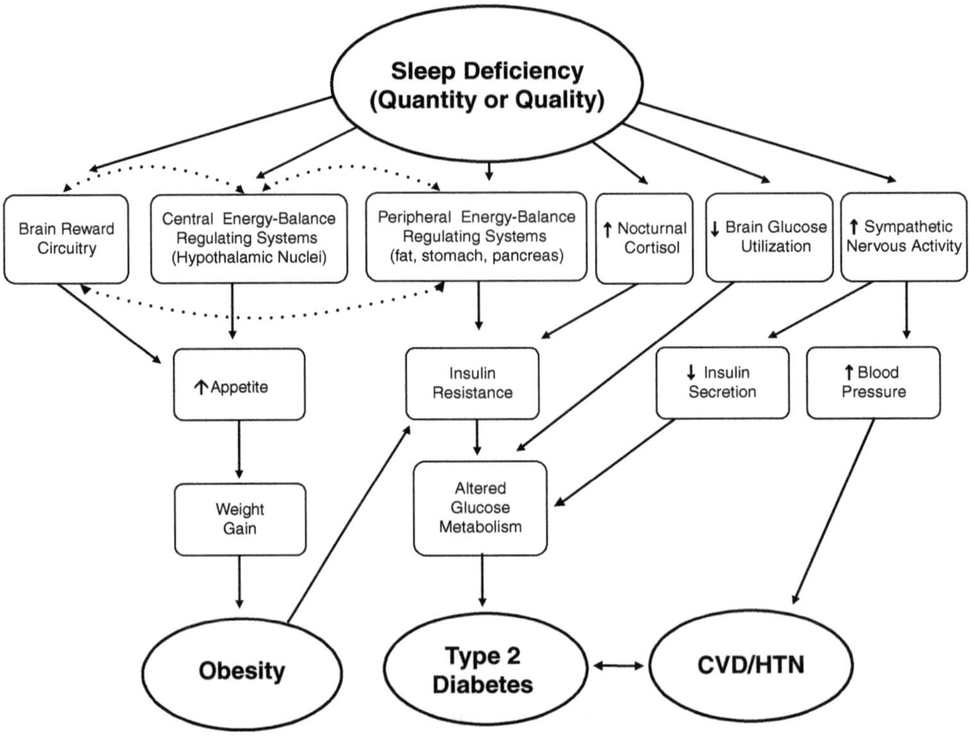

Fig. 10.4 Schematic representation of the potential mechanistic pathways linking sleep deficiency (diminished quantity or quality) to obesity, type II diabetes and cardiovascular disease (CVD) and hypertension (HTN). (Adapted from Knutson [28], with permission from Elsevier)

As shown in Fig. 10.4, the mechanisms by which sleep deficiency may exert its effects on glucose metabolism, energy balance, and feeding behavior include modifications to the periphery, as well as CNS involved in mediating energy, feeding behavior, and reward value. These findings have important implications for public health and well-being. Increased awareness of the deleterious effects of chronic partial sleep loss and poor sleep quality may be important in reducing the prevalence of overweight, obesity, and associated adverse health outcomes.

References

1. Stevens GA, Singh GM, Lu Y, Danaei G, Lin JK, Finucane MM, et al. National, regional, and global trends in adult overweight and obesity prevalences. Popul Health Metr. 2013;10(1):22.
2. Ogden CL, Carroll MD, Curtin LR, McDowell MA, Tabak CJ, Flegal KM. Prevalence of overweight and obesity in the United States, 1999-2004. JAMA. 2006;295(13):1549–55.
3. Danaei G, Finucane MM, Lu Y, Singh GM, Cowan MJ, Paciorek CJ, et al. National, regional, and global trends in fasting plasma glucose and diabetes prevalence since 1980: systematic analysis of health examination surveys and epidemiological studies with 370 country-years and 2.7 million participants. Lancet. 2011;378(9785):31–40.
4. Roger VL, Go AS, Lloyd-Jones DM, Adams RJ, Berry JD, Brown TM, et al. Heart disease and stroke statistics—2011 update: a report from the American Heart Association. Circulation. 2011;123(4):e18–209.
5. McAllister EJ, Dhurandhar NV, Keith SW, Aronne LJ, Barger J, Baskin M, et al. Ten putative contributors to the obesity epidemic. Crit Rev Food Sci Nutr. 2009;49(10):868–913.
6. Bonnet MH, Arand DL. 24-Hour metabolic rate in insomniacs and matched normal sleepers. Sleep. 1995;18(7):581–8.
7. Statistics NCfH. QuickStats: percentage of adults who reported an average of <6 hours of sleep per 24-hour period, by sex and age group—United States, 1985 and 2004. Morb Mortal Wkly Rep. 2005;54:933.
8. Foundation NS. In: Sleep in America Poll: Sleep, Performance and the Workplace. Washington, DC: National Sleep Foundation; 2008.

9. Kripke DF, Mullaney DJ, Atkinson M, Huey LY, Hubbard B. Circadian rhythm phases in affective illnesses. Chronobiologia. 1979;6:365–75.
10. Tune GS. Sleep and wakefulness in normal human adults. Br Med J. 1968;2(5600):269–71.
11. Tune GS. Sleep and wakefulness in a group of shift workers. Br J Ind Med. 1969;26(1):54–8.
12. Hammond EC. Some Preliminary Findings on Physical Complaints from a Prospective Study of 1,064,004 Men and Women. Am J Public Health Nations Health. 1964;54:11–23.
13. Foundation NS. In: Sleep in America Poll. Washington, DC: National Sleep Foundation; 2010.
14. Hale L, Do DP. Racial differences in self-reports of sleep duration in a population-based study. Sleep. 2007;30(9):1096–103.
15. Stamatakis KA, Kaplan GA, Roberts RE. Short sleep duration across income, education, and race/ethnic groups: population prevalence and growing disparities during 34 years of follow-up. Ann Epidemiol. 2007;17(12):948–55.
16. Jean-Louis G, Kripke DF, Ancoli-Israel S, Klauber MR, Sepulveda RS. Sleep duration, illumination, and activity patterns in a population sample: effects of gender and ethnicity. Biol Psychiatry. 2000;47(10):921–7.
17. Lauderdale DS, Knutson KL, Yan LL, Rathouz PJ, Hulley SB, Sidney S, et al. Objectively measured sleep characteristics among early-middle-aged adults: the CARDIA study. Am J Epidemiol. 2006;164(1):5–16.
18. Lauderdale DS, Knutson KL, Rathouz PJ, Yan LL, Hulley SB, Liu K. Cross-sectional and longitudinal associations between objectively measured sleep duration and body mass index: the CARDIA Sleep Study. Am J Epidemiol. 2009;170(7):805–13.
19. Foundation NS. In: Sleep in America Poll: Technology Use and Sleep. Washington, DC: National Sleep Foundation; 2011.
20. Foundation NS. In: Sleep in America poll: transportation workers' sleep. Washington, DC: National Sleep Foundation; 2012.
21. Van Cauter E, Knutson KL. Sleep and the epidemic of obesity in children and adults. Eur J Endocrinol. 2008;159 Suppl 1:S59–66.
22. Patel SR, Hu FB. Short sleep duration and weight gain: a systematic review. Obesity (Silver Spring). 2008;16(3):643–53.
23. Marshall NS, Glozier N, Grunstein RR. Is sleep duration related to obesity? A critical review of the epidemiological evidence. Sleep Med Rev. 2008;12(4):289–98.
24. Patel SR, Blackwell T, Redline S, Ancoli-Israel S, Cauley JA, Hillier TA, et al. The association between sleep duration and obesity in older adults. Int J Obes (Lond). 2008;32(12):1825–34.
25. Chaput JP, Despres JP, Bouchard C, Tremblay A. Longer sleep duration associates with lower adiposity gain in adult short sleepers. Int J Obes (Lond). 2012;36(5):752–6.
26. Taheri S, Lin L, Austin D, Young T, Mignot E. Short sleep duration is associated with reduced leptin, elevated ghrelin, and Increased Body Mass Index. PLoS Med. 2004;1(3):e62.
27. Chaput JP, Despres JP, Bouchard C, Tremblay A. Short sleep duration is associated with reduced leptin levels and increased adiposity: Results from the Quebec family study. Obesity (Silver Spring). 2007;15(1):253–61.
28. Knutson KL. Sleep duration and cardiometabolic risk: a review of the epidemiologic evidence. Best Pract Res Clin Endocrinol Metab. 2010;24(5):731–43.
29. Cappuccio FP, D'Elia L, Strazzullo P, Miller MA. Quantity and quality of sleep and incidence of type 2 diabetes: a systematic review and meta-analysis. Diabetes Care. 2010;33(2):414–20.
30. Xu Q, Song Y, Hollenbeck A, Blair A, Schatzkin A, Chen H. Day napping and short night sleeping are associated with higher risk of diabetes in older adults. Diabetes Care. 2010;33(1):78–83.
31. Cappuccio FP, Cooper D, D'Elia L, Strazzullo P, Miller MA. Sleep duration predicts cardiovascular outcomes: a systematic review and meta-analysis of prospective studies. Eur Heart J. 2011;32(12):1484–92.
32. Knutson KL, Van Cauter E, Rathouz PJ, Yan LL, Hulley SB, Liu K, et al. Association between sleep and blood pressure in midlife: the CARDIA sleep study. Arch Intern Med. 2009;169(11):1055–61.
33. Hanlon EC, Van Cauter E. Quantification of sleep behavior and of its impact on the cross-talk between the brain and peripheral metabolism. Proc Natl Acad Sci U S A. 2011;108 Suppl 3:15609–16.
34. Spiegel K, Leproult R, Van Cauter E. Impact of sleep debt on metabolic and endocrine function. Lancet. 1999;354(9188):1435–9.
35. Leproult R, Van Cauter E. Role of sleep and sleep loss in hormonal release and metabolism. Endocr Dev. 2010;17:11–21.
36. Spiegel K, Leproult R, L'Hermite-Baleriaux M, Copinschi G, Penev PD, Van Cauter E. Leptin levels are dependent on sleep duration: relationships with sympathovagal balance, carbohydrate regulation, cortisol, and thyrotropin. J Clin Endocrinol Metab. 2004;89(11):5762–71.
37. Guilleminault C, Powell NB, Martinez S, Kushida C, Raffray T, Palombini L, et al. Preliminary observations on the effects of sleep time in a sleep restriction paradigm. Sleep Med. 2003;4(3):177–84.
38. Chin-Chance C, Polonsky KS, Schoeller DA. Twenty-four-hour leptin levels respond to cumulative short-term energy imbalance and predict subsequent intake. J Clin Endocrinol Metab. 2000;85(8):2685–91.
39. Nedeltcheva AV, Kessler L, Imperial J, Penev PD. Exposure to recurrent sleep restriction in the setting of high caloric intake and physical inactivity results in increased insulin resistance and reduced glucose tolerance. J Clin Endocrinol Metab. 2009;94(9):3242–50.

40. Buxton OM, Pavlova M, Reid EW, Wang W, Simonson DC, Adler GK. Sleep restriction for 1 week reduces insulin sensitivity in healthy men. Diabetes. 2010;59(9):2126–33.
41. Spiegel K, Tasali E, Penev P, Van Cauter E. Brief communication: Sleep curtailment in healthy young men is associated with decreased leptin levels, elevated ghrelin levels, and increased hunger and appetite. Ann Intern Med. 2004;141(11):846–50.
42. Tasali E, Leproult R, Ehrmann DA, Van Cauter E. Slow-wave sleep and the risk of type 2 diabetes in humans. Proc Natl Acad Sci U S A. 2008;105(3):1044–9.
43. Stamatakis KA, Punjabi NM. Effects of sleep fragmentation on glucose metabolism in normal subjects. Chest. 2010;137(1):95–101.
44. Cizza G, Marincola P, Mattingly M, Williams L, Mitler M, Skarulis M, et al. Treatment of obesity with extension of sleep duration: a randomized, prospective, controlled trial. Clin Trials. 2010;7(3):274–85.
45. Morton GJ, Schwartz MW. Leptin and the central nervous system control of glucose metabolism. Physiol Rev. 2011;91(2):389–411.
46. Aravich PF, Sclafani A. Paraventricular hypothalamic lesions and medial hypothalamic knife cuts produce similar hyperphagia syndromes. Behav Neurosci. 1983;97(6):970–83.
47. Tokunaga K, Fukushima M, Kemnitz JW, Bray GA. Comparison of ventromedial and paraventricular lesions in rats that become obese. American Journal of Physiology. 1986;251(6 Pt 2):R1221–7.
48. van den Pol AN. Lateral hypothalamic damage and body weight regulation: role of gender, diet, and lesion placement. American Journal of Physiology. 1982;242(3):R265–74.
49. Banks WA, Tschop M, Robinson SM, Heiman ML. Extent and direction of ghrelin transport across the blood-brain barrier is determined by its unique primary structure. J Pharmacol Exp Ther. 2002;302(2):822–7.
50. Banks WA. Brain meets body: the blood-brain barrier as an endocrine interface. Endocrinology. 2012;153(9):4111–9.
51. Allen YS, Adrian TE, Allen JM, Tatemoto K, Crow TJ, Bloom SR, et al. Neuropeptide Y distribution in the rat brain. Science. 1983;221(4613):877–9.
52. Khachaturian H, Lewis ME, Haber SN, Akil H, Watson SJ. Proopiomelanocortin peptide immunocytochemistry in rhesus monkey brain. Brain Res Bull. 1984;13(6):785–800.
53. Thim L, Kristensen P, Larsen PJ, Wulff BS. CART, a new anorectic peptide. Int J Biochem Cell Biol. 1998;30(12):1281–4.
54. Wilding JP. Neuropeptides and appetite control. Diabet Med. 2002;19(8):619–27.
55. Stanley BG, Kyrkouli SE, Lampert S, Leibowitz SF. Neuropeptide Y chronically injected into the hypothalamus: a powerful neurochemical inducer of hyperphagia and obesity. Peptides. 1986;7(6):1189–92.
56. Zarjevski N, Cusin I, Vettor R, Rohner-Jeanrenaud F, Jeanrenaud B. Chronic intracerebroventricular neuropeptide-Y administration to normal rats mimics hormonal and metabolic changes of obesity. Endocrinology. 1993;133(4):1753–8.
57. Tomaszuk A, Simpson C, Williams G. Neuropeptide Y, the hypothalamus and the regulation of energy homeostasis. Horm Res. 1996;46(2):53–8.
58. Semjonous NM, Smith KL, Parkinson JR, Gunner DJ, Liu YL, Murphy KG, et al. Coordinated changes in energy intake and expenditure following hypothalamic administration of neuropeptides involved in energy balance. Int J Obes (Lond). 2009;33(7):775–85.
59. Lu D, Willard D, Patel IR, Kadwell S, Overton L, Kost T, et al. Agouti protein is an antagonist of the melanocyte-stimulating-hormone receptor. Nature. 1994;371(6500):799–802.
60. Kelley AE, Baldo BA, Pratt WE, Will MJ. Corticostriatal-hypothalamic circuitry and food motivation: Integration of energy, action and reward. Physiol Behav. 2005;86(5):773–95.
61. Zhang Y, Proenca R, Maffei M, Barone M, Leopold L, Friedman JM. Positional cloning of the mouse obese gene and its human homologue. Nature. 1994;372(6505):425–32.
62. Jequier E. Leptin signaling, adiposity, and energy balance. Ann N Y Acad Sci. 2002;967:379–88.
63. Zigman JM, Elmquist JK. Minireview: From anorexia to obesity–the yin and yang of body weight control. Endocrinology. 2003;144(9):3749–56.
64. Mercer JG, Hoggard N, Williams LM, Lawrence CB, Hannah LT, Trayhurn P. Localization of leptin receptor mRNA and the long form splice variant (Ob-Rb) in mouse hypothalamus and adjacent brain regions by in situ hybridization. FEBS Lett. 1996;387(2–3):113–6.
65. Schwartz MW, Baskin DG, Bukowski TR, Kuijper JL, Foster D, Lasser G, et al. Specificity of leptin action on elevated blood glucose levels and hypothalamic neuropeptide Y gene expression in ob/ob mice. Diabetes. 1996;45(4):531–5.
66. Cheung CC, Clifton DK, Steiner RA. Proopiomelanocortin neurons are direct targets for leptin in the hypothalamus. Endocrinology. 1997; 138(10):4489–92.
67. Fei H, Okano HJ, Li C, Lee GH, Zhao C, Darnell R, et al. Anatomic localization of alternatively spliced leptin receptors (Ob-R) in mouse brain and other tissues. Proc Natl Acad Sci. 1997;94(13):7001–5.
68. Elmquist JK, Bjorbaek C, Ahima RS, Flier JS, Saper CB. Distributions of leptin receptor mRNA isoforms in the rat brain. J Comp Neurol. 1998;395(4): 535–47.
69. Elmquist JK, Ahima RS, Elias CF, Flier JS, Saper CB. Leptin activates distinct projections from the dorsomedial and ventromedial hypothalamic nuclei. Proc Natl Acad Sci U S A. 1998;95(2):741–6.
70. Grill HJ, Schwartz MW, Kaplan JM, Foxhall JS, Breininger J, Baskin DG. Evidence that the caudal brainstem is a target for the inhibitory effect of leptin on food intake. Endocrinology. 2002;143(1): 239–46.

71. Elmquist JK, Coppari R, Balthasar N, Ichinose M, Lowell BB. Identifying hypothalamic pathways controlling food intake, body weight, and glucose homeostasis. J Comp Neurol. 2005;493(1):63–71.
72. Elias CF, Aschkenasi C, Lee C, Kelly J, Ahima RS, Bjorbaek C, et al. Leptin differentially regulates NPY and POMC neurons projecting to the lateral hypothalamic area. Neuron. 1999;23(4):775–86.
73. Spanswick D, Smith MA, Groppi VE, Logan SD, Ashford ML. Leptin inhibits hypothalamic neurons by activation of ATP-sensitive potassium channels. Nature. 1997;390(6659):521–5.
74. Roseberry AG, Liu H, Jackson AC, Cai X, Friedman JM. Neuropeptide Y-mediated inhibition of proopiomelanocortin neurons in the arcuate nucleus shows enhanced desensitization in ob/ob mice. Neuron. 2004;41(5):711–22.
75. Elmquist JK, Elias CF, Saper CB. From lesions to leptin: hypothalamic control of food intake and body weight. Neuron. 1999;22(2):221–32.
76. Friedman JM, Halaas JL. Leptin and the regulation of body weight in mammals. Nature. 1998;395(6704):763–70.
77. O'Rahilly S, Farooqi IS, Yeo GS, Challis BG. Minireview: human obesity-lessons from monogenic disorders. Endocrinology. 2003;144(9):3757–64.
78. Frederich RC, Hamann A, Anderson S, Lollmann B, Lowell BB, Flier JS. Leptin levels reflect body lipid content in mice: evidence for diet-induced resistance to leptin action. Nat Med. 1995;1(12):1311–4.
79. Maffei M, Halaas JL, Ravussin E, Pratley RE, Lee GH, Zhang Y, et al. Leptin levels in human and rodent: measurement of plasma leptin and ob RNA in obese and weight-reduced subjects. Nat Med. 1995;1(11):1155–61.
80. Ahima RS, Prabakaran D, Mantzoros CS, Qu D, Lowell BB, Maratos-Flier E, et al. Role of leptin in the neuroendocrine response to fasting. Nature. 1996;382(6588):250–2.
81. Farooqi IS, Jebb SA, Langmack G, Lawrence E, Cheetham CH, Prentice AM, et al. Effects of recombinant leptin therapy in a child with congenital leptin deficiency. N Engl J Med. 1999;341(12):879–84.
82. Hedbacker K, Birsoy K, Wysocki RW, Asilmaz E, Ahima RS, Farooqi IS, et al. Antidiabetic effects of IGFBP2, a leptin-regulated gene. Cell Metab. 2010;11(1):11–22.
83. Badman MK, Flier JS. The gut and energy balance: visceral allies in the obesity wars. Science. 2005;307(5717):1909–14.
84. Yoshihara F, Kojima M, Hosoda H, Nakazato M, Kangawa K. Ghrelin: a novel peptide for growth hormone release and feeding regulation. Curr Opin Clin Nutr Metab Care. 2002;5(4):391–5.
85. Kojima M, Hosoda H, Date Y, Nakazato M, Matsuo H, Kangawa K. Ghrelin is a growth-hormone-releasing acylated peptide from stomach. Nature. 1999;402(6762):656–60.
86. Date Y, Kojima K, Hosoda H, Sawaguchi A, Mondal MS, Suganuma T, et al. Ghrelin, a novel growth hormone-releasing acylated peptide, is synthesized in a distinct endocrine cell type in the gastrointestinal tracts of rats and humans. Endocrinology. 2000;141(11):4255–61.
87. Mori K, Yoshimoto A, Takaya K, Hosoda K, Ariyasu H, Yahata K, et al. Kidney produces a novel acylated peptide, ghrelin. FEBS Lett. 2000;486(3):213–6.
88. Gualillo O, Caminos J, Blanco M, Garcia-Caballero T, Kojima M, Kangawa K, et al. Ghrelin, a novel placental-derived hormone. Endocrinology. 2001; 142(2):788–94.
89. Korbonits M, Bustin SA, Kojima M, Jordan S, Adams EF, Lowe DG, et al. The expression of the growth hormone secretagogue receptor ligand ghrelin in normal and abnormal human pituitary and other neuroendocrine tumors. Journal of Clinical Endocrinology & Metabolism. 2001;86(2):881–7.
90. Horvath TL, Diano S, Sotonyi P, Heiman M, Tschop M. Minireview: ghrelin and the regulation of energy balance–a hypothalamic perspective. Endocrinology. 2001;142(10):4163–9.
91. Willesen MG, Kristensen P, Romer J. Co-localization of growth hormone secretagogue receptor and NPY mRNA in the arcuate nucleus of the rat. Neuroendocrinology. 1999;70(5):306–16.
92. Dickson SL, Luckman SM. Induction of c-fos messenger ribonucleic acid in neuropeptide Y and growth hormone (GH)-releasing factor neurons in the rat arcuate nucleus following systemic injection of the GH secretagogue, GH-releasing peptide-6. Endocrinology. 1997;138(2):771–7.
93. Hewson AK, Dickson SL. Systemic administration of ghrelin induces Fos and Egr-1 proteins in the hypothalamic arcuate nucleus of fasted and fed rats. J Neuroendocrinol. 2000;12(11):1047–9.
94. Cowley MA, Smith RG, Diano S, Tschop M, Pronchuk N, Grove KL, et al. The distribution and mechanism of action of ghrelin in the CNS demonstrates a novel hypothalamic circuit regulating energy homeostasis. Neuron. 2003;37(4):649–61.
95. Cummings DE, Purnell JQ, Frayo RS, Schmidova K, Wisse BE, Weigle DS. A preprandial rise in plasma ghrelin levels suggests a role in meal initiation in humans. Diabetes. 2001;50(8):1714–9.
96. Toshinai K, Mondal MS, Nakazato M, Date Y, Murakami N, Kojima M, et al. Upregulation of Ghrelin expression in the stomach upon fasting, insulin-induced hypoglycemia, and leptin administration. Biochem Biophys Res Commun. 2001; 281(5):1220–5.
97. Bruning JC, Gautam D, Burks DJ, Gillette J, Schubert M, Orban PC, et al. Role of brain insulin receptor in control of body weight and reproduction. Science. 2000;289(5487):2122–5.
98. Baskin DG, Wilcox BJ, Figlewicz DP, Dorsa DM. Insulin and insulin-like growth factors in the CNS. Trend in Neuroscience. 1988;11(3):107–11.

99. Schwartz MW, Sipols AJ, Marks JL, Sanacora G, White JD, Scheurink A, et al. Inhibition of hypothalamic neuropeptide Y gene expression by insulin. Endocrinology. 1992;130(6):3608–16.
100. Wang J, Leibowitz KL. Central insulin inhibits hypothalamic galanin and neuropeptide Y gene expression and peptide release in intact rats. Brain Res. 1997;777(1–2):231–6.
101. Abe M, Saito M, Ikeda H, Shimazu T. Increased neuropeptide Y content in the arcuato-paraventricular hypothalamic neuronal system in both insulin-dependent and non-insulin-dependent diabetic rats. Brain Res. 1991;539(2):223–7.
102. Woods SC, Lotter EC, McKay LD, Porte D. Chronic intracerebroventricular infusion of insulin reduces food intake and body weight of baboons. Nature. 1979;282(5738):503–5.
103. Chavez M, Kaiyala K, Madden LJ, Schwartz MW, Woods SC. Intraventricular insulin and the level of maintained body weight in rats. Behav Neurosci. 1995;109(3):528–31.
104. Berridge KC, Ho CY, Richard JM, DiFeliceantonio AG. The tempted brain eats: pleasure and desire circuits in obesity and eating disorders. Brain Res. 2010;1350:43–64.
105. Stoeckel LE, Weller RE, Cook 3rd EW, Twieg DB, Knowlton RC, Cox JE. Widespread reward-system activation in obese women in response to pictures of high-calorie foods. Neuroimage. 2008;41(2):636–47.
106. Grabenhorst F, Rolls ET, Parris BA, d'Souza AA. How the brain represents the reward value of fat in the mouth. Cereb Cortex. 2010;20(5):1082–91.
107. Martin LE, Holsen LM, Chambers RJ, Bruce AS, Brooks WM, Zarcone JR, et al. Neural mechanisms associated with food motivation in obese and healthy weight adults. Obesity (Silver Spring). 2010;18(2):254–60.
108. Wang GJ, Volkow ND, Logan J, Pappas NR, Wong CT, Zhu W, et al. Brain dopamine and obesity. Lancet. 2001;357(9253):354–7.
109. Chaput JP, Despres JP, Bouchard C, Tremblay A. The association between short sleep duration and weight gain is dependent on disinhibited eating behavior in adults. Sleep. 2011;34(10):1291–7.
110. Holm SM, Forbes EE, Ryan ND, Phillips ML, Tarr JA, Dahl RE. Reward-related brain function and sleep in pre/early pubertal and mid/late pubertal adolescents. J Adolesc Health. 2009;45(4):326–34.
111. Benedict C, Brooks SJ, O'Daly OG, Almen MS, Morell A, Aberg K, et al. Acute sleep deprivation enhances the brain's response to hedonic food stimuli: an fMRI study. J Clin Endocrinol Metab. 2013;97(3):E443–7.
112. St-Onge MP, McReynolds A, Trivedi ZB, Roberts AL, Sy M, Hirsch J. Sleep restriction leads to increased activation of brain regions sensitive to food stimuli. Am J Clin Nutr. 2012;95(4):818–24.
113. Volkow ND, Wang GJ, Telang F, Fowler JS, Logan J, Wong C, et al. Sleep deprivation decreases binding of [11C]raclopride to dopamine D2/D3 receptors in the human brain. J Neurosci. 2008;28(34):8454–61.
114. Volkow ND, Tomasi D, Wang GJ, Telang F, Fowler JS, Logan J, et al. Evidence that sleep deprivation downregulates dopamine D2R in ventral striatum in the human brain. J Neurosci. 2012;32(19):6711–7.
115. Dalley JW, Fryer TD, Brichard L, Robinson ES, Theobald DE, Laane K, et al. Nucleus accumbens D2/3 receptors predict trait impulsivity and cocaine reinforcement. Science. 2007;315(5816):1267–70.
116. Linnet J, Moller A, Peterson E, Gjedde A, Doudet D. Inverse association between dopaminergic neurotransmission and Iowa Gambling Task performance in pathological gamblers and healthy controls. Scand J Psychol. 2011;52(1):28–34.
117. Volkow ND, Wang GJ, Tomasi D, Kollins SH, Wigal TL, Newcorn JH, et al. Methylphenidate-elicited dopamine increases in ventral striatum are associated with long-term symptom improvement in adults with attention deficit hyperactivity disorder. J Neurosci. 2012;32(3):841–9.
118. Farooqi IS, Bullmore E, Keogh J, Gillard J, O'Rahilly S, Fletcher PC. Leptin regulates striatal regions and human eating behavior. Science. 2007;317(5843):1355.
119. Malik S, McGlone F, Bedrossian D, Dagher A. Ghrelin modulates brain activity in areas that control appetitive behavior. Cell Metab. 2008;7(5):400–9.
120. Irwin M, Thompson J, Miller C, Gillin JC, Ziegler M. Effects of sleep and sleep deprivation on catecholamine and interleukin- 2 levels in humans: clinical implications. J Clin Endocrinol Metab. 1999;84(6):1979–85.
121. Tasali E, Chapotot F, Leproult R, Whitmore H, Ehrmann DA. Treatment of obstructive sleep apnea improves cardiometabolic function in young obese women with polycystic ovary syndrome. J Clin Endocrinol Metab. 2011;96(2):365–74.
122. Leproult R, Copinschi G, Buxton O, Van Cauter E. Sleep loss results in an elevation of cortisol levels the next evening. Sleep. 1997;20(10):865–70.
123. Chapotot F, Buguet A, Gronfier C, Brandenberger G. Hypothalamo-pituitary-adrenal axis activity is related to the level of central arousal: effect of sleep deprivation on the association of high-frequency waking electroencephalogram with cortisol release. Neuroendocrinology. 2001;73(5):312–21.
124. Kumari M, Badrick E, Ferrie J, Perski A, Marmot M, Chandola T. Self-reported sleep duration and sleep disturbance are independently associated with cortisol secretion in the Whitehall II study. J Clin Endocrinol Metab. 2009;94(12):4801–9.
125. Brandenberger G, Gronfier C, Chapotot F, Simon C, Piquard F. Effect of sleep deprivation on overall 24 h growth-hormone secretion. Lancet. 2000;356(9239): 1408.

126. Spiegel K, Leproult R, Colecchia EF, L'Hermite-Baleriaux M, Nie Z, Copinschi G, et al. Adaptation of the 24-h growth hormone profile to a state of sleep debt. Am J Physiol Regul Integr Comp Physiol. 2000;279(3):R874–83.
127. Tsujino N, Sakurai T. Orexin/hypocretin: a neuropeptide at the interface of sleep, energy homeostasis, and reward system. Pharmacol Rev. 2009; 61(2):162–76.
128. Estabrooke IV, McCarthy MT, Ko E, Chou TC, Chemelli RM, Yanagisawa M, et al. Fos expression in orexin neurons varies with behavioral state. J Neurosci. 2001;21(5):1656–62.
129. de Lecea L, Kilduff TS, Peyron C, Gao X, Foye PE, Danielson PE, et al. The hypocretins: hypothalamus-specific peptides with neuroexcitatory activity. Proc Natl Acad Sci U S A. 1998;95(1):322–7.
130. Willie JT, Chemelli RM, Sinton CM, Yanagisawa M. To eat or to sleep? Orexin in the regulation of feeding and wakefulness. Annu Rev Neurosci. 2001;24: 429–58.
131. Harris GC, Wimmer M, Aston-Jones G. A role for lateral hypothalamic orexin neurons in reward seeking. Nature. 2005;437(7058):556–9.
132. Harris GC, Aston-Jones G. Arousal and reward: a dichotomy in orexin function. Trends Neurosci. 2006;29(10):571–7.
133. Bonnavion P, de Lecea L. Hypocretins in the control of sleep and wakefulness. Curr Neurol Neurosci Rep. 2010;10(3):174–9.
134. Sakurai T. The neural circuit of orexin (hypocretin): maintaining sleep and wakefulness. Nat Rev Neurosci. 2007;8(3):171–81.
135. Adamantidis A, de Lecea L. The hypocretins as sensors for metabolism and arousal. J Physiol. 2009;587(Pt 1):33–40.
136. Wu MF, John J, Maidment N, Lam HA, Siegel JM. Hypocretin release in normal and narcoleptic dogs after food and sleep deprivation, eating, and movement. Am J Physiol Regul Integr Comp Physiol. 2002;283(5):R1079–86.
137. Zeitzer JM, Buckmaster CL, Lyons DM, Mignot E. Increasing length of wakefulness and modulation of hypocretin-1 in the wake-consolidated squirrel monkey. Am J Physiol Regul Integr Comp Physiol. 2007;293(4):R1736–42.
138. Sakurai S, Nishijima T, Takahashi S, Yamauchi K, Arihara Z, Takahashi K. Low plasma orexin-A levels were improved by continuous positive airway pressure treatment in patients with severe obstructive sleep apnea-hypopnea syndrome. Chest. 2005;127(3):731–7.
139. Broussard JL, Ehrmann DA, Van Cauter E, Tasali E, Brady MJ. Impaired insulin signaling in human adipocytes after experimental sleep restriction: a randomized, crossover study. Ann Intern Med. 2012;157(8):549–57.
140. Bjornholm M, Al-Khalili L, Dicker A, Naslund E, Rossner S, Zierath JR, et al. Insulin signal transduction and glucose transport in human adipocytes: effects of obesity and low calorie diet. Diabetologia. 2002;45(8):1128–35.
141. Kashiwagi A, Verso MA, Andrews J, Vasquez B, Reaven G, Foley JE. In vitro insulin resistance of human adipocytes isolated from subjects with noninsulin-dependent diabetes mellitus. J Clin Invest. 1983;72(4):1246–54.
142. Jung CM, Melanson EL, Frydendall EJ, Perreault L, Eckel RH, Wright KP. Energy expenditure during sleep, sleep deprivation and sleep following sleep deprivation in adult humans. J Physiol. 2011;589(Pt 1):235–44.
143. Patel SR, Malhotra A, Gottlieb DJ, White DP, Hu FB. Correlates of long sleep duration. Sleep. 2006;29(7):881–9.
144. Zielinski MR, Kline CE, Kripke DF, Bogan RK, Youngstedt SD. No effect of 8-week time in bed restriction on glucose tolerance in older long sleepers. J Sleep Res. 2008;17(4):412–9.

Sleep Deprivation and the Cardiovascular System

11

Ivan Cundrle Jr., Andrew D. Calvin, and Virend K. Somers

Abbreviations

ANP	Atrial natriuretic peptide
CAD	Coronary artery disease
cQTd	Corrected QT dispersion
CRP	C-reactive protein
CSA	Central sleep apnea
DM	Diabetes mellitus
fVII	Factor VII
ICAM-1	Intracellular adhesion molecule-1
IL6	Interleukin-6
LF/HF	Low to high frequency ration
MMAS	Massachusetts Male Aging Study
MSNA	Muscle sympathetic nerve activity
nonREM	Non-rapid eye movement
OSA	Obstructive sleep apnea
QTd	QT dispersion
QT_{max}	QT maximum
REM	Rapid eye movement
SHHS	Sleep Heart Health Study
sTNF-R p55	Soluble tumor necrosis factor-receptor p55
TNF-α	Tumor necrosis factor-alpha
vWF	von Willebrand factor

I. Cundrle, Jr., M.D. • A.D. Calvin, M.D., M.P.H.
V.K. Somers, M.D., Ph.D. (✉)
Division of Cardiovascular Diseases,
Mayo Clinic, Rochester, MN, USA
e-mail: somers.virend@mayo.edu

Introduction

Sleep is an important part of life, occupying about 30 % of each day. With increasing demands on productivity in modern society, sleep time has been diminished to enable more time for other activities, and insufficient sleep has become increasingly prevalent, verging on a public health epidemic [1]. People are now sleeping on average only 6.8 h a day, which is 1.5 h less then a century ago [2, 3]. According to the United States National Sleep Foundation, adults need to sleep 7–9 h each night [1]. Nevertheless, it has been reported that only one third of the population sleeps more than 8 h a day and one third sleeps less than 6 h a day [4].

As the average daily sleep duration declines, there is growing evidence that lack of sleep contributes importantly to cardiovascular disease, including hypertension [5–7], coronary artery disease (CAD) [4, 8, 9], risk of arrhythmia [10, 11], stroke [12, 13], and diabetes mellitus (DM) [14–18].

Nevertheless, it is not only the lack of sleep, but also prolonged sleep duration that has been associated with increased risk [4], suggesting that modulation of the cardiovascular system during sleep is a complex and dynamic process. Finally, while sleep has strong cardiovascular influences, cardiac disease may itself affect sleep, as evident in central sleep apnea [19] developing in patients with heart failure.

M.T. Bianchi (ed.), *Sleep Deprivation and Disease: Effects on the Body, Brain and Behavior*,
DOI 10.1007/978-1-4614-9087-6_11, © Springer Science+Business Media New York 2014

This chapter summarizes the effects of inadequate sleep on the cardiovascular system. It focuses on pathophysiological mechanisms by which sleep influences the cardiovascular system, and also on how the cardiovascular system influences sleep. Furthermore we summarize current knowledge regarding the association between sleep deprivation and specific cardiovascular diseases like hypertension, CAD, arrhythmias, stroke, DM, obesity, metabolic syndrome, and mortality.

Physiological and Pathological Effects of Sleep on the Cardiovascular System

Circadian and diurnal rhythms influence neural circulatory control causing changes in heart rate, vascular tone, and blood pressure. Predominant parasympathetic activity is observed during the night and predominant sympathetic activity during the day, with peak activation in the early morning [20–22].

Autonomic neural circulatory control changes not only in a diurnal pattern, but also fluctuates according to sleep phases. During physiological sleep, rapid eye movement (REM) and non-rapid eye movement (nonREM) phase cycle approximately 5 times per night. NonREM is characterized by an increase in parasympathetic and decrease in sympathetic neural activity, resulting in decreased heart rate, peripheral vascular resistance, blood pressure, cardiac output, and resetting of the arterial baroreflex to a lower pressure set level.

REM sleep is characterized by marked and abrupt fluctuations in sympathetic and parasympathetic drive. REM sleep could be further considered as two stages (tonic and phasic) that affect autonomic tone [23]. Surges of sympathetic activity often occur in the phasic stage, accompanied by changes in muscle tone, rise in blood pressure and heart rate, and regional changes in blood flow [23, 24].

As a consequence of normal sleep physiology, a number of changes occur in the cardiovascular system. Sinus bradycardia, conduction blocks, and vagal-induced atrial fibrillation could occur during sleep [25–27] as well as QT interval changes [28], which may be stage- and gender-specific [29]. Sleep-related QT interval changes may be especially important in patients with prolonged QT intervals, in whom they could conceivably contribute to sudden death [30].

Sleep-associated fluctuations in autonomic drive also influence vascular tone. Brachial artery endothelium-dependent vasodilatation was found to be decreased and coronary artery tone found to be increased in the early morning [31, 32].

Coagulation also seems to have a diurnal rhythm [33–35]. Elevated platelet aggregability [34], tissue plasminogen activator [35], and lower fibrinolytic activity [33] have been reported in the early morning. Nevertheless, these changes seem to be related to body position, occurring only with standing; remaining supine and inactive after waking up is not associated with increased platelet aggregability [34].

High sympathetic tone, impaired vascular function, and enhanced coagulation in the early morning could explain the high incidence of myocardial infarction, ventricular arrhythmias, sudden death, and stroke in this time [36–40].

It is becoming clear that even normal sleep is a complex and dynamic process with profound effects on cardiovascular homeostasis, and with potentially adverse consequences in the setting of a vulnerable cardiovascular substrate.

Mechanisms Linking Insufficient Sleep to Cardiovascular Disease

Sympathetic Nervous System

Insufficient or disrupted sleep is a stressor stimulus that acts through the sympathetic nervous system to elicit changes in blood pressure, heart rate, and baroreflex setpoint. It is important that some of the sympathetic changes are evident even during the daytime and could contribute to increased cardiovascular risk in sleep-deprived subjects. Increased blood pressure is very closely linked to sympathetic activation and will be addressed separately and in detail, later in this chapter.

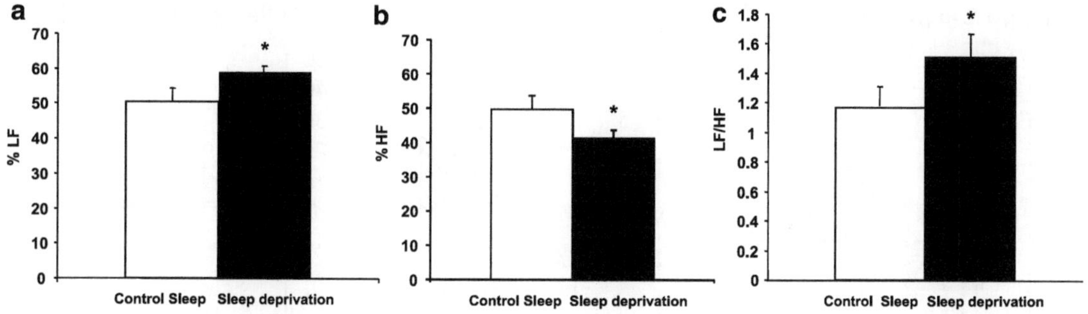

Fig. 11.1 Heart rate variability after control sleep and partial sleep deprivation periods. (a) % Low frequency (LF) component. (b) % High frequency (HF) component. (c) LF-to-HF ratio. $*P<0.05$ vs. control sleep. (Reproduced with permission from Dettoni et al. [42])

Increases in urinary excretion of catecholamines and in the low frequency to high frequency (LF/HF) ratio of heart rate variability were reported in sleep-deprived subjects by Tochikubo et al. [6], and similar changes in the LF/HF ratio were also observed by Zhong et al. [41]. In a recent study, Dettoni et al. [42] found alterations in heart rate variability together with elevated norepinephrine levels and LF/HF ratio after partial sleep deprivation (see Fig. 11.1). Elevated plasma catecholamines with increased heart rate were also noted by Irwin and Ziegler [10] in abstinent alcoholics and in healthy volunteers who underwent partial sleep deprivation [43]. Overall, increased sympathetic activity and heart rate in sleep-deprived subjects were also reported by Lusardi et al. [44], Spiegel et al. [14], and Sauvet et al. [45].

Nevertheless, Kato et al. [7] found no changes in heart rate, muscle sympathetic nerve activity (MSNA), and catecholamines after 1 night of total sleep restriction and Ogawa et al. [5] reported only an increase in blood pressure but a decrease in MSNA. In their study, the change of blood pressure was reported to be caused by baroreflex resetting, which was shifted toward higher values with sleep deprivation. Holmes et al. [46] also proposed resetting of the baroreflex with sleep deprivation as a reason for elevated blood pressure. Sympathetic nerve activity was attenuated in this study as a reflex response to the blood pressure increase.

The different and sometimes conflicting results of these studies could be explained by variations in experimental protocols, especially magnitude and duration of sleep deprivation, and other variables such as body posture, stress, food intake, and ambient conditions.

Inflammation

Cardiovascular risk is primarily driven by atherothrombosis, which seems to be an inflammatory process [47]. As a reflection of this, increased levels of C-reactive protein (CRP) and interleukin-6 (IL6) have been implicated as predictors of cardiovascular disease risk [48, 49]. Both CRP and IL6 have been found to be elevated in both totally and partially sleep-deprived subjects [7, 50–53] (see Fig. 11.2). Furthermore, inflammatory cells such as monocytes and neutrophils were also found to be elevated during acute sleep deprivation [54–57], supporting the concept of sleep deprivation as a pro-inflammatory state. In contrast, however, one study showed no increase, but rather a decrease in IL6 after 1 night of total deprivation [58], and the Wisconsin Sleep Cohort study failed to find a relationship between CRP, self-reported and objectively measured sleep duration [59].

Tumor necrosis factor-alpha (TNF-α) is another important mediator of inflammation that has been linked to cardiovascular risk [60]. Effects of sleep deprivation on TNF-α are not entirely clear. Vgnotzas et al. [52] found significant elevations of TNF-α in partially sleep-deprived men, but not women, and Irwin et al. [61] showed an increase of TNF-α messenger ribonucleic acid

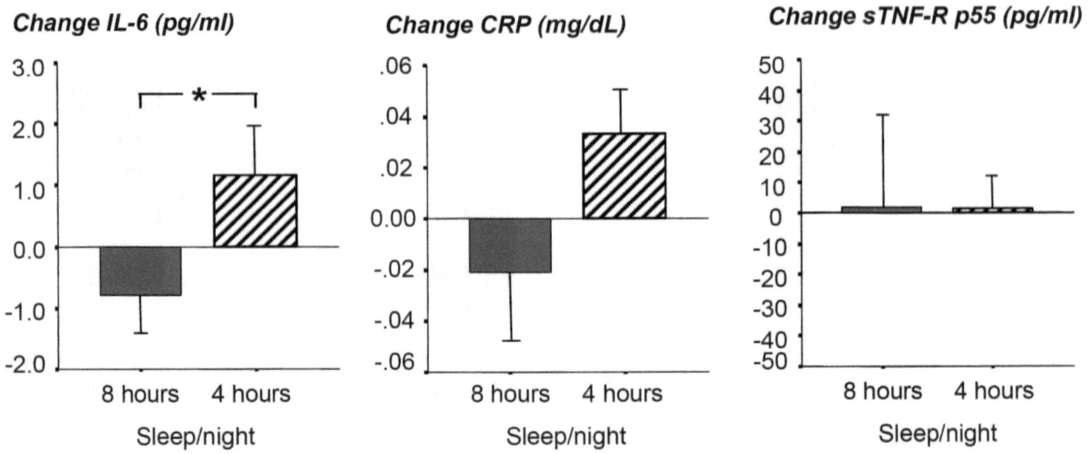

Fig. 11.2 Change of plasma interleukin-6 (IL-6), serum C-reactive protein (CRP), and plasma soluble tumor necrosis factor-receptor (sTNF-R p55) levels from baseline to the 11th day of sleeping either 8 h/night (*grey bar*, $N=8$) or 4 h/night (*hatched bar*, $N=10$ for IL-6, $N=9$ for sTNF-R p55). IL-6, CRP, and sTNF-R p55 were measured every 4 h and averaged across a 24-h period. Original values are presented, and statistics were based on log-transformed values. *Asterisk* indicates significant difference between sleep conditions. (Reproduced with permission from Haack et al. [51])

after a single night of partial sleep deprivation in women but not men. Furthermore, Shearer et al. [50] and Haack et al. [51] were not able to show any increase in TNF-α in partially sleep-deprived subjects.

Discrepancies in these results could be explained in part by different responses of TNF-α receptors to sleep deprivation. It has been proposed that only type 1 TNF-α receptor (but not type 2 TNF-α receptor) is influenced by sleep deprivation [50]. Furthermore the TNF-α response to sleep deprivation may be sex-related [52]. This potential sex difference in inflammatory response is further supported by Irwin et al. [62] who found increased activation of nuclear factor κB in women but not in men. In light of these findings, sex differences in the inflammatory response to insufficient or short sleep were proposed [63].

Endothelial Dysfunction

Endothelial dysfunction correlates with risk of cardiovascular morbidity and mortality [64]. Endothelial dysfunction has been reported after a combination of sleep deprivation and stress. Takase et al. [65] reported blunted endothelial flow-mediated dilatation of the brachial artery in students after a 4-week final exam period, during which they experienced both chronic sleep deprivation (sleep duration < 80 % of that on regular days) and chronic stress. Amir et al. [66] reported similar results in residents and fellows working night shifts.

Increased heart rate, blood pressure, and sympathetic excitation in sleep-deprived subjects could contribute to the endothelial dysfunction [67, 68]. Nevertheless Kato et al. [7] found increased blood pressure without sympathetic nerve activation after 1 night of total sleep deprivation, suggesting that other nonneural factors may contribute to increased blood pressure after sleep deprivation This concept was supported by Sauvet et al. [45], who found that vascular dysfunction preceded both sympathetic activation and elevated blood pressure, after 40 h of total sleep deprivation.

Acute total sleep deprivation has been shown to increase circulating levels of soluble intracellular adhesion molecule-1 (ICAM-1) and E-selectin, but no significant change was found in vascular cell adhesion molecule-1 levels [58]. Also, both pro- and anti-inflammatory cytokines like IL6, interleukin 1β, and TNF-α were found to be elevated during sleep deprivation [52, 57,

58]. Of the above listed measures, IL6, ICAM-1, and E-selectin have been shown to be especially linked with endothelial dysfunction and cardiovascular disease [50, 52, 68].

Coagulation

The balance between coagulation and fibrinolysis is important for proper blood flow, tissue perfusion, and endothelial function. Miller et al. [69] analyzed von Willebrand factor (vWF), fibrinogen, and factor VII (fVII) in a large cohort of 6,400 subjects. They found elevated vWF in men who reported sleeping less than 6 h and those who slept more than 8 h. Interestingly, in women, only in those who reported sleeping longer than 8 h was vWF elevated. There were no differences in fibrinogen or fVII.

Sleep fragmentation has also been associated with elevated vWF and soluble tissue factor, and apnea-related sleep disruptions were related to higher levels of plasminogen activator inhibitor-1 [70].

Hormones

Leptin

Leptin has a broad spectrum of cardiovascular actions. Interpretation of leptin-mediated effects is complicated by differential dose responses and by selective leptin resistance [71]. Leptin may be reduced in amplitude [72] and also peak levels [73] in acute total and partial sleep deprivation. How this may relate to increased cardiovascular risk remains to be clarified.

Leptin has been shown to have vasodilatory effects on coronary arteries [74] and may even be protective against ischemia and reperfusion injury [75]. Leptin was recently found to be stroke-protective [76] and has been shown to down-regulate atrial natriuretic peptide (ANP) expression, without effect on basal ANP secretion [77]. Mice that genetically lack leptin were shown to have blunted release of ANP in reaction to pressure overload making them potentially more prone to development of myocardial hypertrophy. Leptin infusion elevated ANP expression with resulting anti-hypertrophic effects [78]. These recent findings suggest that leptin deficiency due to attenuated leptin release in response to sleep deprivation could contribute to increased risk of stroke and cardiovascular morbidity.

On the other hand, low leptin levels could also have protective effects. Leptin can enhance sympathetic activation [79], worsen left ventricular dysfunction [80], increase platelet activation [81], impair fibrinolysis [82], and have pro-inflammatory effects [83]. Metabolic effects of low leptin could also be relevant, including increased appetite, obesity, and development of metabolic syndrome, which are also connected to increased cardiovascular risk [84].

Thus, taken together, low leptin levels as found during sleep deprivation could have both adverse and protective cardiovascular effects. Further studies are needed to better delineate leptin effects on cardiovascular structure and function in sleep-deprived subjects.

Ghrelin

Ghrelin is a hunger-stimulating hormone that has been reported to be increased in sleep-deprived subjects [85]. Elevated ghrelin levels could contribute to the development of metabolic syndrome and increased cardiovascular risk. On the other hand, ghrelin has been suggested to have possible inotropic effects [86], to cause vasodilatation via nitric oxide synthesis [87], to have cardioprotective effects against ischemia, and to have proliferative and anti-apoptotic effects on cardiomyocytes [88]. Further studies are needed to better understand the overall net effects of ghrelin in mediating consequences of sleep deprivation.

Growth Hormone

Growth hormone secretion has been found to be blunted after sleep deprivation, but appears to be well compensated during the following day, so that the 24 h growth hormone secretion was without change [89]. Growth hormone has beneficial effects in increasing lean body mass and lowers total and low-density lipoprotein cholesterol levels and diastolic blood pressure, but it also reduces insulin sensitivity [90]. The overall cardiovascular effect of changes in growth hormone in sleep-deprived subjects has yet to be determined.

Insulin and Insulin Resistance

DM is clearly linked to cardiovascular risk. The proportion of CVD caused by DM has increased over the past years [91], in accordance with the rise in the prevalence of sleep deprivation. Low glucose tolerance and increased insulin resistance are frequently associated with inadequate sleep. Spiegel et al. [14] reported lower glucose tolerance after 6 nights of 4 h sleep restriction, and the large cross-sectional Sleep Heart Health Study (SHHS) showed a relationship between usual sleep time and DM and impaired glucose tolerance [17]. Furthermore, in the Massachusetts Male Aging Study (MMAS), men without DM were followed for 15 years to evaluate DM development. Those who reported sleeping less than 6 h a day were twice as likely to develop DM, and those sleeping more than 8 h a day were more then three times more likely to develop DM [18]. This U-shaped relation was also evident in the SHHS study [17].

In the MMAS [18], men who developed DM had significantly reduced testosterone levels, suggesting a possible etiologic link between sleep deprivation and insulin resistance, because low levels of testosterone are associated with insulin resistance [92], obesity [93], and DM [94]. Furthermore, apart from testosterone, sympathetic activation, elevated catecholamines, and corticosteroids could contribute to possible DM development in sleep-deprived subjects. The incidence of DM in relation to sleep duration is discussed later in this chapter.

Cortisol

High cortisol levels are associated with stress and may contribute to increased cardiovascular risk [95]. High levels of cortisol cause elevation of blood pressure, obesity, hyperinsulinemia, hyperglycemia, insulin resistance, and dyslipidemia. Elevated levels of cortisol have been found during total [96–98] and even partial sleep deprivation [14].

Thyroid Hormones

Thyroid hormones have a broad range of effects on cardiovascular function and metabolism. They increase metabolic rate, catecholamine sensitivity, cardiac output, and heart rate. Elevated levels of thyroid-stimulating hormone, as well as triiodothyronine and thyroxine, have been found during sleep deprivation [99–103]. Prolonged elevation of these enzymes could lead to adverse cardiovascular effects.

Cardiovascular Diseases Resulting in Sleep Disruption

While sleep disturbances may negatively affect the cardiovascular system via mechanisms described above, cardiovascular disease may also influence sleep, causing further progression of cardiovascular disease. One example of this "vicious cycle" is central sleep apnea (CSA).

Central sleep apnea consists of periodic hyperventilation and apneas [104] during sleep and is common in heart failure patients [19]. The incidence of CSA in heart failure patients ranges from 21 to 40 % [105–107] and CSA is accompanied by increased mortality [108]. Central sleep apnea may lead to significant sleep deprivation because of frequent nocturnal arousals. These may lead to increased sympathetic drive, plasma norepinephrine, and muscle sympathetic nerve activity. Sympathetic activation remains elevated in patients with CSA during wakefulness when compared with those without sleep-disordered breathing [109–111]. However, it is possible that heightened sympathetic drive in heart failure patients with CSA may simply be a consequence of more severe heart failure rather than a direct consequence of CSA [112] or sleep deprivation.

Obstructive sleep apnea (OSA) has also been linked to cardiovascular damage; it stimulates increased sympathetic outflow during wakefulness and sleep, increases left ventricular afterload by inducing hypoxia, increases right ventricular afterload, and increases the risk of myocardial infarction [113]. Improving OSA with successful continuous positive airway pressure therapy can lower blood pressure and attenuate the cardiovascular risk profile [113]. It is possible that at least part of this benefit may be due to a lower number of arousals and enhanced sleep quality.

Cardiovascular Disease and Sleep Deprivation

Hypertension

The link between sleep deprivation and hypertension was first described by Sackner et al. [114] in patients with OSA. Elevated blood pressure after 1 night of partial sleep deprivation has been described by Tochikubo et al. [6] and similar observations were reported by Kato et al. [7]. Ogawa et al. [5] demonstrated elevated diastolic, but not systolic blood pressures, in a small study in six acutely sleep-deprived healthy men.

Gangwisch et al. [67] examined whether the duration of sleep is related to incident hypertension in 4,810 subjects. They found that self-reported sleep duration of less then 5 h a day was significantly associated with increased risk of hypertension but only in subjects aged 32–59 years. Recently, the incidence of hypertension was also examined in a cross-sectional study by Stranges et al. [115], who found increased risk of hypertension in women with self-reported reduced sleep duration. Similarly, other studies have reported that women who reported sleeping less than 5 h had an increased risk of hypertension [116].

Increased risk of hypertension in men and women who objectively slept less than 5 h a night and in those with poor sleep quality was also reported by Vgontzas et al. [117]. However, while Gottlieb et al. [118] reported an increased prevalence of hypertension in subjects reporting more or less than 7–8 h per night, the prevalence was the highest for a sleep time less than 6 h per night. In another study, using actigraphy, short sleep duration was found to be associated with higher propensity to development of hypertension even in young healthy subjects [119].

Two studies using ambulatory blood pressure monitoring for blood pressure evaluation in normotensive [120] and hypertensive [44] subjects showed a rise in blood pressure the day after sleep deprivation. Furthermore, Meier-Ewart et al. [68] found an increased blood pressure after 88 h of total sleep deprivation.

As described earlier, a number of studies have noted that sleep deprivation may be associated with increased sympathetic tone and with high catecholamine levels that may contribute to the development of sustained hypertension. Nevertheless elevated blood pressure after sleep deprivation may also be secondary to other mechanisms, including vascular endothelial dysfunction and increased systemic inflammation [45, 51–53].

Coronary Artery Disease

Ayas et al. [4] found an increased risk of coronary artery disease in those female health professionals who reported sleeping less than 5 h, or more than 9 h a day. This data showed a U-shaped relation between sleep length and coronary vascular events. The American Cancer Society Study [121], the Almeda County study [122], and Partinen et al. [123] also showed an increased risk of CAD in subjects who reported sleeping 4–6 h a day.

Interestingly, Janszky et al. [124] noted that the incidence of acute myocardial infarction is significantly increased (by about 5 %) for the first 3 weekdays after the switch to daylight saving time (loss of an hour of sleep) in the spring and is actually lower (also by about 5 %) on the first weekday after the transition out of daylight saving time in the autumn, when an extra hour of sleep time is possible (see Fig. 11.3).

King et al. [8] found a higher incidence of coronary calcification in subjects with shorten sleep duration and Shankar et al. [125] found both short and long self-reported sleep durations to be positively associated with CAD-related mortality. This association was independent of smoking, alcohol intake, and body mass index. When compared with subjects sleeping 7 h, the relative risk of coronary heart disease mortality for a sleep duration less than 5 h was 1.57 (95 % CI of 1.32–1.88) and for a sleep duration more than 9 h 1.79 (95 % CI of 1.48–2.17). Similar U-shaped patterns for coronary heart disease have been shown by other investigators [126–128].

However, an increase in coronary disease only in those with self-reported short sleep duration

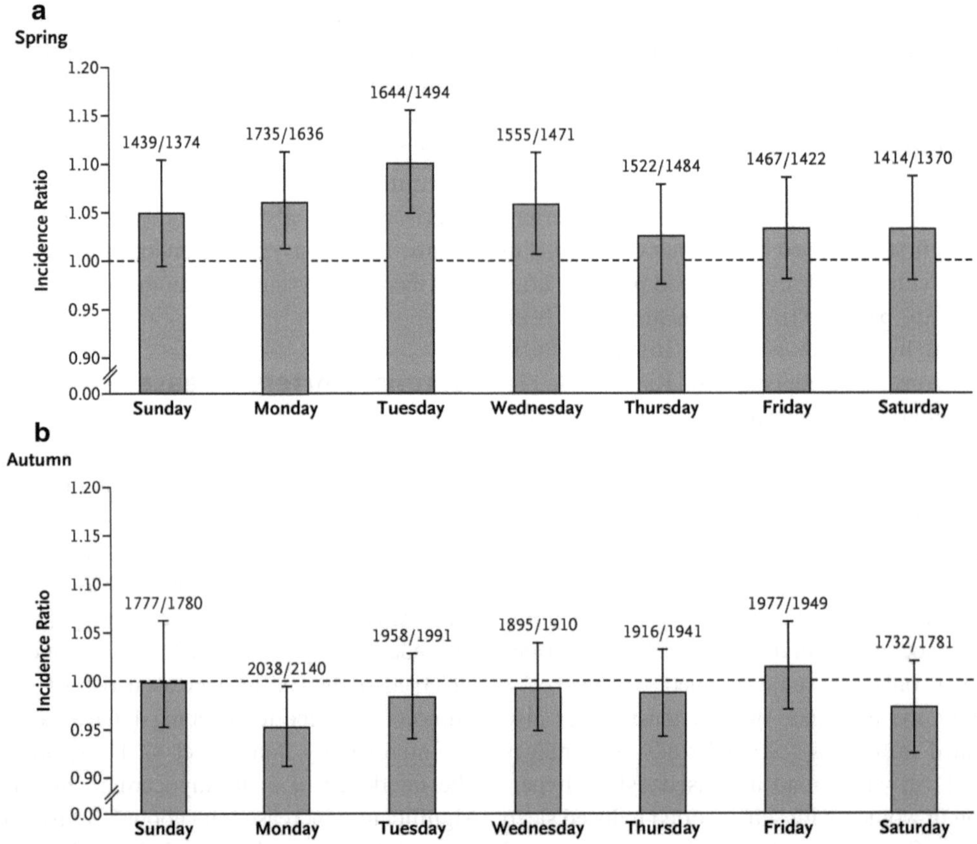

Fig. 11.3 Incidence ratios of acute myocardial infarction on the first 7 days after the spring and autumn clock shifts for Daylight Saving Time. The incidence is represented by the ratio of the number of acute myocardial infarctions (as the main diagnosis) on the given day after the shift to the mean number on the corresponding days 2 weeks earlier and 2 weeks later (both *numbers* given above the *bars*). *I bars* denote 95 % confidence intervals. (Reproduced with permission from Janszky et al. [124])

was reported by Heslop et al. [129] and Meisinger et al. [130], and only for longer sleep by Kripke et al. [131] and Mallon et al. [132]. A tendency to increased incidence of coronary disease was also noted in persons who reported sleeping more than 8 h, compared with those who slept between 6 and 8 h [133].

Interestingly, one study [134] found an increased risk of coronary disease only for subjects with sleep duration shorter than 6 h accompanied by some sleep disturbances. In subjects who did not report any sleep disturbances, the coronary disease risk was not increased. These findings are consistent with two studies by Eksted et al. [135, 136], who showed increased blood pressure, cortisol, and blood lipids in subjects with a high frequency of arousals and normal sleep time, suggesting the importance of not only the length but also quality of the sleep [130].

Prolonged working time was also found to be associated with increased risk of myocardial infarction [137–141]; nevertheless these studies did not point directly to sleep deprivation and involved many confounding factors. Liu et al. [9] distinguished between working hours and sleep duration reporting that those working more then 60 h a week had a twofold higher risk of having a myocardial infarction. Those subjects who slept less than 5 h a day had a 2.3 higher risk of having a myocardial infarction.

Stroke

Ruiter et al. [142] very recently published data from nearly 6,000 working adults from the Reasons for Geographic and Racial Differences in Stroke (REGARDS) study. This was a well phenotyped cohort without stroke and OSA. They found that self-reported sleep duration of less than 6 hours was strongly associated with a greater incidence of stroke symptoms (hazard ratio 4.54).

Cappuccio et al. [12], in a meta-analysis of 15 studies involving nearly 500,000 participants, demonstrated that self-reported short sleep duration (≤5–6 h) was associated with a greater risk of developing or dying of stroke (relative risk 1.15). Interestingly, and consistent with other studies of risks of prolonged sleep time, long duration of sleep (>8–9 h) was associated with an even greater risk of developing or dying of stroke (relative risk 1.65).

Qureshi et al. [133] found an increased risk of stroke in persons who reported sleeping greater than 8 h compared with persons who slept between 6 and 8 h. Daytime somnolence was also associated with stroke incidence in this study. Similarly, Chen et al. [143] reported an increased relative risk for ischemic stroke for women reporting ≤6 h of sleep—relative risk 1.14 (95 % CI of 0.97–1.33) and ≥9 h of sleep—relative risk 1.70 (95 % CI of 1.32–2.21). Finally, shorter sleep duration (<7.5 h) has been independently associated with the increased risk of stroke in patients with hypertension and especially in those with imaging evidence of silent cerebral infarction [144].

Arrhythmias

Ozer et al. [11] investigated the association between acute sleep deprivation and various measurements of QT interval (maximum QT interval (QT_{max}), QT dispersion (QTd), and corrected QT dispersion (cQTd), which may be good predictors of atrial fibrillation, ventricular arrhythmias, and sudden death. They obtained ECG recordings from 37 healthy volunteers after a night of normal sleep and after a night of sleep deprivation (approximately 2 h of sleep) and found that after a night of sleep deprivation, subjects had significantly higher values of QT_{max}, QTd, and cQTd. These changes could conceivably contribute to the development of recurrent arrhythmias in sleep-deprived subjects.

Irwin et al. [10] concluded in their study of sleep-deprived alcoholic men that sleep deprivation may contribute to triggering cardiac arrhythmias by increasing the sympathetic activation and catecholamine secretion.

Sari and colleagues [145] examined electrocardiograms from 37 healthy young subjects after a night of regular sleep and after a night of sleep deprivation. They evaluated P wave changes and found P minimum positively and P maximum and P dispersion negatively correlated with sleep time. This finding is important as P wave duration and dispersion may be predictors of atrial fibrillation [146].

Metabolic Syndrome and Obesity

Both the metabolic syndrome and obesity are known cardiovascular disease risk factors [84, 147]. Self-reported short (≤5 h) and long (≥8 h) sleep durations have been associated with metabolic syndrome [148]. Hall et al. [149] also reported increased risk of having the metabolic syndrome (45 %) in both short (<6 h) and long time (>8 h) sleepers, compared with those sleeping 7–8 h per night.

Van der Berg et al. [150] found, using actigraphy, a U-shaped relationship between sleep duration and obesity in an elderly population. Furthermore, subjects with high sleep fragmentation and short sleep duration were at higher risk of obesity.

In a large study of more than 35,000 Japanese workers, self-reported short sleep duration was significantly associated with weight gain and obesity after 1-year follow-up in men, but not in women [151]. However, in another study, objectively measured sleep duration less than 5 h was found to be associated with increased body mass index in both men and women [152].

The effect of sleep duration on body fat distribution was examined by Park et al. [153].

Self-reported short sleep duration (<5 h) in this study of nearly 9,000 adults was significantly associated with both abdominal (odds ratio 1.24) and general obesity (odds ratio 1.25). Finally, a large meta-analysis of cross-sectional studies [154], including more than 600,000 subjects, concluded that self-reported short sleep duration is associated with increased risk of obesity in children and adults.

Diabetes Mellitus

DM is a major risk factor for cardiovascular disease [155] and in the past decade several studies reported sleep duration as a risk factor for DM.

In experimental conditions, Buxton et al. [156] recently demonstrated that sleep restriction (5 h/night) lasting 1 week significantly reduces insulin sensitivity. Similar findings were reported by Donga et al. [157] even after just one night of partial sleep deprivation.

Chaput et al. [158] reported a significant association between self-reported short and long sleep duration with DM/impaired glucose toleration. The odds ratio was 1.58 (95 % CI of 1.13–2.31) for those reporting 9–10 h of sleep and 2.09 (95 % CI of 1.34–2.98) for those with 5–6 h of sleep. Similar findings were reported by Tuomilehto et al. [159] who found an association between self-reported short (≤6 h) or long sleep duration (≥8 h) and an increased risk of DM in middle-aged women but not in men. In contrast to these studies, Rafalson and coworkers found that fasting glucose was not impaired in long duration sleepers [160].

Recent data have suggested that self-reported day napping and short night sleeping confer a higher risk of DM [161]. Interestingly, it was the combination of ≥1 h of napping and both long or short sleeping that was associated with the higher DM risk. In the subjects with no napping, only short night sleeping was significantly associated with a higher incidence of DM.

Sleep disturbances have also been associated with DM. Kawakami et al. [162] noted that subjects with self-reported sleep disturbances had a 2–3 times higher risk of DM onset. The observed association was independent of other known DM risk factors. The authors concluded that the increased sympathetic activity associated with sleep disturbances could contribute to the impaired glucose intolerance and increased DM risk. These findings are supportive of those reported by Rafalson et al. [160], who showed insulin resistance in short time sleepers.

Mortality

Finally, sleep duration has been shown to also have an effect on mortality. Wingard et al. [122] reported that both short and long time sleepers have an increased mortality risk. Subjects included in this study, who reported sleeping less than 7 h or more than 8 h, had a 30 % greater mortality risk than those sleeping 7–8 h. Similar findings were reported by Patel et al. [163] who found an increased relative mortality risk for women who reported sleeping 5 or less hours [relative risk 1.15; (95 % CI of 1.02–1.29)] and also for women sleeping 9 or more hours [relative risk 1.42; (95 % CI of 1.27–1.58)].

These findings are consistent with a large study of 1.1 million American Cancer Society volunteers by Kripke et al. [131], who found an even greater mortality risk in subjects with self-reported prolonged sleep duration than in subjects with reduced sleep duration. The minimum mortality risk in this study was reported for those who slept 7 h per night supporting the findings of Wingard et al. [122].

Conclusion

While the study of cardiovascular risk associated with inadequate sleep is still in its early stages, there is increasing evidence that sleep deprivation may contribute to heightened likelihood of cardiovascular disease. Advancing the science in this area is of some urgency, given the high and rising prevalence of inadequate sleep in the population at large. Especially concerning is the fact that teenagers and young adults are exposed to increasing levels of inadequate sleep, in large part because of the advent of smart phones and social media, with many young people occupying traditional sleep time by communicating with peers. Any enhanced cardiometabolic risk as a result of consequent inadequate sleep would likely present as early onset of obesity, hypertension, glucose intolerance, and DM, thus exacerbating the overall social and economic burden of these increasingly prevalent chronic disease conditions.

References

1. CDC Data & Statistics|Feature: Insufficient sleep is a public health epidemic [Internet]. [Cited 2012 Aug 21]. Available from: http://www.cdc.gov/features/dsSleep/
2. Bonnet MH, Arand DL. We are chronically sleep deprived. Sleep. 1995;18(10):908–11.
3. Nagai M, Hoshide S, Kario K. Sleep duration as a risk factor for cardiovascular disease—a review of the recent literature. Curr Cardiol Rev. 2010;6(1):54–61.
4. Ayas NT, White DP, Manson JE, Stampfer MJ, Speizer FE, Malhotra A, et al. A prospective study of sleep duration and coronary heart disease in women. Arch Intern Med. 2003;163(2):205–9.
5. Ogawa Y, Kanbayashi T, Saito Y, Takahashi Y, Kitajima T, Takahashi K, et al. Total sleep deprivation elevates blood pressure through arterial baroreflex resetting: a study with microneurographic technique. Sleep. 2003;26(8):986–9.
6. Tochikubo O, Ikeda A, Miyajima E, Ishii M. Effects of insufficient sleep on blood pressure monitored by a new multibiomedical recorder. Hypertension. 1996;27(6):1318–24.
7. Kato M, Phillips BG, Sigurdsson G, Narkiewicz K, Pesek CA, Somers VK. Effects of sleep deprivation on neural circulatory control. Hypertension. 2000;35(5):1173–5.
8. King CR, Knutson KL, Rathouz PJ, Sidney S, Liu K, Lauderdale DS. Short sleep duration and incident coronary artery calcification. JAMA. 2008;300(24):2859–66.
9. Liu Y, Tanaka H. Overtime work, insufficient sleep, and risk of non-fatal acute myocardial infarction in Japanese men. Occup Environ Med. 2002;59(7):447–51.
10. Irwin MR, Ziegler M. Sleep deprivation potentiates activation of cardiovascular and catecholamine responses in abstinent alcoholics. Hypertension. 2005;45(2):252–7.
11. Ozer O, Ozbala B, Sari I, Davutoglu V, Maden E, Baltaci Y, et al. Acute sleep deprivation is associated with increased QT dispersion in healthy young adults. Pacing Clin Electrophysiol. 2008;31(8):979–84.
12. Cappuccio FP, Cooper D, D'Elia L, Strazzullo P, Miller MA. Sleep duration predicts cardiovascular outcomes: a systematic review and meta-analysis of prospective studies. Eur Heart J [Internet]. 2011 Feb 7 [cited 2012 Aug 3]; Available from: http://eurheartj.oxfordjournals.org/content/early/2011/02/03/eurheartj.ehr007
13. Shahar E, Whitney CW, Redline S, Lee ET, Newman AB, Javier Nieto F, et al. Sleep-disordered breathing and cardiovascular disease: cross-sectional results of the Sleep Heart Health Study. Am J Respir Crit Care Med. 2001;163(1):19–25.
14. Spiegel K, Leproult R, Van Cauter E. Impact of sleep debt on metabolic and endocrine function. Lancet. 1999;354(9188):1435–9.
15. Spiegel K, Knutson K, Leproult R, Tasali E, Cauter EV. Sleep loss: a novel risk factor for insulin resistance and Type 2 diabetes. J Appl Physiol. 2005; 99(5):2008–19.
16. Chaput J-P, Després J-P, Bouchard C, Astrup A, Tremblay A. Sleep duration as a risk factor for the development of type 2 diabetes or impaired glucose tolerance: analyses of the Quebec Family Study. Sleep Med. 2009;10(8):919–24.
17. Gottlieb DJ, Punjabi NM, Newman AB, Resnick HE, Redline S, Baldwin CM, et al. Association of sleep time with diabetes mellitus and impaired glucose tolerance. Arch Intern Med. 2005;165(8):863–7.
18. Yaggi HK, Araujo AB, McKinlay JB. Sleep duration as a risk factor for the development of Type 2 diabetes. Diabetes Care. 2006;29(3):657–61.
19. Wolk R, Kara T, Somers VK. Sleep-disordered breathing and cardiovascular disease. Circulation. 2003;108(1):9–12.
20. Cooke-Ariel H. Circadian variations in cardiovascular function and their relation to the occurrence and timing of cardiac events. Am J Health Syst Pharm. 1998;55 Suppl 3:S5–11.
21. Furlan R, Guzzetti S, Crivellaro W, Dassi S, Tinelli M, Baselli G, et al. Continuous 24-hour assessment of the neural regulation of systemic arterial pressure and RR variabilities in ambulant subjects. Circulation. 1990;81(2):537–47.
22. Yasue H, Touyama M, Kato H, Tanaka S, Akiyama F. Prinzmetal's variant form of angina as a manifestation of alpha-adrenergic receptor-mediated coronary artery spasm: documentation by coronary arteriography. Am Heart J. 1976;91(2):148–55.
23. Verrier RL, Muller JE, Hobson JA. Sleep, dreams, and sudden death: the case for sleep as an autonomic stress test for the heart. Cardiovasc Res. 1996; 31(2):181–211.
24. Somers VK, Dyken ME, Mark AL, Abboud FM. Sympathetic-nerve activity during sleep in normal subjects. N Engl J Med. 1993;328(5):303–7.
25. Guilleminault C, Pool P, Motta J, Gillis AM. Sinus arrest during REM sleep in young adults. N Engl J Med. 1984;311(16):1006–10.

26. Nevins DB. First- and second-degree A-V heart block with rapid Eye movement sleep. Ann Intern Med. 1972;76(6):981–3.
27. Singh J, Mela T, Ruskin J. Images in cardiovascular medicine. Sleep (vagal)-induced atrial fibrillation. Circulation. 2004;110(4):e32–3.
28. Molnar J, Zhang F, Weiss J, Ehlert FA, Rosenthal JE. Diurnal pattern of QTc interval: how long is prolonged? Possible relation to circadian triggers of cardiovascular events. J Am Coll Cardiol. 1996; 27(1):76–83.
29. Lanfranchi PA, Shamsuzzaman ASM, Ackerman MJ, Kara T, Jurak P, Wolk R, et al. Sex-selective QT prolongation during rapid eye movement sleep. Circulation. 2002;106(12):1488–92.
30. Schwartz PJ, Priori SG, Spazzolini C, Moss AJ, Vincent GM, Napolitano C, et al. Genotype-phenotype correlation in the long-QT syndrome: gene-specific triggers for life-threatening arrhythmias. Circulation. 2001;103(1):89–95.
31. Otto ME, Svatikova A, Barretto RB de Mattos, Santos S, Hoffmann M, Khandheria B, et al. Early morning attenuation of endothelial function in healthy humans. Circulation. 2004;109(21): 2507–10.
32. Quyyumi AA, Panza JA, Diodati JG, Lakatos E, Epstein SE. Circadian variation in ischemic threshold. A mechanism underlying the circadian variation in ischemic events. Circulation. 1992;86(1):22–8.
33. Rosing DR, Brakman P, Redwood DR, Goldstein RE, Beiser GD, Astrup T, et al. Blood fibrinolytic activity in man. Diurnal variation and the response to varying intensities of exercise. Circ Res. 1970;27(2):171–84.
34. Tofler GH, Brezinski D, Schafer AI, Czeisler CA, Rutherford JD, Willich SN, et al. Concurrent morning increase in platelet aggregability and the risk of myocardial infarction and sudden cardiac death. N Engl J Med. 1987;316(24):1514–8.
35. Andreotti F, Davies GJ, Hackett DR, Khan MI, De Bart AC, Aber VR, et al. Major circadian fluctuations in fibrinolytic factors and possible relevance to time of onset of myocardial infarction, sudden cardiac death and stroke. Am J Cardiol. 1988; 62(9):635–7.
36. Rocco MB, Barry J, Campbell S, Nabel E, Cook EF, Goldman L, et al. Circadian variation of transient myocardial ischemia in patients with coronary artery disease. Circulation. 1987;75(2):395–400.
37. Muller JE, Stone PH, Turi ZG, Rutherford JD, Czeisler CA, Parker C, et al. Circadian variation in the frequency of onset of acute myocardial infarction. N Engl J Med. 1985;313(21):1315–22.
38. Willich SN, Linderer T, Wegscheider K, Leizorovicz A, Alamercery I, Schröder R. Increased morning incidence of myocardial infarction in the ISAM Study: absence with prior beta-adrenergic blockade. ISAM Study Group. Circulation. 1989; 80(4):853–8.
39. Marler JR, Price TR, Clark GL, Muller JE, Robertson T, Mohr JP, et al. Morning increase in onset of ischemic stroke. Stroke. 1989;20(4):473–6.
40. Argentino C, Toni D, Rasura M, Violi F, Sacchetti ML, Allegretta A, et al. Circadian variation in the frequency of ischemic stroke. Stroke. 1990; 21(3):387–9.
41. Zhong X, Hilton HJ, Gates GJ, Jelic S, Stern Y, Bartels MN, et al. Increased sympathetic and decreased parasympathetic cardiovascular modulation in normal humans with acute sleep deprivation. J Appl Physiol. 2005;98(6):2024–32.
42. Dettoni JL, Consolim-Colombo FM, Drager LF, Rubira MC, de Souza SBP C, Irigoyen MC, et al. Cardiovascular effects of partial sleep deprivation in healthy volunteers. J Appl Physiol. 2012;113(2): 232–6.
43. Irwin M, Thompson J, Miller C, Gillin JC, Ziegler M. Effects of sleep and sleep deprivation on catecholamine and interleukin-2 levels in humans: clinical implications. J Clin Endocrinol Metab. 1999;84(6):1979–85.
44. Lusardi P, Zoppi A, Preti P, Pesce RM, Piazza E, Fogari R. Effects of insufficient sleep on blood pressure in hypertensive patients: a 24-h study. Am J Hypertens. 1999;12(1 Pt 1):63–8.
45. Sauvet F, Leftheriotis G, Gomez-Merino D, Langrume C, Drogou C, Van Beers P, et al. Effect of acute sleep deprivation on vascular function in healthy subjects. J Appl Physiol. 2010;108(1):68–75.
46. Holmes AL, Burgess HJ, Dawson D. Effects of sleep pressure on endogenous cardiac autonomic activity and body temperature. J Appl Physiol. 2002;92(6): 2578–84.
47. Ridker PM. Testing the inflammatory hypothesis of atherothrombosis: scientific rationale for the cardiovascular inflammation reduction trial (CIRT). J Thromb Haemost. 2009;7 Suppl 1:332–9.
48. Ridker PM, Rifai N, Stampfer MJ, Hennekens CH. Plasma concentration of interleukin-6 and the risk of future myocardial infarction among apparently healthy men. Circulation. 2000;101(15):1767–72.
49. Ridker PM. High-sensitivity C-reactive protein potential adjunct for global risk assessment in the primary prevention of cardiovascular disease. Circulation. 2001;103(13):1813–8.
50. Shearer WT, Reuben JM, Mullington JM, Price NJ, Lee BN, Smith EO, et al. Soluble TNF-alpha receptor 1 and IL-6 plasma levels in humans subjected to the sleep deprivation model of spaceflight. J Allergy Clin Immunol. 2001;107(1):165–70.
51. Haack M, Sanchez E, Mullington JM. Elevated inflammatory markers in response to prolonged sleep restriction Are associated with increased pain experience in healthy volunteers. Sleep. 2007;30(9): 1145–52.
52. Vgontzas AN, Zoumakis E, Bixler EO, Lin H-M, Follett H, Kales A, et al. Adverse effects of modest sleep restriction on sleepiness, performance, and

inflammatory cytokines. J Clin Endocrinol Metab. 2004;89(5):2119–26.
53. Larkin EK, Rosen CL, Kirchner HL, Storfer-Isser A, Emancipator JL, Johnson NL, et al. Variation of C-reactive protein levels in adolescents: association with sleep-disordered breathing and sleep duration. Circulation. 2005;111(15):1978–84.
54. Born J, Lange T, Hansen K, Mölle M, Fehm HL. Effects of sleep and circadian rhythm on human circulating immune cells. J Immunol. 1997;158(9): 4454–64.
55. Bøyum A, Wiik P, Gustavsson E, Veiby OP, Reseland J, Haugen AH, et al. The effect of strenuous exercise, calorie deficiency and sleep deprivation on white blood cells, plasma immunoglobulins and cytokines. Scand J Immunol. 1996;43(2):228–35.
56. Kuhn E, Brodan V, Brodanová M, Rysánek K. Metabolic reflection of sleep deprivation. Act Nerv Super (Praha). 1969;11(3):165–74.
57. Dinges DF, Douglas SD, Zaugg L, Campbell DE, McMann JM, Whitehouse WG, et al. Leukocytosis and natural killer cell function parallel neurobehavioral fatigue induced by 64 hours of sleep deprivation. J Clin Invest. 1994;93(5):1930–9.
58. Frey DJ, Fleshner M, Wright Jr KP. The effects of 40 hours of total sleep deprivation on inflammatory markers in healthy young adults. Brain Behav Immun. 2007;21(8):1050–7.
59. Taheri S, Austin D, Lin L, Nieto FJ, Young T, Mignot E. Correlates of serum C-reactive protein (CRP)—no association with sleep duration or sleep disordered breathing. Sleep. 2007;30(8):991–6.
60. Sarzi-Puttini P, Atzeni F, Doria A, Iaccarino L, Turiel M. Tumor necrosis factor-alpha, biologic agents and cardiovascular risk. Lupus. 2005; 14(9):780–4.
61. Irwin MR, Wang M, Campomayor CO, Collado-Hidalgo A, Cole S. Sleep deprivation and activation of morning levels of cellular and genomic markers of inflammation. Arch Intern Med. 2006;166(16): 1756–62.
62. Irwin MR, Wang M, Ribeiro D, Cho HJ, Olmstead R, Breen EC, et al. Sleep loss activates cellular inflammatory signaling. Biol Psychiatry. 2008; 64(6):538–40.
63. Mullington JM, Haack M, Toth M, Serrador JM, Meier-Ewert HK. Cardiovascular, inflammatory, and metabolic consequences of sleep deprivation. Prog Cardiovasc Dis. 2009;51(4):294–302.
64. Bonetti PO, Lerman LO, Lerman A. Endothelial dysfunction a marker of atherosclerotic risk. Arterioscler Thromb Vasc Biol. 2003;23(2):168–75.
65. Takase B, Akima T, Uehata A, Ohsuzu F, Kurita A. Effect of chronic stress and sleep deprivation on both flow-mediated dilation in the brachial artery and the intracellular magnesium level in humans. Clin Cardiol. 2004;27(4):223–7.
66. Amir O, Alroy S, Schliamser JE, Asmir I, Shiran A, Flugelman MY, et al. Brachial artery endothelial function in residents and fellows working night shifts. Am J Cardiol. 2004;93(7):947–9.
67. Gangwisch JE, Heymsfield SB, Boden-Albala B, Buijs RM, Kreier F, Pickering TG, et al. Short sleep duration as a risk factor for hypertension: analyses of the first National Health and Nutrition Examination Survey. Hypertension. 2006;47(5):833–9.
68. Meier-Ewert HK, Ridker PM, Rifai N, Regan MM, Price NJ, Dinges DF, et al. Effect of sleep loss on C-reactive protein, an inflammatory marker of cardiovascular risk. J Am Coll Cardiol. 2004;43(4):678–83.
69. Miller MA, Kandala N-B, Kumari M, Marmot MG, Cappuccio FP. Relationships between sleep duration and von Willebrand factor, factor VII, and fibrinogen: Whitehall II study. Arterioscler Thromb Vasc Biol. 2010;30(10):2032–8.
70. Von Kanel R, Loredo JS, Ancoli-Israel S, Mills PJ, Natarajan L, Dimsdale JE. Association between polysomnographic measures of disrupted sleep and prothrombotic factors. Chest. 2007;131(3):733–9.
71. Wolk R, Somers VK. Leptin and vascular function: friend or foe? Eur Heart J. 2006;27(19):2263–5.
72. Mullington JM, Chan JL, Van Dongen HPA, Szuba MP, Samaras J, Price NJ, et al. Sleep loss reduces diurnal rhythm amplitude of leptin in healthy men. J Neuroendocrinol. 2003;15(9):851–4.
73. Spiegel K, Tasali E, Penev P, Cauter EV. Brief communication: sleep curtailment in healthy young men is associated with decreased leptin levels, elevated ghrelin levels, and increased hunger and appetite. Ann Intern Med. 2004;141(11):846–50.
74. Matsuda K, Teragawa H, Fukuda Y, Nakagawa K, Higashi Y, Chayama K. Leptin causes nitric-oxide independent coronary artery vasodilation in humans. Hypertens Res. 2003;26(2):147–52.
75. Smith CCT, Dixon RA, Wynne AM, Theodorou L, Ong S-G, Subrayan S, et al. Leptin-induced cardioprotection involves JAK/STAT signaling that may be linked to the mitochondrial permeability transition pore. Am J Physiol Heart Circ Physiol. 2010; 299(4):H1265–70.
76. Zhang F, Wang S, Signore AP, Chen J. Neuroprotective effects of leptin against ischemic injury induced by oxygen-glucose deprivation and transient cerebral ischemia. Stroke. 2007;38(8):2329–36.
77. Yuan K, Yu J, Shah A, Gao S, Kim SY, Kim SZ, et al. Leptin reduces plasma ANP level via nitric oxide-dependent mechanism. Am J Physiol Regul Integr Comp Physiol. 2010;298(4):R1007–16.
78. Mascareno E, Beckles D, Dhar-Mascareno M, Siddiqui MAQ. Enhanced hypertrophy in ob/ob mice due to an impairment in expression of atrial natriuretic peptide. Vascul Pharmacol. 2009;51(2–3):198–204.
79. Eikelis N, Schlaich M, Aggarwal A, Kaye D, Esler M. Interactions between leptin and the human sympathetic nervous system. Hypertension. 2003;41(5): 1072–9.
80. Purdham DM, Rajapurohitam V, Zeidan A, Huang C, Gross GJ, Karmazyn M. A neutralizing leptin

receptor antibody mitigates hypertrophy and hemodynamic dysfunction in the postinfarcted rat heart. Am J Physiol Heart Circ Physiol. 2008;295(1): H441–6.
81. Elbatarny HS, Maurice DH. Leptin-mediated activation of human platelets: involvement of a leptin receptor and phosphodiesterase 3A-containing cellular signaling complex. Am J Physiol Endocrinol Metab. 2005;289(4):E695–702.
82. Thøgersen AM, Söderberg S, Jansson J-H, Dahlén G, Boman K, Nilsson TK, et al. Interactions between fibrinolysis, lipoproteins and leptin related to a first myocardial infarction. Eur J Cardiovasc Prev Rehabil. 2004;11(1):33–40.
83. Loffreda S, Yang SQ, Lin HZ, Karp CL, Brengman ML, Wang DJ, et al. Leptin regulates proinflammatory immune responses. FASEB J. 1998;12(1):57–65.
84. Hu G, Qiao Q, Tuomilehto J. The metabolic syndrome and cardiovascular risk. Curr Diabetes Rev. 2005;1(2):137–43.
85. Taheri S, Lin L, Austin D, Young T, Mignot E. Short sleep duration is associated with reduced leptin, elevated ghrelin, and increased body mass index. PLoS Med. 2004;1(3):e62.
86. Korbonits M, Grossman AB. Ghrelin: update on a novel hormonal system. Eur J Endocrinol. 2004;151 Suppl 1:S67–70.
87. Xu X, Sook Jhun B, Hoon Ha C, Jin Z-G. Molecular mechanisms of ghrelin-mediated endothelial nitric oxide synthase activation. Endocrinology. 2008; 149(8):4183–92.
88. Isgaard J, Barlind A, Johansson I. Cardiovascular effects of ghrelin and growth hormone secretagogues. Cardiovasc Hematol Disord Drug Targets. 2008;8(2):133–7.
89. Brandenberger G, Gronfier C, Chapotot F, Simon C, Piquard F. Effect of sleep deprivation on overall 24 h growth-hormone secretion. Lancet. 2000;356(9239): 1408.
90. Maison P, Griffin S, Nicoue-Beglah M, Haddad N, Balkau B, Chanson P. Impact of growth hormone (GH) treatment on cardiovascular risk factors in GH-deficient adults: a metaanalysis of blinded, randomized, placebo-controlled trials. J Clin Endocrinol Metab. 2004;89(5):2192–9.
91. Fox CS, Coady S, Sorlie PD, D'Agostino RB, Pencina MJ, Vasan RS, et al. Increasing cardiovascular disease burden due to diabetes mellitus the Framingham Heart Study. Circulation. 2007;115(12): 1544–50.
92. Haffner SM, Karhapää P, Mykkänen L, Laakso M. Insulin resistance, body fat distribution, and sex hormones in men. Diabetes. 1994;43(2):212–9.
93. Barrett-Connor E, Khaw KT. Endogenous sex hormones and cardiovascular disease in men. A prospective population-based study. Circulation. 1988;78(3):539–45.
94. Stellato RK, Feldman HA, Hamdy O, Horton ES, McKinlay JB. Testosterone, sex hormone-binding globulin, and the development of type 2 diabetes in middle-aged men: prospective results from the Massachusetts male aging study. Diabetes Care. 2000;23(4):490–4.
95. Whitworth JA, Williamson PM, Mangos G, Kelly JJ. Cardiovascular consequences of cortisol excess. Vasc Health Risk Manag. 2005;1(4):291–9.
96. Mullington J, Hermann D, Holsboer F, Pollmächer T. Age-dependent suppression of nocturnal growth hormone levels during sleep deprivation. Neuroendocrinology. 1996;64(3):233–41.
97. Späth-Schwalbe E, Uthgenannt D, Voget G, Kern W, Born J, Fehm HL. Corticotropin-releasing hormone-induced adrenocorticotropin and cortisol secretion depends on sleep and wakefulness. J Clin Endocrinol Metab. 1993;77(5):1170–3.
98. Weitzman ED, Zimmerman JC, Czeisler CA, Ronda J. Cortisol secretion is inhibited during sleep in normal man. J Clin Endocrinol Metab. 1983;56(2):352–8.
99. Gary KA, Winokur A, Douglas SD, Kapoor S, Zaugg L, Dinges DF. Total sleep deprivation and the thyroid axis: effects of sleep and waking activity. Aviat Space Environ Med. 1996;67(6):513–9.
100. Radomski MW, Hart LE, Goodman JM, Plyley MJ. Aerobic fitness and hormonal responses to prolonged sleep deprivation and sustained mental work. Aviat Space Environ Med. 1992;63(2):101–6.
101. Palmblad J, Akerstedt T, Fröberg J, Melander A, Von Schenck H. Thyroid and adrenomedullary reactions during sleep deprivation. Acta Endocrinol. 1979;90(2):233–9.
102. Goichot B, Brandenberger G, Saini J, Wittersheim G, Follenius M. Nycthemeral patterns of thyroid hormones and their relationships with thyrotropin variations and sleep structure. J Endocrinol Invest. 1994;17(3):181–7.
103. Sadamatsu M, Kato N, Iida H, Takahashi S, Sakaue K, Takahashi K, et al. The 24-hour rhythms in plasma growth hormone, prolactin and thyroid stimulating hormone: effect of sleep deprivation. J Neuroendocrinol. 1995;7(8):597–606.
104. Bradley TD, Floras JS. Sleep apnea and heart failure. Part II: central sleep apnea. Circulation. 2003; 107(13):1822–6.
105. Sin DD, Fitzgerald F, Parker JD, Newton G, Floras JS, Bradley TD. Risk factors for central and obstructive sleep apnea in 450 men and women with congestive heart failure. Am J Respir Crit Care Med. 1999;160(4):1101–6.
106. Wang H, Parker JD, Newton GE, Floras JS, Mak S, Chiu K-L, et al. Influence of obstructive sleep apnea on mortality in patients with heart failure. J Am Coll Cardiol. 2007;49(15):1625–31.
107. Javaheri S, Parker TJ, Liming JD, Corbett WS, Nishiyama H, Wexler L, et al. Sleep apnea in 81 ambulatory male patients with stable heart failure

types and their prevalences, consequences, and presentations. Circulation. 1998;97(21):2154–9.
108. Naughton MT, Bradley TD. Sleep apnea in congestive heart failure. Clin Chest Med. 1998;19(1): 99–113.
109. Naughton MT, Benard DC, Liu PP, Rutherford R, Rankin F, Bradley TD. Effects of nasal CPAP on sympathetic activity in patients with heart failure and central sleep apnea. Am J Respir Crit Care Med. 1995;152(2):473–9.
110. Van de Borne P, Oren R, Abouassaly C, Anderson E, Somers VK. Effect of Cheyne-Stokes respiration on muscle sympathetic nerve activity in severe congestive heart failure secondary to ischemic or idiopathic dilated cardiomyopathy. Am J Cardiol. 1998;81(4): 432–6.
111. Spaak J, Egri ZJ, Kubo T, Yu E, Ando S-I, Kaneko Y, et al. Muscle sympathetic nerve activity during wakefulness in heart failure patients with and without sleep apnea. Hypertension. 2005;46(6): 1327–32.
112. Mansfield D, Kaye DM, Brunner La Rocca H, Solin P, Esler MD, Naughton MT. Raised sympathetic nerve activity in heart failure and central sleep apnea is due to heart failure severity. Circulation. 2003;107(10):1396–400.
113. Somers VK, White DP, Amin R, Abraham WT, Costa F, Culebras A, et al. Sleep apnea and cardiovascular disease: An American Heart Association/American College of Cardiology Foundation Scientific Statement From the American Heart Association Council for High Blood Pressure Research Professional Education Committee, Council on Clinical Cardiology, Stroke Council, and Council on Cardiovascular Nursing In Collaboration With the National Heart, Lung, and Blood Institute National Center on Sleep Disorders Research (National Institutes of Health). Circulation. 2008;118(10):1080–111.
114. Sackner MA, Landa J, Forrest T, Greeneltch D. Periodic sleep apnea: chronic sleep deprivation related to intermittent upper airway obstruction and central nervous system disturbance. Chest. 1975; 67(2):164–71.
115. Stranges S, Dorn JM, Cappuccio FP, Donahue RP, Rafalson LB, Hovey KM, et al. A population-based study of reduced sleep duration and hypertension: the strongest association may be in premenopausal women. J Hypertens. 2010;28(5):896–902.
116. Stang A, Moebus S, Möhlenkamp S, Erbel R, Jöckel KH. Gender-specific associations of short sleep duration with prevalent hypertension. Hypertension. 2008;51(3):e15–6.
117. Vgontzas AN, Liao D, Bixler EO, Chrousos GP, Vela-Bueno A. Insomnia with objective short sleep duration is associated with a high risk for hypertension. Sleep. 2009;32(4):491–7.
118. Gottlieb DJ, Redline S, Nieto FJ, Baldwin CM, Newman AB, Resnick HE, et al. Association of usual sleep duration with hypertension: the Sleep Heart Health Study. Sleep. 2006;29(8):1009–14.
119. Javaheri S, Storfer-Isser A, Rosen CL, Redline S. Sleep quality and elevated blood pressure in adolescents. Circulation. 2008;118(10):1034–40.
120. Lusardi P, Mugellini A, Preti P, Zoppi A, Derosa G, Fogari R. Effects of a restricted sleep regimen on ambulatory blood pressure monitoring in normotensive subjects. Am J Hypertens. 1996;9(5):503–5.
121. Kripke DF, Simons RN, Garfinkel L, Hammond EC. Short and long sleep and sleeping pillsis increased mortality associated? Arch Gen Psychiatry. 1979; 36(1):103–16.
122. Wingard DL, Berkman LF. Mortality risk associated with sleeping patterns among adults. Sleep. 1983; 6(2):102–7.
123. Partinen M, Putkonen PT, Kaprio J, Koskenvuo M, Hilakivi I. Sleep disorders in relation to coronary heart disease. Acta Med Scand Suppl. 1982; 660:69–83.
124. Janszky I, Ljung R. Shifts to and from daylight saving time and incidence of myocardial infarction. N Engl J Med. 2008;359(18):1966–8.
125. Shankar A, Koh W-P, Yuan J-M, Lee H-P, Yu MC. Sleep duration and coronary heart disease mortality among Chinese adults in Singapore: a population-based cohort study. Am J Epidemiol. 2008; 168(12):1367–73.
126. Amagai Y, Ishikawa S, Gotoh T, Doi Y, Kayaba K, Nakamura Y, et al. Sleep duration and mortality in Japan: the Jichi Medical School Cohort Study. J Epidemiol. 2004;14(4):124–8.
127. Empana J-P, Dauvilliers Y, Dartigues J-F, Ritchie K, Gariepy J, Jouven X, et al. Excessive daytime sleepiness is an independent risk indicator for cardiovascular mortality in community-dwelling elderly: the three city study. Stroke. 2009;40(4):1219–24.
128. Ferrie JE, Shipley MJ, Cappuccio FP, Brunner E, Miller MA, Kumari M, et al. A prospective study of change in sleep duration: associations with mortality in the Whitehall II Cohort. Sleep. 2007;30(12):1659–66.
129. Heslop P, Smith GD, Metcalfe C, Macleod J, Hart C. Sleep duration and mortality: the effect of short or long sleep duration on cardiovascular and all-cause mortality in working men and women. Sleep Med. 2002;3(4):305–14.
130. Meisinger C, Heier M, Löwel H, Schneider A, Döring A. Sleep duration and sleep complaints and risk of myocardial infarction in middle-aged men and women from the general population: the MONICA/KORA Augsburg Cohort Study. Sleep. 2007;30(9):1121–7.
131. Kripke DF, Garfinkel L, Wingard DL, Klauber MR, Marler MR. Mortality associated with sleep duration and insomnia. Arch Gen Psychiatry. 2002; 59(2):131–6.
132. Mallon L, Broman JE, Hetta J. Sleep complaints predict coronary artery disease mortality in males: a

12-year follow-up study of a middle-aged Swedish population. J Intern Med. 2002;251(3):207–16.
133. Qureshi AI, Giles WH, Croft JB, Bliwise DL. Habitual sleep patterns and risk for stroke and coronary heart disease: a 10-year follow-up from NHANES I. Neurology. 1997;48(4):904–10.
134. Chandola T, Ferrie JE, Perski A, Akbaraly T, Marmot MG. The effect of short sleep duration on coronary heart disease risk is greatest among those with sleep disturbance: a prospective study from the Whitehall II cohort. Sleep. 2010;33(6):739–44.
135. Ekstedt M, Akerstedt T, Söderström M. Microarousals during sleep are associated with increased levels of lipids, cortisol, and blood pressure. Psychosom Med. 2004;66(6):925–31.
136. Ekstedt M, Söderström M, Akerstedt T, Nilsson J, Søndergaard H-P, Aleksander P. Disturbed sleep and fatigue in occupational burnout. Scand J Work Environ Health. 2006;32(2):121–31.
137. Buell P, Breslow L. Mortality from coronary heart disease in California men who work long hours. J Chronic Dis. 1960;11(6):615–26.
138. Falger PR, Schouten EG. Exhaustion, psychological stressors in the work environment, and acute myocardial infarction in adult men. J Psychosom Res. 1992;36(8):777–86.
139. Netterstrom B, Nielsen FE, Kristensen TS, Bach E, Moller L. Relation between job strain and myocardial infarction: a case–control study. Occup Environ Med. 1999;56(5):339–42.
140. Theorell T, Rahe RH. Behavior and life satisfactions characteristics of Swedish subjects with myocardial infarction. J Chronic Dis. 1972;25(3):139–47.
141. Sokejima S, Kagamimori S. Working hours as a risk factor for acute myocardial infarction in Japan: case–control study. BMJ. 1998;317(7161):775–80.
142. Ruiter M, Howard VJ, Letter AJ, Kleindorfer D. Short sleep predicts stroke symptoms in persons of normal weight. SLEEP 2012; June 11, 2012; Boston, MA. Abstract 0829.
143. Chen J-C, Brunner RL, Ren H, Wassertheil-Smoller S, Larson JC, Levine DW, et al. Sleep duration and risk of ischemic stroke in postmenopausal women. Stroke. 2008;39(12):3185–92.
144. Eguchi K, Hoshide S, Ishikawa S, Shimada K, Kario K. Short sleep duration is an independent predictor of stroke events in elderly hypertensive patients. J Am Soc Hypertens. 2010;4(5):255–62.
145. Sari I, Davutoglu V, Ozbala B, Ozer O, Baltaci Y, Yavuz S, et al. Acute sleep deprivation is associated with increased electrocardiographic P-wave dispersion in healthy young men and women. Pacing Clin Electrophysiol. 2008;31(4):438–42.
146. Dilaveris PE, Gialafos JE. P-wave dispersion: a novel predictor of paroxysmal atrial fibrillation. Ann Noninvasive Electrocardiol. 2001;6(2):159–65.
147. Poirier P, Giles TD, Bray GA, Hong Y, Stern JS, Pi-Sunyer FX, et al. Obesity and cardiovascular disease: pathophysiology, evaluation, and effect of weight loss an update of the 1997 American Heart Association Scientific Statement on Obesity and Heart Disease From the Obesity Committee of the Council on Nutrition, Physical Activity, and Metabolism. Circulation. 2006;113(6):898–918.
148. Choi KM, Lee JS, Park HS, Baik SH, Choi DS, Kim SM. Relationship between sleep duration and the metabolic syndrome: Korean National Health and Nutrition Survey 2001. Int J Obes (Lond). 2008; 32(7):1091–7.
149. Hall MH, Muldoon MF, Jennings JR, Buysse DJ, Flory JD, Manuck SB. Self-reported sleep duration is associated with the metabolic syndrome in midlife adults. Sleep. 2008;31(5):635–43.
150. Van den Berg JF, Knvistingh Neven A, Tulen JHM, Hofman A, Witteman JCM, Miedema HME, et al. Actigraphic sleep duration and fragmentation are related to obesity in the elderly: the Rotterdam Study. Int J Obes (Lond). 2008;32(7):1083–90.
151. Watanabe M, Kikuchi H, Tanaka K, Takahashi M. Association of short sleep duration with weight gain and obesity at 1-year follow-up: a large-scale prospective study. Sleep. 2010;33(2):161–7.
152. Patel SR, Blackwell T, Redline S, Ancoli-Israel S, Cauley JA, Hillier TA, et al. The association between sleep duration and obesity in older adults. Int J Obes (Lond). 2008;32(12):1825–34.
153. Park SE, Kim HM, Kim DH, Kim J, Cha BS, Kim DJ. The association between sleep duration and general and abdominal obesity in Koreans: data from the Korean National Health and Nutrition Examination Survey, 2001 and 2005. Obesity (Silver Spring). 2009;17(4):767–71.
154. Cappuccio FP, Taggart FM, Kandala N-B, Currie A, Peile E, Stranges S, et al. Meta-analysis of short sleep duration and obesity in children and adults. Sleep. 2008;31(5):619–26.
155. Mellitus D. A major risk factor for cardiovascular disease: A Joint Editorial Statement by the American Diabetes Association; the National Heart, Lung, and Blood Institute; the Juvenile Diabetes Foundation International; the National Institute of Diabetes and Digestive and Kidney Diseases; and the American Heart Association. Circulation. 1999;100(10): 1132–3.
156. Buxton OM, Pavlova M, Reid EW, Wang W, Simonson DC, Adler GK. Sleep restriction for 1 week reduces insulin sensitivity in healthy men. Diabetes. 2010;59(9):2126–33.
157. Donga E, Van Dijk M, Van Dijk JG, Biermasz NR, Lammers G-J, Van Kralingen KW, et al. A single night of partial sleep deprivation induces insulin resistance in multiple metabolic pathways in healthy subjects. J Clin Endocrinol Metab. 2010;95(6): 2963–8.
158. Chaput J-P, Després J-P, Bouchard C, Tremblay A. Association of sleep duration with type 2 diabetes and impaired glucose tolerance. Diabetologia. 2007;50(11):2298–304.

159. Tuomilehto H, Peltonen M, Partinen M, Seppä J, Saaristo T, Korpi-Hyövälti E, et al. Sleep duration is associated with an increased risk for the prevalence of type 2 diabetes in middle-aged women—The FIN-D2D survey. Sleep Med. 2008;9(3):221–7.
160. Rafalson L, Donahue RP, Stranges S, Lamonte MJ, Dmochowski J, Dorn J, et al. Short sleep duration is associated with the development of impaired fasting glucose: the Western New York Health Study. Ann Epidemiol. 2010;20(12):883–9.
161. Xu Q, Song Y, Hollenbeck A, Blair A, Schatzkin A, Chen H. Day napping and short night sleeping are associated with higher risk of diabetes in older adults. Diabetes Care. 2010;33(1):78–83.
162. Kawakami N, Takatsuka N, Shimizu H. Sleep disturbance and onset of type 2 diabetes. Diabetes Care. 2004;27(1):282–3.
163. Patel SR, Ayas NT, Malhotra MR, White DP, Schernhammer ES, Speizer FE, et al. A prospective study of sleep duration and mortality risk in women. Sleep. 2004;27(3):440–4.

Sleep Deprivation and Rheumatologic Disease

12

Vivien C. Abad and Christian Guilleminault

Introduction

Our 24/7 world demands longer work hours, longer work shifts, constant connectivity, and a culture of sleep machismo. It is not surprising, therefore, that the prevalence of sleep deprivation is rising. Over the past 40 years, nocturnal sleep duration has decreased from over 8 h/night to 6.22 h per night [1]. In a cross-sectional survey of 110,411 adults from 2004 to 2007, 28.3 % self-reported sleeping ≤6 h per night. Measures of poor health, including pain, increased the odds of short sleep [2]. The percentage of Americans not meeting their sleep needs more than doubled from 29 % in 2009 to 63 % in 2011 [3]. What constitutes optimal sleep duration? The amount of sleep required varies depending upon age, gender, prior sleep amounts, genetic, and physiological factors. Most adults sleep between 7 and 8 h per night. Sleep durations that are shorter or longer than 7–8 h in a 24-h period have been associated with increased risks for cardiovascular disease, cognitive problems with learning and memory, depression, diabetes, increased accident risks, and excess mortality [4–11].

Sleep deprivation occurs when sleep obtained is insufficient to support adequate alertness, maintain performance, and support health. Sleep deprivation can be total or partial. Total sleep deprivation in humans is mainly seen in the experimental setting, but long-term total sleep deprivation is not ethically feasible. Partial sleep deprivation is more common in the clinical setting. Partial sleep deprivation occurs in one of three ways: (1) sleep fragmentation disrupting the normal progression of sleep, (2) selective sleep-stage deprivation, and (3) sleep restriction through reduced sleep duration. Sleep fragmentation is associated with painful conditions and various sleep disorders, while selective sleep-stage deprivation can be associated with medication use. Sleep restriction is more common as part of lifestyle changes.

The hypothesized restorative properties of sleep are crucial in combating the effects of illness and enhancing a sense of well-being. Sleep deprivation can be detrimental in the setting of underlying rheumatologic diseases, many of which have arthritis as a prominent complaint/finding. Short sleep (less than 6 h per night) is more prevalent in adults with arthritis (15 %) compared to those without arthritis (11 %) [3]. Since arthritis affects at least 46.4 million Americans [12], improving sleep in this population could have a significant impact. In this chapter, we explore what is known about the relationship between sleep deprivation and various rheumatologic diseases and identify what needs further study.

V.C. Abad, M.D., M.B.A. (✉) • C. Guilleminault, M.D., D.M., D.Biol.
Division of Sleep Medicine, Department of Psychiatry and Behavioral Sciences, Stanford University School of Medicine, Redwood City, CA, USA
e-mail: vcabad@gmail.com

M.T. Bianchi (ed.), *Sleep Deprivation and Disease: Effects on the Body, Brain and Behavior*, DOI 10.1007/978-1-4614-9087-6_12,

Cytokines, Sleep Deprivation, Inflammation, and Rheumatologic Diseases

Role of Cytokines

Central to the immune response are cytokines, a large family of proteins, peptides, and glycoproteins that act as messengers between cells within the immune system and between immune system cells and host tissue cells. Cytokines are involved in cell-to-cell signaling, coordinating B-cell and T-cell immune interactions and amplifying immune reactivity. Cytokines bind to receptors that subsequently send signals to recipient cells, thereby altering the function or phenotype of those cells. Following activation, the subset of T cells known as CD4 T cells develops into different T helper (Th) cell subsets with characteristic cytokine profiles and distinct effector functions. The first Th subsets identified were termed Th1 and Th2 cells, depending on the cytokines they produce. Th1 cytokines, which include interleukin (IL)-1β, tumor necrosis factor (TNF)-α, and IL-6, are pro-inflammatory and trigger the acute phase response (APR). Th2 cytokines, which include interferon (IFN)-α, IFN-β, IL-4, and IL-10, are anti-inflammatory and down-regulate the APR, in addition to modulating the sleep response. More recently, another subset of Th cells called Th17 has been characterized. Th17 cells induce tissue reactions by producing IL-17, IL-17F, and IL-22. Th17 cells also secrete IL-21, which produce inflammatory mediators including TNF-α and IL-6. These cytokines play a key role in the pathogenesis of inflammatory arthritis (see Table 12.1), and most of the recent progress in treating these disorders has involved modulation of specific cytokines (see Tables 12.2 and 12.3).

Table 12.1 Rheumatologic disorders and cytokines

Rheumatologic disorder	Cytokines
Rheumatoid arthritis	↑ IL-1, IL-1Ra, IL-2, IL-4, IL-6, IL-8, IL-10, IL-12, IL-13, IL-15, IL-17, IL-18, IL-23, IL-29, IL-32, IL-33, IFN-β, MCP-1, TGF-β, TNF, EGF, bFGF levels in synovial fluid [128–131].
Juvenile idiopathic arthritis	↑ IL1-β, IL-6, IL-8, IL-17, IL-18, TNF-α in serum [131, 132] ↑ IL-22 and IL-17in serum in juvenile psoriasis variant [132]
Seronegative spondyloarthropathies	
Ankylosing spondylitis	↑ IL-6, IL-17, TGF-β, IFN-γ in synovium [133] ↑ TNF-α, ↓TGF-β in sacroiliac joints [131]
Psoriatic arthritis	↑ IL-1β, IL-2, IL-10, IL-12, IL-15, IL-17, IL-18, IL-23, and TNF in synovium [67]
Systemic lupus erythematosus	↑ IL-4, IL-6, IL-10 and IL-18 in serum [131]; disease activity correlates with IL-18 levels [131] ↑ IL-1α, IL-8, CXCR1, CXCR2 in PBMC [129] ↓ IL-16, CCR7 in PBMC [129]
Sjögren's syndrome	↑ IL-2, IFN-γ, IL-4, IL-5, IL-13 and slight ↑ in IL-17, IL-6, IL-23, and TGF-β in salivary glands [134] ↑ IL-1, IL6, IL12, IL-18, TNF in salivary ductal epithelium [134]
Scleroderma	↑ IL-4, IL-6, IL-8, IL-13 levels in serum and IL-1α in epidermal keratinocytes [135]. ↑ IL-17 serum levels stimulates IL-1β and IL-6 expression by endothelial cells [131]
Behcet's disease	↑ IL-1, IL-6, IL-8, IL-10, IL-12, IL-17, IL-18, TNF levels in serum [131, 136]

IFN Interferon, *IL* interleukin, *PBMC* peripheral blood mononuclear cell, *CCR7* chemokine receptor 7, *CXCR1* chemokine receptor, *CXCR2* chemokine receptor, *EGF* epidermal growth factor, *bFGF* basic fibroblast growth factor, *TNF* tumor necrosis factor

Table 12.2 Biologic and new DMARD agents used to treat rheumatic disorders

Agent	Description
TNF Inhibitors	
Adalimumab (Humira)	Human anti-TNF monoclonal antibody that binds soluble TNF
Certolizumab (Cimzia)	Pegylated, humanized anti-TNF Fab' fragment
Etanercept (Enbrel)	Human IgG-TNF receptor fusion protein
Golimumab (Simponi)	Human anti-TNF monoclonal antibody
Infliximab (Remicade)	Chimeric (mouse-human) anti-TNF monoclonal antibody
Other biologic agents	
Abatacept (Orencia)	Human IgG-CTLA4 (Cytotoxic T-Lymphocyte Antigen-4) fusion protein that inhibits costimulation of T cells by antigen-presenting cells.
Anakinra (Kineret)	Human IL-1 receptor antagonist protein
Belimumab (Benlysta)	Human monoclonal antibody to B-cell lymphocyte stimulator (BLys)
Canakinumab (Ilaris)	Human monoclonal antibody to IL-1β
Rituximab (Rituxan)	Chimeric (mouse-human) monoclonal antibody to the pan-B-cell marker CD-20
Tocilizumab (Actemra)	Humanized monoclonal antibody to IL-6 receptor
New DMARD agent	
Tofacitinib (Xeljanz)	Janus kinase (JAK) inhibitor that interferes with cytokine signaling

Table 12.3 Rheumatologic disorders and biologic response modifiers

Rheumatologic disorder	TNF inhibitors	Other biologic and new DMARD agents
Rheumatoid arthritis	Adalimumab	Abatacept
	Certolizumab	
	Etancercept	Anakinra
	Golimumab	
	Infliximab	Rituximab
		Tocilizumab
		Tofacitinib
Juvenile idiopathic arthritis	Adalimumab	Abatacept
	Etancercept	
		Tocilizumab
		Canakinumab
Seronegative spondyloarthropathies		
Ankylosing spondylitis	Adalimumab	
	Etancercept	
	Golimumab	
	Infliximab	
	Adalimumab Etancercept	
	Golimumab	Abatacept (off-label)
	Infliximab	
Psoriatic arthritis		
Systemic lupus erythematosus		Belimumab
Sjögren's syndrome		Rituximab (off-label)
Scleroderma		
Behcet's disease		Rituximab (off-label)

Source: Data from refs. [33, 119–121, 137–139]

Sleep Deprivation and the Immune Response

Levels of cytokines can be affected by many factors. Stress, infection, and tissue damage result in release of inflammatory cytokines. Likewise, disruption of the normal sleep wake cycle via sleep deprivation can significantly alter immune function and host defense mechanisms.

Following 40 h of total sleep deprivation in healthy volunteers under constant routine conditions, the pro-inflammatory markers E-selectin, intracellular adhesion molecule (ICAM)-1, and IL-1β increased [4]. The anti-inflammatory marker interleukin-1 receptor antagonist (IL-1Ra) also increased, whereas levels of the acute phase proteins IL-6 and C-reactive protein (CRP) decreased. Levels of pro-inflammatory VCAM did not change [13]. This study shows that total sleep deprivation may elicit a mixed response with an increase in some pro-inflammatory markers, but a decrease or no change in others and an increase in an anti-inflammatory marker. Others have reported that total sleep deprivation of healthy volunteers for 4 nights increases plasma levels of soluble TNF-α receptor 1 (sTNFR1) on days 2–4 and increases plasma levels of IL-6 on day 4 [14]. In another study, following 2 nights of total sleep deprivation in healthy adult men, neutrophils and CD4 T cells increased, and the increase in CD4 T cells persisted even after sleep recovery [15]. However, in this study, levels of studied cytokines (IL-1β, IL-2, IL-4, IL-6, IL-10, TNF-α, and IL-6) did not change. The reasons for the discrepant cytokine levels among these studies are uncertain, but factors may include the difference in duration of total sleep deprivation and methodological differences (circadian phase, blood sampling frequency, limits of assay sensitivity), any local inflammatory reaction to indwelling catheter, and differences in subjects (BMI).

In healthy adults, partial sleep deprivation (4 h [16] to 6 h [17] sleep time/night) decreases the proportion of natural killer (NK) cells, reduces lymphokine-activated killer cell activity, and lowers interleukin IL-2 production [16, 17]. In contrast, partial sleep deprivation (4 h sleep time/night) in healthy adults increases peripheral mononuclear cells, including B lymphocytes, and increases levels of IL-1β, IL-6, IL-17, TNF-α, and CRP [14, 18–20]. After recovery sleep, NK cells and B cells recover almost completely, though IL-17 remains elevated [18].

Partial sleep deprivation also activates nuclear factor (NF)-κβ transcription control [21], which plays a critical role in controlling cellular expression of pro-inflammatory genes [22]. In contrast to total sleep deprivation, partial sleep deprivation of healthy volunteers for 4 nights does not increase plasma levels of sTNFR1 or IL-6, suggesting that these changes during total sleep deprivation are due to the homeostatic drive [14].

Gender differences in response to sleep deprivation may help explain the differential risk profile for inflammatory disorders, such as arthritis, where more women are affected compared to men. With sleep deprivation, activation of NF-κβ occurs primarily in females, rather than males. In the Whitehall II study [23], women who slept longer had lower IL-6 levels and lower bedtime CRP levels compared to women who had shorter sleep. In men, there was no relationship between sleep duration and IL-6 levels or bedtime CRP levels [23]. In a study of moderate sleep restriction (sleep was reduced by 2 h/night from 8 to 6 h) in healthy men and women, 24-h secretion of IL-6 was increased in both sexes, while TNF-α was increased only in men [17]. Peak cortisol secretion was lower after sleep restriction than at baseline, and this difference was more pronounced in men [17]. After a night of partial sleep deprivation (4 h sleep time/night) in 26 healthy adults, both sexes showed a marked increase in lipopolysaccharide-stimulated production of IL-6 and TNF-α in the morning. Production of these cytokines increased during the early and late evening in women, while levels decreased in men, indicating that women had greater cellular immune alteration than men [21].

Does recovery sleep correct the abnormalities induced by sleep deprivation? One night of recovery sleep does not allow full recovery of a number of these systemic immune and inflammatory markers [24]. Does napping help? In healthy males subjected to a night of severe sleep restriction (2 h sleep time/night), leukocytes, especially neutrophils, increased and IL-8 levels increased. These effects persisted after 8-h recovery sleep. However, in subjects who napped (2 h) or who had a longer recovery sleep (10 h), these values returned nearly to baseline [25].

Clinical Correlation

Many of the rheumatologic diseases involving joint and/or muscle inflammation are associated with pain, fatigue, depression, and disturbed sleep. Sleep deprivation can enhance pain, induce or worsen fatigue, and contribute to depression. In our 2008 review of the interrelationship between sleep and rheumatologic disorders [26], we highlighted what was known and not known about sleep and rheumatologic disorders and underscored the need for more research into these issues. Many reports have been published since then elucidating these various aspects. However, there are still aspects that await further clarification. The question as to whether sleep restriction versus sleep fragmentation contributes to increased pain remains controversial. In a study of normal subjects [27], sleep continuity disturbance, but not simple sleep restriction, impaired endogenous pain-inhibitory function and increases spontaneous pain, thereby supporting the theory that sleep continuity is important. However, in a study in patients with rheumatoid arthritis (RA), it appeared that sleep duration is the more important factor, since these patients did not have evidence for sleep fragmentation [28].

As discussed earlier in the section on sleep deprivation, studies have shown that sleep loss can influence the inflammatory and immune responses, which could potentially lead to deleterious effects in patients with arthritis. The above studies also showed improvement in some immune and inflammatory markers following recovery sleep/napping. These findings lend credence to claims by fatigued patients with arthritis and poor sleep quality at night that napping during the day helps "recharge" their energy supply. What has not been clearly established are answers to the following: (1) Does napping benefit all arthritis patients or does it benefit only patients with inflammatory arthritis? (2) Does napping benefit only those with poor sleep quality and/or insufficient sleep quantity? (3) What is the optimum timing for naps? (4) What is the optimum duration of the nap? (5) Does napping affect disease activity, fatigue, depression, and does it worsen insomnia? The answers to these various questions await further investigation.

Rheumatologic Diseases

Rheumatoid Arthritis

RA, a systemic autoimmune disease characterized by symmetric polyarthritis, affects 1.3 million adults in the United States [12]. About 54–70 % of adult RA subjects complain of difficulty falling sleep, poor quality sleep, multiple awakenings at night, non-restorative sleep, early morning awakenings, daytime sleepiness, and fatigue [29–35]. Various studies have reported short total sleep time, suggesting partial sleep deprivation [29–39], but this issue is still not completely settled. Although self-reported measures of short total sleep time and daytime symptoms suggest partial sleep deprivation, differences between self-report and objective measures, together with absence of significant differences during polysomnography (PSG) in recorded total sleep time between controls and subjects [30, 31, 36], lack of PSG changes suggestive of prior sleep deprivation, and reports of sleep state misperception in RA subjects confuse the issue [39]. Diary-recorded mean sleep time was shorter at 6.85 h ± 1.32 compared to actigraphy-recorded mean sleep time of 7.23 h ± 1.08, in a study of 25 women with RA [40]. Many RA patients focus on poor sleep quality and sleep fragmentation rather than duration of sleep. Sixty-two percent of RA participants ($n = 145$) surveyed reported poor sleep quality, with fragmented sleep as the most common abnormality [41]. The two most commonly cited reasons for awakening were the need to use the bathroom (51 %) and pain (33 %) [41].

PSG studies have shown normal sleep architecture with normal total sleep time, REM sleep time, non-REM sleep stages, and normal number of sleep cycles [30, 31, 36]. NREM sleep latency is usually normal [30, 36], although prolonged sleep latencies may occur associated with disease flares [31, 36, 37]. Alpha intrusions and/or sleep fragmentation may account for poor sleep quality, with PSG and actigraphy demonstrating increased number of awakenings per hour, prolonged wake after sleep onset (WASO), increased movement index, and reduced sleep efficiency [31–33, 36, 37, 41]. Actigraphy performed in a small number of RA patients has demonstrated a positive correlation between increased nocturnal pain and body movements at night and a negative correlation between nocturnal pain and sleep efficiency [33].

The number of nocturnal awakenings also positively correlated with the intensity of morning pain [33]. Alpha intrusion into NREM sleep has been reported in RA subjects [30–32, 36], but this could represent either a non-specific epiphenomenon or arousal intrusions disrupting sleep.

The role of disease activity in impairing sleep has been explored. Questionnaire-based studies with large sample sizes ($n=200$ [42], $n=8{,}676$ [38]) have reported positive correlations between disease activity and sleep complaints, while a study with 19 RA subjects did not show any correlation [31]. PSG studies of RA patients in flare ($n=5$) demonstrated more sleep fragmentation, frequent nocturnal awakenings, and reduced sleep efficiency compared to non-flare subjects ($n=10$) with positive correlations between sleep fragmentation and fatigue ($r=0.42$) and pain ($r=0.91$) in the flare group [37]. Increased disease markers (morning stiffness, joint pain, joint tenderness) positively correlated with slow wave sleep and Stage Wake and negatively correlated with Stage 2 NREM sleep [30]. The increase in slow wave sleep is postulated to reflect the need for restorative sleep in these patients. In 38 RA patients who were followed longitudinally for a mean of 175.8 ± 70.9 days from the baseline polysomnographic study, deterioration in disease activity was associated with increased time in Stage 1 NREM sleep, SWS, and Stage Wake and reduced time in Stage 2 NREM sleep on repeat PSG [34].

Treatment with anti-TNF-α therapy (etanercept in 9, adalimumab in 1) significantly improved pain, fatigue, disease activity index, and modified health assessment questionnaire scores in ten RA subjects [41]. PSG showed significant improvement in sleep efficiency, reduction in WASO minutes, and a trend toward reduction in sleep latency. Sleep-stage transitions/hours slightly decreased, SWS % slightly decreased, and REM % slightly increased, but these did not significantly vary from the control group [41]. Various studies [37, 41, 43] indicate that sleep impairment is associated with disease flare and that response to anti-TNF-α therapy [44] can improve sleep and reduce pain and fatigue. In a study of six RA patients, 1 day after the first infusion with infliximab, sleep efficiency increased, sleep latency decreased, and the number of sleep-stage transitions significantly decreased, although the number of swollen and tender joints or joint stiffness had not improved [43]. Median (IR) for SWS % increased from 9.5 (10) to 31 (30) and REM sleep % increased from 2 (10) to 11.5 (8) [43]. Since the improvement in sleep parameters appeared unrelated to amelioration of joint discomfort, the authors postulated a central effect through inhibition of circulating TNF levels.

Sleep deprivation and altered cytokine levels are associated with increased sensitivity to pain. Animal studies have shown hyperalgesic effects from paradoxic sleep deprivation [45]. Prior human sleep deprivation studies have not yielded consistent results as far as the effects of sleep deprivation on pain modulation. Data from five studies showed hyperalgesic changes from sleep deprivation, while three studies did not show any effect on pain, with the combined evidence from these studies suggesting that SWS deprivation induces a hyperalgesic state, while the effects of REM sleep deprivation in humans are less clear [46]. In 59 female RA patients who underwent pressure pain threshold testing assessing hyperalgesia at joint and non-joint sites, sleep problems were associated with low pain threshold at joint and non-joint sites, suggesting both peripheral and central mechanisms [47]. Conversely, pain has been a significant predictor of subsequent sleep disturbances in RA patients [30, 34, 48, 49].

The presence of pain in some patients despite treatment with nonsteroidal anti-inflammatory drugs (NSAIDs), disease-modifying antirheumatic drugs (DMARDs), or biologic agents suggests that factors other than inflammation influence pain. In a cross-sectional analysis of 12,090 RA patients conducted over a 6-year period, pain levels were almost constant over RA duration and were increased in women, ethnic minorities, smokers, and less educated individuals [50]. A biphasic pain response was shown in a longitudinal study conducted over 5 years in 882 RA patients: pain levels decreased during the first 3 years, but then subsequently increased over time [51]. The initial improvement in pain was attributed to reduced inflammation, with the subsequent resurgence attributed to other pain pathways [51]. Local inflammation in the joints incites release of inflammatory mediators that activate primary afferent nociceptive neurons and result in peripheral sensitization [52]. Central augmentation of pain via central sensitization and/or loss of descending analgesia has also been suggested [53]. Repetitive noxious stimuli evoked enhanced cortical responses in RA patients, compared to control subjects, suggesting changes in modulation of pain centrally [54]. Functional magnetic resonance imaging in 31 RA patients revealed increased gray matter content in the basal ganglia [55]. These basal ganglia changes may result from altered motor control or prolonged pain processing in RA patients [55]. The peripheral and central sensitization triggered by repetitive bombardment by painful stimuli highlights the importance of addressing pain issues promptly and effectively, in addition to treating the primary illness. Another study showed improvement in polysomnographic parameters with increased sleep efficiency and reduced minutes of WASO (compared to baseline PSG) associated with improvement in pain as well as in disease parameters [44].

In addition to its hyperalgesic effects, sleep deprivation can counteract analgesic effects of pharmacological treatments involving opioidergic and serotoninergic mechanisms of action [56]. The descending pain-inhibitory control systems contain opioidergic and monoaminergic links, which can be influenced by sleep deprivation through changes in the pre-synaptic and post-synaptic serotoninergic systems or inhibition of opioid synthesis or reduced affinity of mu- and delta-opioid receptors. A study in rats comparing analgesic effects of three doses of morphine, each administered to three categories of rats—(1) rats deprived of sleep for 96 h (2) rats which had 24-h recovery after partial sleep deprivation, and (3) normal controls [57]—showed that the usual analgesic dose of morphine was effective in the control group, but both groups of sleep-deprived rats did not respond except to the highest dose of morphine [57]. This could suggest that painful conditions in sleep-deprived patients may require higher opiate doses for analgesic effect.

With the focus on poor quality sleep, attention has slipped away from adequate sleep duration. A study of partial sleep deprivation (4 h sleep time/night) comparing 27 RA subjects with normal controls showed that measures of sleep fragmentation were similar in both groups [28]. However, RA patients reported higher pain symptoms and disease-specific activity parameters (as indexed by joint pain severity and self-reported number of painful joints) were worse. Mood symptoms including fatigue, depression, and anxiety were increased in RA patients. The effects of sleep loss on pain symptoms were independent of changes in mood symptoms and the increases in mood symptoms in response to sleep loss did not appear to mediate increases in self-reported pain responses [28]. Partial sleep loss in this study was associated with increased joint symptoms and raises the issue that recurrent nights of sleep loss with repeated elevations of RA-specific joint pain might exacerbate RA symptomatology.

Healthcare outcomes are being identified for many chronic diseases. These results may vary depending upon the manner in which patients are queried. Among 23 desired outcomes identified in RA patient-focus groups, staying independent (39 %), reducing pain (36 %), and keeping mobile (34 %) were the top three selected outcomes. Among seven domains identified by professionals, a patient panel weighted them as follows: pain (21 %), functional disability (16 %), fatigue (15 %), emotional well-being (12 %), sleep (12 %), coping (12 %), and physical well-being (12 %) [58].

In summary, RA patients complain of pain, depression, and fatigue. Sleep architecture is usually normal, but sleep is fragmented with increased arousals. Poor sleep quality has been linked to sleep fragmentation. Pain is cited as a significant cause of sleep fragmentation and sleep deprivation can exacerbate pain pathways. Sleep deprivation can contribute to inflammation and cytokine release. Anti-TNF therapy can improve pain, fatigue, disease activity parameters, and improve sleep. Duration of sleep is also important and this should be emphasized in patient education.

Juvenile Idiopathic Arthritis

Juvenile idiopathic arthritis (JIA), a heterogenous group of inflammatory joint diseases with symptom onset before age 16 years and duration ≥6 weeks, includes pauciarticular, polyarticular (rheumatoid factor positive and rheumatoid factor negative), and systemic subsets previously known as juvenile rheumatoid arthritis (JRA) in addition to enthesis-related and psoriatic arthritis. In 2007, the Center for Disease Control and Prevention estimated that approximately 300,000 children in the United States are affected with arthritis or other rheumatic conditions.

Forty-four percent of 92 JIA subjects (oligoarticular $n=31$, polyarticular $n=33$, systemic $n=28$) reported disturbed sleep (Child Sleep Health Questionnaire >41), despite mostly low to moderate disease activity and low number of swollen or painful joints [59]. Two-thirds reported low to moderate pain, while one-third reported no pain; self-reported pain was higher in the polyarticular-onset type. There was no correlation between disease activity and the severity of the sleep disturbance. Pain and fatigue were correlated. "Worst pain" was modestly correlated with sleep disturbance and patient-reported sleep disturbance correlated moderately with pain and fatigue. Subjects treated with NSAIDS had a lower CSHQ score when adjusted for pain, but CSHQ did not differ between subjects taking DMARDS, biologics, or prednisone.

Similar findings were present in another study of 70 children with JIA (oligoarticular $n=26$, polyarticular $n=40$, systemic $n=4$) compared with normal control subjects [60]. JIA subjects had significantly higher overall sleep disturbance scores on CSHQ with mean of 45.0 ± 7.3 [60]. Total sleep duration did not differ from the control group, with JIA group mean sleep duration of 9.27 ± 0.54 h. Significantly higher scores for sleep-onset delay, night awakenings, and parasomnias were present in the JIA group. Although scores for bedtime resistance, sleep duration, sleep anxiety, sleep disordered breathing, and daytime sleepiness subscales were slightly higher in children with JIA, they did not significantly differ from the control group [60]. There was no difference in neurobehavioral performance. However, regardless of group, children with clinically significant sleep disturbances had slower mean simple reaction time and mean 5-choice reaction time compared to those below the cutoff score [60].

PSG in 16 patients with JIA documented sleep fragmentation [61]. JIA patients had 90 % more arousals and awakenings and the median length of uninterrupted sleep in NREM Stages 2 and 3 and REM sleep was 60 % shorter than in normal controls [61]. More sleep-stage shifts occurred (23.5 ± 10.8 events in patients compared to 14.9 ± 4.0 in controls). Alpha delta sleep occurred in 15 % of JIA subjects compared to <1 % in controls [61]. Similar findings were seen in 20 JIA children when compared to normal controls. The periodic limb movement (PLM) index was significantly higher, and isolated leg movements, arousals, and increased alpha activity in NREM sleep were present in JIA subjects. Pain symptoms and disability were related to sleep fragmentation [62].

Seventy children with JIA, ages 6–11 years ($n=38$ with active JIA, $n=32$ with inactive JIA), reported symptoms via questionnaire and completed 2 nights of PSG [63]. Pain and fatigue were significantly higher in children with active compared to inactive disease, although PSG and self-reported sleep variables were not different. All children showed longer sleep latency and reduced sleep efficiency on night 1, consistent with first night effect. Younger children with active disease slept more quickly than older children (sleep latency 13 ± 4.0 vs. 23.3 ± 3.3 min) with active disease and sleep duration was longer (563 ± 9.6 vs. 537 ± 8.0 min). The PLM Index was normal. The mean apnea–hypopnea index (AHI) was similar (1.8 ± 3) between the active group and the inactive group (1.3 ± 0.8) [63].

Normative data from multiple sleep latency tests (MSLTs) in children have shown that normal, pre-pubertal, school-aged children rarely fall asleep during standard 20-min daytime nap opportunities and that older (Tanner stages 3–5) adolescents are sleepier on MSLT [64]. MSLTs in children with JIA vary in results. In a study of 16 JIA subjects (ages 12 ± 4 years) compared to normal controls, MSLTs performed in 7/16 JIA subjects showed mean sleep latency of 10.3 ± 2.6 min [61]. In this study, JIA children were sleepier and reported longer afternoon naps of 1.8 ± 1.3 h compared to 0.3 ± 0.8 h in controls. In another study, MSLTs were performed on 70 children with JIA, 6–11 years of age [65]. Children with active JIA ($n = 38$) had slightly shorter mean sleep latencies (14.9 ± 5.9) than children with inactive JIA ($n = 32$) with mean sleep latency of 16.5 ± 5.5 min [65]. The difference in mean sleep latency results from these studies could be due to sample size, difference in ages, and disease status of the subjects.

In summary, sleep disturbances are common in JIA and are associated with pain and daytime fatigue. Sleep duration did not differ from normal controls, but sleep is fragmented with more arousals and stage shifts, more frequent reports of parasomnia, more PLMS, and more sleep disordered breathing. Pain symptoms and disability are associated with sleep fragmentation. Addressing pain issues and treating symptomatic periodic leg movements of sleep and sleep disordered breathing may help consolidate sleep. Longitudinal outcome studies with objective measures for sleep, to demonstrate the effects of interventions that improve sleep on disease activity, fatigue, depression, disability, would help enhance our understanding of JIA.

Seronegative Spondyloarthropathies

These disorders affect the spine, sacroiliac joints, and peripheral joints, with pathologic changes that affect the enthesis (ligamentous insertion into the bone) in addition to the synovium. Seronegative spondyloarthropathies affect about 0.6–1.9 % of the US population. Five subtypes include psoriatic arthritis (PsA), ankylosing spondylitis (AS), reactive arthritis, arthritis with inflammatory bowel disease, and undifferentiated types.

Psoriatic Arthritis

Between 5.8 and 7.5 million Americans have cutaneous psoriasis, according to National Psoriasis Foundation (NPF) surveys from 2003 to 2006 [66]. Thirty percent of psoriasis patients surveyed by NPF in 2011 reported symptoms of arthritis. The exact prevalence and incidence of PsA are unknown due to lack of widely accepted diagnostic criteria [67]. The reported prevalence of PsA ranges from 0.056 to 0.28 % in a US-based population study, while the reported incidence has varied from 3 to 23 cases per 100,000 [67]. PsA is an inflammatory, peripheral, or axial arthritis that usually affects adults between ages 33–55 years, but also represents up to 20 % of childhood arthritis cases (juvenile PsA). NPF surveys from 2003 to 2006 reported that in patients with cutaneous psoriasis, 48 % had sleep problems at least once a month and 11.3 % had sleep problems more than 15 days/month.

Using 2005 NPF survey data ($n = 405$), Duffin et al. [68] reported that PsA was the most significant predictor of sleep interference in patients with psoriasis, with odds ratio of 3.27 (95 % CI 1.77–6.05, $P < 0.001$). Other predictors were itching, with odds ratio of 1.24 (95 % CI 1.11–1.39, $P < 0.001$) and physical pain/ soreness with odds ratio of 1.12 (95 % CI 1.00–1.25, $P < 0.01$) [68]. The impact of cutaneous psoriasis on emotional well-being also predicted sleep interference, with odds ratio of 1.19 (95 % CI 1.02–1.40, $P < 0.05$) [68].

Pruritus is an important cause of sleep disruption. In a study of 101 patients with psoriasis, pruritus was reported in 84 %, occurring daily in

77 % of cases and weekly in 18 %. Sixty-nine percent of patients with pruritus had difficulty falling asleep and 66 % reported nocturnal awakenings; only 6 % used soporific medications. Pruritus was described as painful by 17 % of subjects [69].

Pain and depression are known disruptors of sleep and may contribute to poor quality sleep in PsA [69]. Sleep apnea is another potential disruptor of sleep. A study of 33 PsA subjects [70] showed 54.5 % prevalence of sleep apnea, but study participants were overweight, five patients were hypertensive, sample size was small, and there was no control group. Given the study limitations, the true prevalence of sleep apnea in patients with PsA remains uncertain. Although some PSG parameters were reported [70], these did not include total sleep time, sleep efficiency, arousal indices, or sleep stage shifts to assess whether sleep disruption was present.

PsA not only impairs sleep but also worsens quality of life (QOL). In a study comparing 799 patients with inflammatory rheumatic diseases to normal controls, patients with PsA ($n=65$ axial PsA, $n=101$ peripheral PsA) had worse scores in the Physical and Mental Component Summaries of the SF-36 scales [71]. The physical component scores were associated with high disease activity and comorbidity, while poor mental functioning was correlated with the severity of the psoriatic lesions. Bodily pain scores on visual analogue scales (VAS) were also worse for PsA subjects than normal controls [71].

Impaired sleep in PsA can improve with adalimumab therapy. A group of 152 patients with chronic plaque psoriasis and suboptimal response to prior therapy (etanercept, methotrexate, or narrowband ultraviolet B phototherapy) were treated with adalimumab [72]. Mean sleep duration (self-reported) prior to treatment was 6.6 ± 1.2 h. Using Medical Outcomes Study Sleep Scales scores, sleep quality improved by 15 % compared to pretreatment scores. PsA pain scores using VAS also improved [72]. The improvement in sleep was partially explained by improvements in objectively measured psoriasis signs [72].

In summary, significant predictors for sleep impairment in patients with psoriasis are PsA, pruritus, pain, and depression. The role of sleep apnea is to be determined further. Additional studies are needed with subjective parameters (scales), objective sleep parameters (actigraphy, PSG), and disease activity parameters to determine how pruritus, pain, depression, sleep disordered breathing, and sleep influence each other.

Ankylosing Spondylitis

Approximately 2.7 million Americans suffer from AS, a chronic, progressive inflammatory disease of the axial skeleton, entheses, and sacroiliac joints. In various studies, sleep disturbances in patients with AS have ranged from 54.1 % ($n=175$) to 58.6 % ($n=314$) to 68.8 % ($n=125$) [73–75]. More AS patients perceived insufficient sleep when compared to normal controls, especially among women with AS (80.8 %) compared to men (50 %) [76]. In addition, 32 % of women with AS reported prolonged wakefulness ≥ 1 h compared to 15 % of men with AS [76].

In 125 AS patients, mean sleep duration was short at 6.5 ± 1.5 h and mean sleep efficiency was reduced at 79.5 ± 17 %, consistent with sleep restriction [75]. Almost half (49.6 %) of AS subjects reported difficulties in falling asleep with mean sleep-onset latency of 31 min. Eleven percent reported sleep latencies greater than 60 min [75]. Sleep continuity was impaired, with 66.4 % reporting waking up ≥ 3 times/week [75]. Sleep was disrupted by pain (36 %), socio-psychological factors including stress (17 %), and other factors including snoring and awakenings by children (9 %) [76]. Pain at bedtime and during the night disturbs sleep and correlates with daytime fatigue [76]. A longer sleep latency and total sleep duration have been positively correlated with disease activity, functional status, depressed mood, and perceived stress [75]. Sleep quality was rated as fairly bad to very bad by 41.6 % of AS patients, with mean global PSQI score of 8.7 ± 5, which is highly indicative of poor sleep quality [75]. Poor sleep quality (PSQI > 5) positively correlates with increased pain, poor QOL, depressed mood, higher disease activity, and mobility restrictions [77]. In this study, however, although subjective sleep quality and habitual sleep efficiency were worse compared to controls, sleep latency, sleep duration, sleep disturbance, use of sleeping medication, and daytime dysfunction domains did not significantly differ [77]. Other prevalent QOL issues for AS patients are stiffness (90.2 %), pain (83.1 %), and fatigue (62.4 %) [73]. Fatigued patients complained of waking up more than three times each night, and 41 % reported sleep disturbances compared to 26 % in the non-fatigued group [78]. Pain, functional disability, and stiffness were significantly correlated with fatigue [78].

For most patients with inflammatory arthritis, pain is rated as a top priority for improvement by patients, regardless of whether they have RA, PsA, JIA, or AS. What is different is that AS patients rate improvement of sleep disturbances as a top priority compared to patients with other inflammatory arthropathies, as shown in a study of 2,138 adults [79]. Similarly, JIA patients rated improvement of fatigue higher than patients with other types of arthritis [79].

In summary, a high proportion of AS patients suffer from sleep disturbances including sleep onset and sleep maintenance insomnia. Sleep fragmentation and awakenings are associated with pain, psychological stress, and other factors. Daytime fatigue correlates with sleep disturbances and pain. Addressing sleep issues is an important priority for AS patients. We need outcome studies for interventions addressing insomnia (sleep onset and sleep maintenance), pain, fatigue, and disease activity, correlated with subjective and objective measures to assess sleep and QOL measures.

Systemic Lupus Erythematosus

Systemic lupus erythematosus (SLE) is an autoimmune disorder that affects 1.5 million Americans, with peak incidence between 15 and 45 years of age. It is more prevalent in women, African-Americans, Hispanics, Asians, and Native Americans.

Fifty-six to 72 % of SLE patients report moderate to severe sleep disturbances and poor sleep quality [80–82]. Compared to working control subjects, SLE patients ($n=172$) have worse ratings for total sleep time, sleep-onset latency, WASO, and sleep efficiency [83]. Depressed mood, steroid use, and lack of exercise contributed to poor sleep quality in 56/100 women with SLE [80]. The sleep deficit (difference between perceived need for sleep and actual sleep time) in SLE women (0.8 ± 0.9 h) did not significantly differ from normal controls (0.4 ± 0.8 h) [84], but there were more awakenings due to pain (including headache, muscular pain, joint pain), palpitations, sweating, and feeling breathless and there were longer periods of wakefulness in SLE patients.

In a group of 120 SLE patients, 81 % reported abnormal fatigue, while 60 % reported poor sleep quality. Fatigue scores were up to 33 % higher in patients with active disease, using the systemic lupus activity measure (SLAM), compared to patients with inactive disease [81]. Fatigue significantly correlates with sleep quality [81, 85], disease activity [81, 85], anxiety or depression [81, 82, 85], and pain [82]. Higher physical fatigue scores are associated with greater disease damage and activity, depressed mood, sleep disturbance, and less participation in physical activities, while mental fatigue is significantly influenced by depressed mood.

PSG findings in 35 SLE patients [86] compared to healthy controls showed impaired sleep efficiency, increased number of arousals, increased N1 sleep percentage, and reduced slow wave sleep percentage. Seventy-seven percent had increased alpha EEG intrusions [86]. Twenty-six percent of patients had sleep apnea and 23 % had PLM disorder. Fifty-one percent of patients had excessive sleepiness documented on ESS and mean sleep latency tests (MSLT), which was not related to sleep restriction. No correlation occurred between pathological sleepiness and neuropsychiatric SLE, disease activity, medications, or fibromyalgia. Although the group as a whole had mild to moderate depression scores, fewer of the sleepy patients were depressed [86]. Similar findings were seen in 14 SLE patients without fibromyalgia—there was more sleep fragmentation with more arousals and sleep state transitions [87]. Patients with active disease (AD,

$n = 6$) differed significantly from SLE patients with inactive disease (ID, $n = 8$) in the following parameters: (1) reduced mean sleep efficiency in AD patients (85.52 ± 8.60) compared to (92.21 ± 3.9) in ID patients; (2) less slow wave sleep percentage (9.58 ± 3.88) in AD compared to (17.54 ± 6.55) in ID patients; (3) more awakenings of <1 min in AD (21.30 ± 10.13) compared to ID (13.13 ± 7.7) patients. In this set of patients, 50 % of patients had mild to moderate sleep apnea and 50 % also had PLMs of sleep [87].

In an experimental mouse model of SLE, Palma et al. demonstrated that increased disease activity was associated with increased number of sleep-stage transitions and microarousals; during this time, pain threshold was also lower [88]. These findings are similar to what has been reported in human studies. Of interest is an earlier experiment by Palma et al., also in a mouse model of SLE, that showed that mice subjected to sleep deprivation had earlier onset of the disease [89]. This raises the question as to whether poor sleep in predisposed individuals could accelerate the onset of SLE.

In summary, SLE patients experience poor quality fragmented sleep, fatigue, pain, and depression [90]. PSG findings confirm sleep fragmentation and also document a higher prevalence of comorbid sleep disorders (sleep apnea, PLM disorder) that may contribute to sleep fragmentation and perceived poor sleep. Addressing sleep deprivation in SLE patients would include treating underlying comorbid sleep disorders in addition to addressing pain, depression, and disease parameters. Outcome studies with objective sleep parameters showing the results of these interventions on fatigue, pain, depression, disease activity, and QOL are needed.

Sjögren's Syndrome

About four million Americans have Sjögren's syndrome (SS), and 90 % of those affected are women. Fifty percent have primary Sjögren's syndrome (pSS), a systemic autoimmune disorder that affects exocrine glands, while the other 50 % have SS coexisting with a connective tissue disease.

Sleep is severely impaired in pSS patients, with 75 % complaining of moderate to severe sleep disturbances [91]. Compared to RA patients ($n = 42$) and healthy controls ($n = 60$), pSS patients ($n = 40$) had longer self-rated sleep latencies and significantly reduced sleep time (5.2 ± 0.3 h), while describing shorter need for sleep [79]. Compared to RA patients, pSS patients complained of significantly more difficulty falling asleep (33.3 % vs. 0 %), increased muscular tension (45 % vs. 12 %), increased "creeping sensation in the legs" (24 % vs. 2 %), increased pain (59 % vs. 38 %), and increased racing thoughts (28 % vs. 10 %) [92]. pSS patients also were significantly more fatigued, sleepier during the day, and felt more unrefreshed after sleep. PSG findings in 10 of pSS patients showed total sleep time of 358 min, reduced sleep efficiency ($n = 8$, mean SE of 70 %), increased number of awakenings ($n = 5$), prolonged WASO ($n = 9$), and increased alpha sleep ($n = 5$) [92]. Sleep fragmentation and nocturnal awakenings in pSS patients have been attributed to pain, headache, shortness of breath, and palpitations [93].

Poor sleep, fatigue, anxiety, and depression are prominent complaints by pSS patients [40, 93–95]. Sleep disturbances during the night correlate with overall fatigue levels [94]. Poor quality sleep and fatigue impair their QOL. Fatigue is perceived as the worst biopsychological stressor and a reason to seek treatment [40]. Fatigue worsens as the day progresses for patients with pSS, RA, and SLE [40, 94, 95]. There may be abatement in fatigue in the first hour after awakening in RA and SLE patients [94], or midmorning [95], but not in pSS patients [94]. Understanding the factors contributing to fatigue generation is an important part of treating patients with pSS [40, 95, 96].

Data collected from sleep diaries, questionnaires, and actigraphy over 35 consecutive days in 14 pSS and 35 RA subjects has shown that, in both groups, somatic and mental fatigue increased as the day progressed [40]. Women who had more severe discomfort and worse sleep also reported more severe fatigue. Evening discomfort predicted both somatic and mental fatigue the following afternoon and, on sleep disturbed nights, the association between evening discomfort and greater fatigue the next afternoon was stronger [40].This is similar to findings from another study which demonstrated that greater pain predicted fatigue the next day in patients with RA, OA, and fibromyalgia [97].

Daytime fatigue in pSS subjects is predicted by anxiety and nightly awakenings due to pain [96]. Restless legs syndrome (RLS), depression, and sicca symptoms also contribute to perception of fatigue [96]. Since RLS symptoms, nocturnal pain, depression, and sicca symptoms also lead to sleep fragmentation, addressing these predisposing factors could reduce disruption of sleep and improve fatigue. pSS patients experience significant functional disability compared to normal controls, and impaired function in these patients is associated with symptoms such as pain, fatigue, and depression, as well as disease activity [98]. It would seem appropriate that optimal management would encompass treatment of all of these aspects of the disease.

Symptomatic therapy addressing keratoconjunctivitis sicca and oral sicca symptoms as well as treatment for systemic complaints is well described in Vitali's review [99]. Rebamipide has been used systemically for oral sicca symptoms with inconclusive results [100]. In pSS patients with associated fibromyalgia and/or depression, tricyclic antidepressants should be avoided, but selective serotonin reuptake inhibitors may be utilized. Peripheral neuropathy can occur in 10–20 % of patients with pSS and may respond to immunosuppressive therapy [99]. Anti-TNF-α therapy with infliximab did not improve joint pain, fatigue, or sicca symptoms in pSS patients. Similarly, treatment with etanercept did not benefit pSS patients [99]. Studies of rituximab showed some benefit, but 10–20 % of patients developed serum sickness [99]. Treatment with IL-1 inhibitor (anakinra) in 26 pSS patients did not show a significant reduction in fatigue (accessed via fatigue severity scales and VAS) at week 4 compared to baseline [101]. Post-hoc analysis showed significantly more patients on the drug reached a 50 % reduction in fatigue on VAS compared to placebo, suggesting that IL-1 inhibition might affect fatigue [101].

In summary, pSS is associated with moderate to severe sleep disturbances with fatigue, pain, depression, and insomnia. PSG findings show reduced total sleep time, reduced sleep efficiency, sleep fragmentation, increased number of awakenings, increased WASO, and increased alpha sleep. PLMS is increased. Recent studies have highlighted the impairment of QOL, the high prevalence of depression, anxiety, fatigue, and sleep impairment in pSS patients. What is not currently available are outcomes data on the effects of combined symptomatic therapy for sicca symptoms, pain control, optimization of sleep duration, treatment of underlying insomnia or RLS, treatment of depression/anxiety, and disease activity on various parameters (QOL, pain, depression, anxiety, fatigue, sleep quality/ quantity, disease activity).

Scleroderma or Systemic Sclerosis

Scleroderma or systemic sclerosis (SSc) has a prevalence of 240 cases per million adults in the USA. Women are four times more likely to develop systemic scleroderma than men, with symptom onset usually between ages 30–40 years. SSc is characterized by tightening of the skin, Raynaud's phenomenon, cutaneous telangiectasias, polyarthritis, skeletal muscle atrophy, endothelial lesions, and visceral fibrosis.

In a study of 446 SSc subjects, 76 % complained of difficulty sleeping and that sleep difficulties moderately impacted their daily activities [102]. Other common symptoms reported were: fatigue (89 %), Raynaud's phenomenon (86 %), hand stiffness (81 %), and joint pain (81 %) [102]. Symptoms related to joint pain included skin tightening (72 %), muscle pain (71 %), and tender joints (71 %) [102]. Fatigue was one of the top three complaints in another study [103]. Fatigue was associated with poor sleep quality, pain, depressive symptoms, and worse physical function [103]. However, fatigue has less impact on physical function than pain.

Although reported mean sleep duration of 7.1 ± 1.73 h/night parallels that of the US general population, SSc patients score worse in four out of six scales for sleep [104]. The presence of reflux, new or recent worsening of dyspnea, and depressed mood are independent predictors of poor sleep [104]. Interestingly, patient-reported pain, physician assessment of disease severity, and demographics did not predict sleep disturbances [104].

Sleep in SSc patients is disrupted with mean sleep disruption score of 38.5 ± 29.9, using a 100-mm sleep disruption VAS. Results are similar to those of RA subjects, and both are higher compared to the general population [105]. In this study, pain was a significant disruptor of sleep. Breathing problems, gastrointestinal symptoms, smoking, and depression were associated with sleep scores in bivariate analysis, but not in multivariate analysis when pain was included, leading the authors to hypothesize that pain is the mediator between these SSc symptoms and sleep [105].

PSG in 27 patients with SSc showed reduced sleep efficiency (mean 82 ± 12.3 %), reduced REM sleep percentage (mean 13.1 ± 5.6 %), increased arousal index (26.1 ± 13 arousals/hours), and increased slow wave sleep percentage (25.7 ± 9.7 %). PLMI was also increased in 48 % of patients, and 22 % of patients had restless legs symptoms [106]. Poor sleep was significantly associated with esophageal dyskinesia, dyspnea, and restless leg symptoms [106]. PSG documented sleep fragmentation.

Addressing pain issues improves sleep. A SSc patient with severely painful ischemic ulcers, who had previously failed oral opioids, had 90–100 % pain relief with intrathecal pain management. As pain improved, her self-reported nocturnal sleep duration increased from 2 h/night to 7–8 h/night [107]. Twenty-nine SSc patients who had severe pain due to skin ulcers were treated with oxycodone 10–20 mg twice a day [108]. After a month of therapy, pain improved and VAS for pain decreased significantly from 93.8 ± 8.72 to 56.7 ± 10.4 with better sleep quality and significantly increased self-reported total hours of sleep from (3.68 ± 1.28 to 5.27 ± 0.75) hours. These parameters improved further after 3 months of therapy and remained stable during the 7.9 ± 3.2 months of follow-up and dosage of oxycodone remained unchanged.

Esophageal dyskinesia and dyspnea have been listed as factors for sleep disruption [106]. Thirty percent of patients with aperistaltic esophagus (n = 13, 7/13 had scleroderma) had severe reflux [109]. In 19 % of the reflux events, there was sleep disruption, while in 81 % of the reflux events, the patients either returned to sleep or did not awaken despite severe reflux [109]. Esophageal dyskinesia and prolonged reflux events may contribute to pulmonary fibrosis (PF). Studies of patients with SSc [110, 111] have demonstrated higher incidence of PF. In 18/40 (45 %) [111], PF was associated with significantly lower pressure at the lower esophageal sphincter, more esophageal acid exposure, more total and proximal reflux events, and a higher percentage of proximal reflux episodes compared to those without fibrosis.

Targeted interventions previously had limited outcome measures specific to the underlying medical issue: for instance, treatment outcomes for interstitial lung disease associated with SSc had disease outcome measures (stabilization of forced vital capacity, biomarkers). Since the publication of our review article in 2008, in addition to standard health assessment questionnaires (HAQ) [112], various outcome measures for monitoring SSc patients have been published, including two new instruments—Patient-Reported Outcomes Measurement Information System 29-item Health Profile (PROMIS-29) and the Functional Assessment of Chronic Illness Therapy-Dyspnea short form (FACIT-Dyspnea) [113, 114]. Validation of these outcome measurements has been the recent focus of publications. With these validated instruments, what is still missing are the results of targeted and combined systematic interventions not only on disease markers, but to incorporate measures that address well-defined problems—fatigue, pain, poor sleep quality, anxiety/depression, dyspnea, and esophageal dysmotility.

Behcet's Disease

Behcet's disease (BD) is a recurrent systemic inflammatory disorder of unknown origin that affects approximately 6.6 individuals per 100,000 in the United States. Apthous oral and genital ulcers, uveitis, and skin lesions characterize BD. Systemic vasculitis can involve large vessels, the central nervous system, and gastrointestinal tract and can be life-threatening. Joint involvement occurs in 41 % of patients, with asymmetric oligoarthritis as the most characteristic form [115]. Pain intensity is higher in BD patients with arthritis than those without arthritis [115]. The QOL scores for general health, physical functioning, and role emotional domains of SF-36 are significantly worse than in patients without arthritis [116].

Depression is an important concern for BD patients. A study comparing BD patients ($n=30$) to RA patients ($n=30$) showed a greater ratio of BD patients with high depression scores. Disease activity and joint involvement as assessed by BD patients were found to be factors related to the depression score [117]. Fatigue, sedation, and insomnia are common in BD patients, as demonstrated in a study of 95 BD patients who were either in placebo or thalidomide treatment groups [118].

In a study of 51 BD patients without neurological involvement [119] the prevalence of sleep apnea (32.5 %) and RLS (35.3 %) was higher compared to normal controls. Insomnia was present in 49 % of BD patients [119]. Fatigue, anxiety, depression scores, and subjective sleep quality were worse compared to control subjects. Fatigue was more prominent in BD patients with RLS or with sleep apnea associated with nocturnal desaturation. Compared to normal control subjects, PSG in BD patients demonstrated reduced sleep efficiency index (75.87 ± 15.87 % vs. 85.36 ± 9.42 %), reduced sleep continuity index (80.83 ± 14.27 % vs. 89.63 ± 8.13 %), and WASO was longer (91.97 ± 68.71 min vs. 47.17 ± 37.99 min). Disease activity did not correlate with either sleep disorders or PSG findings [119].

In summary, BD patients experience pain, depression, fatigue, sedation, and insomnia. The prevalence of sleep apnea and RLS is higher in BD patients, and fatigue is more prominent in these affected patients. Sleep fragmentation and reduced sleep efficiency were documented during PSG. What is needed are outcome studies that show the effects of interventions to reduce pain/arthralgias, fatigue, and depression on sleep quality, QOL measures, and disease activity.

Osteoarthritis

Osteoarthritis (OA) is the most common articular disease of older adults. Approximately 20 million US adults are affected, with no gender preference until after age 55, when females are more frequently affected.

Sixty-seven percent of OA patients report poor sleep quality and fragmented sleep, with need to use the bathroom and pain as the top two reasons for awakening [41]. Symptomatic hip or knee OA is associated with increased odds of having any sleep problem (OR 1.25, 95 % CI 1.02–1.54), insomnia (OR 1.29, 95 % CI 1.07–1.56), and insufficient sleep (OR 1.35, 95 % CI 1.12–1.62) [120]. Among 429 patients with knee OA, 31 % experienced sleep-onset difficulties, 81 % had difficulties with sleep continuity, and 51 % had early morning awakenings occurring at least twice a week [121]. Greater sleep disturbances correlated with more arthritis and knee pain, poorer self-rated health, poorer physical functioning, and depressive symptoms [121]. PSG carried out on 2 nights in 14 OA patients showed significantly increased Stage 1 NREM Sleep and significantly reduced Stage 2 NREM sleep compared to 16 normal subjects. Sleep latency, sleep efficiency, number of awakenings, and duration of awakenings did not significantly differ between OA and normal subjects [122].

Fatigue in OA correlates with sleep disturbance and depression [123]. Compared to RA subjects ($n=103$), OA subjects ($n=103$) reported greater pain, disability, depression, and sleeplessness [123]. In a study of women ($n=2,225$) correlating Western Ontario and McMaster Universities (WOMAC) hip pain severity score and objective sleep measures using actigraphy, the greatest predictor of sleep fragmentation was hip pain while sitting or lying [124]. WASO for ≥90 min was more likely for every 5-point increase in WOMAC score. Standing pain was associated with more WASO minutes, independent of pain while in bed. For women with hip pain, sleep disturbances increased significantly after the first 2 h of sleep [124]. Greater arthritis severity, depressed mood, and RLS symptoms were independent correlates of poor sleep [125]. Poor sleep was significantly associated with greater fatigue and napping did not improve this. Identifying the cause(s) of the sleep disturbance is important in devising a treatment plan.

Pain and sleep have a dual relationship. Through peripheral and central quantitative sensory testing of OA subjects, Lee et al. demonstrated low pain thresholds locally at affected sites and low pain thresholds in a widespread distribution, in addition to dysfunctional central pain mechanisms, which included loss of descending analgesia (conditioned pain modulation), temporal summation, and expanded areas of hyperalgesia [53]. Loss of descending analgesic activity is contingent upon the chronic pain state and is potentially reversible if the painful stimulus is removed, for example, via hip surgery [53]. For OA patients with fibromyalgia, the use of serotonin-norepinephrine reuptake inhibitors (SNRIs), such as duloxetine or milnacipram, could modulate the descending serotonin-norepinephrine pathways involved in central pain inhibiting mechanisms [53]. Duloxetine 60–120 mg daily significantly reduced mean 24-h pain scores in patients with OA and also significantly improved Western Ontario and McMasters physical function scores. Long-acting opioid analgesics simultaneously improved pain control and improved sleep quality in OA subjects by reducing the awakenings from pain, increasing the duration of sleep, and improving sleep quality [126]. Cognitive behavioral therapy for insomnia has improved immediate and long-term self-reported sleep and pain in OA patients with comorbid insomnia [127].

In summary, OA of the hip and knee is associated with poor sleep quality and sleep fragmentation. Sleep deprivation in this subgroup appears to be rooted in pain and depression. Pain disrupts sleep and treating pain effectively improves sleep. Fatigue correlates with sleep disturbance and depression. Napping does not appear to improve fatigue. Addressing depression/pain through SNRI's or surgical interventions to address painful joints improves sleep.

Conclusion

Sleep deprivation is a common occurrence in our current society. Quantity and quality of sleep are both important. Surveys suggest that sleep duration is short, but many of the studies do not list sleep duration as a parameter. Perceived adequacy of sleep is a surrogate parameter in QOL scales. Objective measures of sleep duration (actigraphy) and sleep quality (PSG) are needed to correlate with the QOL scales, depression/anxiety scales, fatigue scales, sleepiness scales, and specific disease activity parameters. For the specific interventions and combined interventions for the different types of arthritis, we need to measure results of these interventions using disease activity, QOL measures, and effects on fatigue, sleepiness, insomnia, depression, anxiety, and disability. Longitudinal studies that evaluate the effects of interventions that improve sleep by optimizing sleep duration, addressing insomnia (either pharmacologically or by cognitive behavioral therapy), nocturnal pain, pruritus, ocular/oral sicca symptoms, depression, PLMs of sleep, and sleep disordered breathing should also have baseline and follow-up subjective and objective measures to see the effects on disease activity, QOL scales, fatigue, depression/anxiety. By having these data, we can then formulate a more systematic approach to treating these diseases.

References

1. Jean-Louis G, Kripke DF, Ancoli-Israel S. Sleep and quality of well-being. Sleep. 2000;23(8):1115–21.
2. Krueger PM, Friedman EM. Sleep duration in the United States: a cross-sectional population-based study. Am J Epidemiol. 2009;169(9):1052–63.
3. National Sleep Foundation [internet]. Portland, OR: The Foundation; c 2011 [cited 2013 May 23]. Sleep in America polls. Available from: http://www.sleepfoundation.org/category/article-type/sleep-america-polls/.
4. Açar G, Akçakoyun M, Sari I, et al. Acute sleep deprivation in healthy adults is associated with a

reduction in left atrial early diastolic strain rate. Sleep Breath. 2012;17(3):975–83 [Epub ahead of print].
5. Kerkhofs M, Boudjeltia KZ. From total sleep deprivation to cardiovascular disease: a key role for the immune system? Sleep. 2012;35(7):895–6.
6. Nagai M, Hoshide S, Kario K. Sleep duration as a risk factor for cardiovascular disease—a review of the recent literature. Curr Cardiol Rev. 2010;6(1): 54–61.
7. Ayas NT, White DP, Manson JE, et al. A prospective study of sleep duration and coronary heart disease in women. JAMA. 2003;163:205–9.
8. Liu Y, Tanaka H, Group TFHS. Overtime work, insufficient sleep, and risk of non-fatal acute myocardial infarction in Japanese men. J Occup Environ Med. 2002;59:447–51.
9. Luyster FS, Strollo PJ, Zee PC, Walsh JK. Sleep: a health imperative. Sleep. 2012;35(6):727–34.
10. Gruber R, Wiebe S, Montecalvo L, Brunetti B, Amsel R, Carrier J. Impact of sleep restriction on neurobehavioral functioning of children with attention deficit hyperactivity disorder. Sleep. 2011;34(3): 315–23.
11. Kripke DF, Garfinkel L, Wingard DL, Klauber MR, Marler MR. Mortality associated with sleep duration and insomnia. Arch Gen Psychiatry. 2002;59:131–6.
12. Helmick CG, Felson DT, Lawrence RC. Estimates of the prevalence of arthritis and other rheumatic conditions in the United States. Arthritis Rheum. 2008;58(1):15–25.
13. Frey DJ, Fleshner M, Wright Jr KP. The effects of 40 hours of total sleep deprivation on inflammatory markers in healthy young adults. Brain Behav Immun. 2007;21(8):1050–7.
14. Shearer WT, Reuben JM, Mullington JM, Price NJ, Lee BN, Smith EO, Szuba MP, Van Dongen HP, Dinges DF. Soluble TNF-alpha receptor 1 and IL-6 plasma levels in humans subjected to the sleep deprivation model of spaceflight. J Allergy Clin Immunol. 2001;107:165–70.
15. Ruiz FS, Andersen ML, Martins RC, Zager A, Lopes JD, Tufik S. Immune alterations after selective rapid eye movement or total sleep deprivation in healthy male volunteers. Innate Immun. 2012;18(1):44–54.
16. Irwin MR, Wang M, Campomayor CO, et al. Sleep deprivation and activation of morning levels of cellular and genomic markers of inflammation. Arch Intern Med. 2006;166:1756–62.
17. Vgontzas AN, Zoumakis E, Bixler EO, et al. Adverse effects of modest sleep restriction on sleepiness, performance, and inflammatory cytokines. J Clin Endocrinol Metab. 2004;89:2119–26.
18. van Leeuwen WM, Lehto M, Karisola P, Lindholm H, Luukkonen R, Sallinen M, Härmä M, Porkka-Heiskanen T, Alenius H. Sleep restriction increases the risk of developing cardiovascular diseases by augmenting proinflammatory responses through IL-17 and CRP. PLoS One. 2009;4(2):e4589.
19. Irwin M, Rinetti G, Redwine L, Motivala S, Dang J, Ehlers C. Nocturnal proinflammatory cytokine-associated sleep disturbances in abstinent African American alcoholics. Brain Behav Immun. 2004;18(4):349–60.
20. Meier-Ewert HK, Ridker PM, Rifai N, Regan MM, Price NJ, Dinges DF, Mullington JM. Effect of sleep loss on C-reactive protein, an inflammatory marker of cardiovascular risk. J Am Coll Cardiol. 2004;43(4):678–83.
21. Irwin MR, Wang M, Ribeiro D, Cho HJ, Olmstead R, Breen EC, Martinez-Maza O, Cole S. Sleep loss activates cellular inflammatory signaling. Biol Psychiatry. 2008;64:538–40.
22. Pascual G, Glass CK. Nuclear receptors versus inflammation: mechanisms of transrepression. Trends Endocrinol Metab. 2006;17:321–7.
23. Miller MA, Kandala NB, Kivimaki M, Kumari M, Brunner EJ, Lowe GD, Marmot MG, Cappuccio FP. Gender differences in the cross-sectional relationships between sleep duration and markers of inflammation: Whitehall II study. Sleep. 2009;32(7):857–64.
24. Faraut B, Boudjeltia KZ, Vanhamme L, Kerkhofs M. Immune, inflammatory and cardiovascular consequences of sleep restriction and recovery. Sleep Med Rev. 2012;16(2):137–49.
25. Faraut B, Boudjeltia KZ, Dyzma M, Rousseau A, David E, Stenuit P, Franck T, Van Antwerpen P, Vanhaeverbeek M, Kerkhofs M. Benefits of napping and an extended duration of recovery sleep on alertness and immune cells after acute sleep restriction. Brain Behav Immun. 2011;25(1):16–24.
26. Abad VC, Sarinas PS, Guilleminault C. Sleep and rheumatologic disorders. Sleep Med Rev. 2008;12(3):211–28.
27. Smith MT, Haythornthwaite JA. How do sleep disturbance and chronic pain inter-relate? Insights from the longitudinal and cognitive-behavioral clinical trials literature. Sleep Med Rev. 2004;8(2):119–32.
28. Irwin MR, Olmsted R, Carrillo C, Sadeghi N, Fitzgerald JD, Ranganath VK, Nicassio PM. Sleep loss exacerbates fatigue, depression and pain in rheumatoid arthritis. Sleep. 2012;35(4):537–43.
29. Bourguignon C, Taibi D, Taylor AG. Sleep disturbances, fatigue, depression, and heart rate variability in menopausal women with and without RA. Sleep. 2005;28:302.
30. Drewes AM, Svendsen L, Taagholt SJ, et al. Sleep in rheumatoid arthritis: a comparison with healthy subjects and studies of sleep/wake interactions. Br J Rheumatol. 1998;37:71–81.
31. Hirsch M, Carlander B, Verge M, et al. Objective and subjective sleep disturbances in patients with rheumatoid arthritis. A reappraisal. Arthritis Rheum. 1994;37:41–9.
32. Moldofsky H, Lue FA, Smythe HA. Alpha EEG sleep and morning symptoms in rheumatoid arthritis. J Rheumatol. 1983;10:373–9.
33. Lavie P, Epstein R, Tzischinsky O, et al. Actigraphic measurements of sleep in rheumatoid arthritis: comparison of patients with low back pain and healthy controls. J Rheumatol. 1992;19:362–5.

34. Drewes AM, Nielsen KD, Hansen B, et al. A longitudinal study of clinical symptoms and sleep parameters in rheumatoid arthritis. Rheumatology (Oxford). 2000;39:1287–9.
35. Walsh JK, Muehlbach MJ, Lauter SA, et al. Effects of triazolam on sleep, daytime sleepiness, and morning stiffness in patients with rheumatoid arthritis. J Rheumatol. 1996;23:245–52.
36. Mahowald MW, Mahowald ML, Bundlie SR, Ytterberg SR. Sleep fragmentation in rheumatoid arthritis. Arthritis Rheum. 1989;32:974–83.
37. Crosby LJ. Factors which contribute to fatigue associated with rheumatoid arthritis. J Adv Nurs. 1991;16:974–81.
38. Wolfe F, Michaud K, Li T. Sleep disturbance in patients with rheumatoid arthritis: evaluation by medical outcomes study and visual analog sleep scales. J Rheumatol. 2006;33:1942–51.
39. Mahowald ML, Sing JA, Mahowald MW. Sleep misperception in patients with rheumatoid arthritis (abstract). Sleep Med. 2005;6:S89.
40. Goodchild CE, Treharne GJ, Booth DA, Bowman SJ. Daytime patterning of fatigue and its associations with the previous night's discomfort and poor sleep among women with primary Sjögren's syndrome or rheumatoid arthritis. Musculoskeletal Care. 2010;8(2):107–17.
41. Taylor-Gjevre RM, Gjevre JA, Nair B, Skomro R, Lim HJ. Components of sleep quality and sleep fragmentation in rheumatoid arthritis and osteoarthritis. Musculoskeletal Care. 2011.
42. Houssien DA, McKenna SP, Scott DL. The Nottingham Health Profile as a measure of disease activity and outcome in rheumatoid arthritis. Br J Rheumatol. 1997;36(1):69–73.
43. Zamarron C, Maceiras F, Mera A, Gomez-Reino JJ. Effect of the first infliximab infusion on sleep and alertness in patients with active rheumatoid arthritis. Ann Rheum Dis. 2004;63:88–90.
44. Taylor-Gjevre RM, Gjevre JA, Nair BV, Skomro RP, Lim HJ. Improved sleep efficiency after anti-tumor necrosis factor α therapy in rheumatoid arthritis patients. Ther Adv Musculoskelet Dis. 2011;3(5):227–33.
45. Neto J, Lira F, Venancio D, et al. Sleep deprivation affects inflammatory marker expression in adipose tissue. Lipids Health Dis. 2010;9:125. doi:10.1186/1476-511X-9-125.
46. Lautenbacher S, Kundermann B, Krieg JC. Sleep deprivation and pain perception. Sleep Med Rev. 2006;10(5):357–69.
47. Lee YC, Chibnik LB, Lu B, Wasan AD, Edwards RR, Fossel AH, Helfgott SM, Solomon DH, Clauw DJ, Karlson EW. The relationship between disease activity, sleep, psychiatric distress and pain sensitivity in rheumatoid arthritis: a cross-sectional study. Arthritis Res Ther. 2009;11(5):R160.
48. Nicassio PM, Wallston KA. Longitudinal relationships among pain, sleep problems, and depression in rheumatoid arthritis. J Abnorm Psychol. 1992;101(3):514–20.
49. Nicassio PM, Ormseth SR, Kay M, Custodio M, Irwin MR, Olmstead R, Weisman MH. The contribution of pain and depression to self-reported sleep disturbance in patients with rheumatoid arthritis. Pain. 2012;153(1):107–12.
50. Wolfe F, Michaud K. Assessment of pain in rheumatoid arthritis: minimal clinically significant difference, predictors, and the effect of anti-tumor necrosis factor therapy. J Rheumatol. 2007;34(8):1674–83.
51. Rupp I, Boshuizen HC, Roorda LD, Dinant HJ, Jacobi CE, van den Bos G. Course of patient-reported health outcomes in rheumatoid arthritis: comparison of longitudinal and cross-sectional approaches. J Rheumatol. 2006;33(2):228–33.
52. Meeus M, Vervisch S, De Clerck LS, Moorkens G, Hans G, Nijs J. Central sensitization in patients with rheumatoid arthritis: a systematic literature review. Semin Arthritis Rheum. 2012;41(4):556–67.
53. Lee YC, Nassikas NJ, Clauw DJ. The role of the central nervous system in the generation and maintenance of chronic pain in rheumatoid arthritis, osteoarthritis and fibromyalgia. Arthritis Res Ther. 2011;13(2):211.
54. Wendler J, Hummel T, Reissinger M, Manger B, Pauli E, Kalden JR, Kobal G. Patients with rheumatoid arthritis adapt differently to repetitive painful stimuli compared to healthy controls. J Clin Neurosci. 2001;8(3):272–7.
55. Wartolowska K, Hough MG, Jenkinson M, Andersson J, Wordsworth BP, Tracey I. Structural changes of the brain in rheumatoid arthritis. Arthritis Rheum. 2012;64(2):371–9. doi:10.1002/art.33326.
56. Kundermann B, Krieg JC, Schreiber W, Lautenbacher S. The effect of sleep deprivation on pain. Pain Res Manag. 2004 Spring;9(1):25–32.
57. Nascimento DC, Andersen ML, Hipólide DC, Nobrega JN, Tufik S. Pain hypersensitivity induced by paradoxical sleep deprivation is not due to altered binding to brain mu-opioid receptors. Behav Brain Res. 2007;178(2):216–20.
58. Sanderson T, Morris M, Calnan M, Richards P, Hewlett S. Patient perspective of measuring treatment efficacy: the rheumatoid arthritis patient priorities for pharmacologic interventions outcomes. Arthritis Care Res (Hoboken). 2010;62(5):647–56.
59. Butbul Aviel Y, Stremler R, Benseler SM, Cameron B, Laxer RM, Ota S, Schneider R, Spiegel L, Stinson JN, Tse SM, Feldman BM. Sleep and fatigue and the relationship to pain, disease activity and quality of life in juvenile idiopathic arthritis and juvenile dermatomyositis. Rheumatology (Oxford). 2011;50(11):2051–60. Epub 2011 Aug 25.
60. Ward TM, Ringold S, Metz J, Archbold K, Lentz M, Wallace CA, Landis CA. Sleep disturbances and neurobehavioral functioning in children with and without juvenile idiopathic arthritis. Arthritis Care Res (Hoboken). 2011;63(7):1006–12. doi:10.1002/acr.20469.

61. Zamir G, Press J, Tal A, Tarasiuk A. Sleep fragmentation in children with juvenile rheumatoid arthritis. J Rheumatol. 1998;25(6):1191–7.
62. Passarelli CM, Roizenblatt S, Len CA, Moreira GA, Lopes MC, Guilleminault C, Tufik S, Hilario MO. A case–control sleep study in children with polyarticular juvenile rheumatoid arthritis. J Rheumatol. 2006;33(4):796–802. Epub 2006 Mar 1.
63. Ward TM, Brandt P, Archbold K, Lentz M, Ringold S, Wallace CA, Landis CA. Polysomnography and self-reported sleep, pain, fatigue, and anxiety in children with active and inactive juvenile rheumatoid arthritis. J Pediatr Psychol. 2008;33(3):232–41.
64. Kotagal S, Nichols CD, Grigg-Damberger MM, et al. Non-respiratory indications for polysomnography and related procedures in children: an evidence-based review. Sleep. 2012;35(11):1451–66.
65. Ward TM, Archbold K, Lentz M, Ringold S, Wallace CA, Landis CA. Sleep disturbance, daytime sleepiness, and neurocognitive performance in children with juvenile idiopathic arthritis. Sleep. 2010; 33(2):252–9.
66. National Psoriasis Foundation. Psoriasis and comorbid conditions issue brief executive Summary [internet].National Psoriasis Foundation; Portland, OR: 2012 [cited 2013 May 23]. Available from: http://www.psoriasis.org/document.doc?id=793.
67. Fitzgerald O. Psoriatic Arthritis. In: Firestein GS, Budd RC, Gabriel SE, McInnes IB, O'Dell JR, editors. Kelley's textbook of rheumatology. 9th ed. Philadelphia: Elsevier Saunders; 2013. p. 1232–50.
68. Callis Duffin K, Wong B, Horn EJ, Krueger GG. Psoriatic arthritis is a strong predictor of sleep interference in patients with psoriasis. J Am Acad Dermatol. 2009;60(4):604–8.
69. Yosipovitch G, Goon A, Wee J, Chan YH, Goh CL. The prevalence and clinical characteristics of pruritus among patients with extensive psoriasis. Br J Dermatol. 2000;143(5):969–73.
70. Karaca S, Fidan F, Erkan F, Nural S, Pinarcı T, Gunay E, Unlu M. Might psoriasis be a risk factor for obstructive sleep apnea syndrome? Sleep Breath. 2013;17(1):275–80 [Epub ahead of print].
71. Salaffi F, Carotti M, Gasparini S, Intorcia M, Grassi W. The health-related quality of life in rheumatoid arthritis, ankylosing spondylitis, and psoriatic arthritis: a comparison with a selected sample of healthy people. Health Qual Life Outcomes. 2009;7:25.
72. Strober BE, Sobell JM, Duffin KC, Bao Y, Guérin A, Yang H, Goldblum O, Okun MM, Mulani PM. Sleep quality and other patient-reported outcomes improve after patients with psoriasis with suboptimal response to other systemic therapies are switched to adalimumab: results from PROGRESS, an open-label Phase IIIB trial. Br J Dermatol. 2012; 167(6):1374–81.
73. Ward MM. Health-related quality of life in ankylosing spondylitis: a survey of 175 patients. Arthritis Care Res. 1999;12(4):247–55.
74. Li Y, Zhang S, Zhu J, Du X, Huang F. Sleep disturbances are associated with increased pain, disease activity, depression, and anxiety in ankylosing spondylitis: a case–control study. Arthritis Res Ther. 2012;14(5):R215.
75. Da Costa D, Zummer M, Fitzcharles MA. Determinants of sleep problems in patients with spondyloarthropathy. Musculoskeletal Care. 2009;7(3):143–61.
76. Hultgren S, Broman JE, Gudbjörnsson B, Hetta J, Lindqvist U. Sleep disturbances in outpatients with ankylosing spondylitisa questionnaire study with gender implications. Scand J Rheumatol. 2000; 29(6):365–9.
77. Batmaz I, Sarıyıldız MA, Dilek B, Bez Y, Karakoç M, Cevik R. Sleep quality and associated factors in ankylosing spondylitis: relationship with disease parameters, psychological status and quality of life. Rheumatol Int. 2013;33(4):1039–45 [Epub ahead of print].
78. Jones SD, Koh WH, Steiner A, Garrett SL, Calin A. Fatigue in ankylosing spondylitis: its prevalence and relationship to disease activity, sleep, and other factors. J Rheumatol. 1996;23(3):487–90.
79. Heiberg T, Lie E, van der Heijde D, Kvien TK. Sleep problems are of higher priority for improvement for patients with ankylosing spondylitis than for patients with other inflammatory arthropathies. Ann Rheum Dis. 2011;70(5):872–3 [Epub 2010 Nov 24].
80. Costa DD, Bernatsky S, Dritsa M, Clarke AE, Dasgupta K, Keshani A, Pineau C. Determinants of sleep quality in women with systemic lupus erythematosus. Arthritis Rheum. 2005;53(2):272–8.
81. Tench CM, McCurdie I, White PD, D'Cruz DP. The prevalence and associations of fatigue in systemic lupus erythematosus. Rheumatology (Oxford). 2000;39(11):1249–54.
82. Huang HC, Chou CT, Lin KC, Chao YF. The relationships between disability level, health-promoting lifestyle, and quality of life in outpatients with systemic lupus erythematosus. J Nurs Res. 2007; 15(1):21–32.
83. Greenwood KM, Lederman L, Lindner HD. Self-reported sleep in systemic lupus erythematosus. Clin Rheumatol. 2008;27(9):1147–51 [Epub 2008 Apr 12].
84. Gudbjörnsson B, Hetta J. Sleep disturbances in patients with systemic lupus erythematosus: a questionnaire-based study. Clin Exp Rheumatol. 2001; 19(5):509–14.
85. Ad Hoc Committee on Systemic Lupus Erythematosus Response Criteria for Fatigue. Measurement of fatigue in systemic lupus erythematosus: a systematic review. Arthritis Rheum. 2007; 57(8):1348–57.
86. Iaboni A, Ibanez D, Gladman DD, Urowitz MB, Moldofsky H. Fatigue in systemic lupus erythematosus: contributions of disordered sleep, sleepiness, and depression. J Rheumatol. 2006;33(12):2453–7.

87. Valencia-Flores M, Resendiz M, Castaño VA, Santiago V, Campos RM, Sandino S, Valencia X, Alcocer J, Ramos GG, Bliwise DL. Objective and subjective sleep disturbances in patients with systemic lupus erythematosus. Arthritis Rheum. 1999;42(10):2189–93.
88. Palma BD, Tufik S. Increased disease activity is associated with altered sleep architecture in an experimental model of systemic lupus erythematosus. Sleep. 2010;33(9):1244–8.
89. Palma BD, Gabriel Jr A, Colugnati FA, Tufik S. Effects of sleep deprivation on the development of autoimmune disease in an experimental model of systemic lupus erythematosus. Am J Physiol Regul Integr Comp Physiol. 2006;291(5):R1527–32 [Epub 2006 Jun 29].
90. Mckinley PS, Quellette SC, Winkel GH. The contributions of disease activity, sleep patterns, and depression to fatigue in systemic lupus erythematosus. A proposed model. Arthritis Rheum. 1995;38(6):826–34.
91. Tishler M, Barak Y, Paran D, Yaron M. Sleep disturbances, fibromyalgia and primary Sjögren's syndrome. Clin Exp Rheumatol. 1997;15(1):71–4.
92. Gudbjörnsson B, Broman JE, Hetta J, Hällgren R. Sleep disturbances in patients with primary Sjögren's syndrome. Br J Rheumatol. 1993;32(12):1072–6.
93. Valtýsdóttir ST, Gudbjörnsson B, Lindqvist U, Hällgren R, Hetta J. Anxiety and depression in patients with primary Sjögren's syndrome. J Rheumatol. 2000;27(1):165–9.
94. van Oers ML, Bossema ER, Thoolen BJ, Hartkamp A, Dekkers JC, Godaert GL, Kruize AA, Derksen RH, Bijlsma JW, Geenen R. Variability of fatigue during the day in patients with primary Sjögren's syndrome, systemic lupus erythematosus, and rheumatoid arthritis. Clin Exp Rheumatol. 2010;28(5):715–21.
95. Godaert GL, Hartkamp A, Geenen R, Garssen A, Kruize AA, Bijlsma JW, Derksen RH. Fatigue in daily life in patients with primary Sjögren's syndrome and systemic lupus erythematosus. Ann N Y Acad Sci. 2002;966:320–6.
96. Theander L, Strömbeck B, Mandl T, Theander E. Sleepiness or fatigue? Can we detect treatable causes of tiredness in primary Sjögren's syndrome? Rheumatology (Oxford). 2010;49(6):1177–83 [Epub 2010 Mar 2].
97. Zautra AJ, Fasman R, Parish BP, Davis MC. Daily fatigue in women with osteoarthritis, rheumatoid arthritis, and fibromyalgia. Pain. 2007;128(1–2):128–35 [Epub 2006 Oct 20].
98. Hackett KL, Newton JL, Frith J, Elliott C, Lendrem D, Foggo H, Edgar S, Mitchell S, Ng WF. Impaired functional status in primary Sjögren's syndrome. Arthritis Care Res (Hoboken). 2012;64(11):1760–4. doi:10.1002/acr.21738.
99. Vitali C, Palombi G, Cataleta P. Treating Sjögren's syndrome: insights for the clinician. Ther Adv Musculoskelet Dis. 2010;2(3):155–66.
100. Sugai S, Takahashi H, Ohta S, et al. Efficacy and safety of rebamipide for the treatment of dry mouth symptoms in patients with Sjögren's syndrome: a double-blind placebo-controlled multicenter trial. Mod Rheumatol. 2009;19(2):114–24.
101. Norheim KB, Harboe E, Gøransson LG, Omdal R. Interleukin-1 inhibition and fatigue in primary Sjögren's syndrome—a double blind, randomised clinical trial. PLoS One. 2012;7(1):e30123. doi:10.1371/journal.pone.0030123.
102. Bassel M, Hudson M, Taillefer SS, Schieir O, Baron M, Thombs BD. Frequency and impact of symptoms experienced by patients with systemic sclerosis: results from a Canadian National Survey. Rheumatology (Oxford). 2011;50(4):762–7 [Epub 2010 Dec 11].
103. Sandusky SB, McGuire L, Smith MT, Wigley FM, Haythornthwaite JA. Fatigue: an overlooked determinant of physical function in scleroderma. Rheumatology (Oxford). 2009;48(2):165–9 [Epub 2008 Dec 23].
104. Frech T, Hays RD, Maranian P, Clements PJ, Furst DE, Khanna D. Prevalence and correlates of sleep disturbance in systemic sclerosis—results from the UCLA scleroderma quality of life study. Rheumatology (Oxford). 2011;50(7):1280–7 [Epub 2011 Feb 15].
105. Milette K, Razykov I, Pope J, Hudson M, Motivala SJ, Baron M, Thombs BD. Clinical correlates of sleep problems in systemic sclerosis: the prominent role of pain. Rheumatology (Oxford). 2011;50(5):921–5 [Epub 2010 Dec 17].
106. Prado GF, Allen RP, Trevisani VM, Toscano VG, Earley CJ. Sleep disruption in systemic sclerosis (scleroderma) patients: clinical and polysomnographic findings. Sleep Med. 2002;3(4):341–5.
107. Lundborg CN, Nitescu PV, Appelgren LK, Curelaru ID. Progressive systemic sclerosis: intrathecal pain management. Reg Anesth Pain Med. 1999; 24(1):89–93.
108. Giuggioli D, Manfredi A, Colaci M, Ferri C. Oxycodone in the long-term treatment of chronic pain related to scleroderma skin ulcers. Pain Med. 2010;11(10):1500–3.
109. Shoenut JP, Yamashiro Y, Orr WC, Kerr P, Micflikier AB, Kryger MH. Effect of severe gastroesophageal reflux on sleep stage in patients with aperistaltic esophagus. Dig Dis Sci. 1996;41(2):372–6.
110. Marie I, Dominique S, Levesque H, et al. Esophageal involvement and pulmonary manifestations in systemic sclerosis. Arthritis Rheum. 2001;45:346–54.
111. Savarino E, Bazzica M, Zentilin P, et al. Gastroesophageal reflux and pulmonary fibrosis in scleroderma: a study using pH- impedance monitoring. Am J Respir Crit Care Med. 2009;179:408–13.
112. Pincus T, Swearingen C, Wolfe F. Toward a multidimensional Health Assessment Questionnaire (MDHAQ): assessment of advanced activities of daily living and psychological status in the patient-

friendly health assessment questionnaire format. Arthritis Rheum. 1999;42(10):2220–30.
113. Hinchcliff M, Beaumont JL, Thavarajah K, Varga J, Chung A, Podlusky S, Carns M, Chang RW, Cella D. Validity of two new patient-reported outcome measures in systemic sclerosis: Patient-Reported Outcomes Measurement Information System 29-item Health Profile and Functional Assessment of Chronic Illness Therapy-Dyspnea short form. Arthritis Care Res (Hoboken). 2011;63(11):1620–8.
114. Pope J. Measures of systemic sclerosis (scleroderma): Health Assessment Questionnaire (HAQ) and Scleroderma HAQ (SHAQ), physician- and patient-rated global assessments, Symptom Burden Index (SBI), University of California, Los Angeles, Scleroderma Clinical Trials Consortium Gastrointestinal Scale (UCLA SCTC GIT) 2.0, Baseline Dyspnea Index (BDI) and Transition Dyspnea Index (TDI) (Mahler's Index), Cambridge Pulmonary Hypertension Outcome Review (CAMPHOR), and Raynaud's Condition Score (RCS). Arthritis Care Res (Hoboken). 2011;63 Suppl 11:S98–111.
115. Gur A, Sarac AJ, Burkan YK, Nas K, Cevik R. Arthropathy, quality of life, depression, and anxiety in Behcet's disease: relationship between arthritis and these factors. Clin Rheumatol. 2006; 25(4):524–31.
116. Ertam I, Kitapcioglu G, Aksu K, Keser G, Ozaksar A, Elbi H, Unal I, Alper S. Quality of life and its relation with disease severity in Behçet's disease. Clin Exp Rheumatol. 2009;27(2 Suppl 53):S18–22.
117. Melikoglu MA, Melikoglu M. The relationship between disease activity and depression in patients with Behcet disease and rheumatoid arthritis. Rheumatol Int. 2010;30(7):941–6.
118. Hamuryudan V, Mat C, Saip S, Ozyazgan Y, Siva A, Yurdakul S, Zwingenberger K, Yazici H. Thalidomide in the treatment of the mucocutaneous lesions of the Behçet syndrome. A randomized, double-blind, placebo-controlled trial. Ann Intern Med. 1998;128(6):443–50.
119. Tascilar NF, Tekin NS, Ankarali H, Sezer T, Atik L, Emre U, Duysak S, Cinar F. Sleep disorders in Behçet's disease, and their relationship with fatigue and quality of life. J Sleep Res. 2012;21(3):281–8.
120. Allen KD, Renner JB, Devellis B, Helmick CG, Jordan JM. Osteoarthritis and sleep: the Johnston County Osteoarthritis Project. J Rheumatol. 2008;35(6):1102–7 [Epub 2008 May 15].
121. Wilcox S, Brenes GA, Levine D, Sevick MA, Shumaker SA, Craven T. Factors related to sleep disturbance in older adults experiencing knee pain or knee pain with radiographic evidence of knee osteoarthritis. J Am Geriatr Soc. 2000;48(10):1241–51.
122. Leigh TJ, Hindmarch I, Bird HA, Wright V. Comparison of sleep in osteoarthritic patients and age and sex matched healthy controls. Ann Rheum Dis. 1988;47(1):40–2.
123. Stebbings S, Herbison P, Doyle TC, Treharne GJ, Highton J. A comparison of fatigue correlates in rheumatoid arthritis and osteoarthritis: disparity in associations with disability, anxiety and sleep disturbance. Rheumatology (Oxford). 2010;49(2):361–7. Epub 2009 Dec 10.
124. Parimi N, Blackwell T, Stone KL, Lui LY, Ancoli-Israel S, Tranah GJ, Hillier TA, Nevitt ME, Lane NE. Study of Osteoporotic Fractures Study Group. Hip pain while using lower extremity joints and sleep disturbances in elderly white women: results from a cross-sectional analysis. Arthritis Care Res (Hoboken). 2012;64(7):1070–8.
125. Hawker GA, French MR, Waugh EJ, Gignac MA, Cheung C, Murray BJ. The multidimensionality of sleep quality and its relationship to fatigue in older adults with painful osteoarthritis. Arthritis Care Res (Hoboken). 2012;64(7):1070–8. doi:10.1002/acr.21630.
126. Turk DC, Cohen MJ. Sleep as a marker in the effective management of chronic osteoarthritis pain with opioid analgesics. Semin Arthritis Rheum. 2010;39(6):477–90. Epub 2009 Jan 10. Review.
127. Vitiello MV, Rybarczyk B, Von Korff M, Stepanski EJ. Cognitive behavioral therapy for insomnia improves sleep and decreases pain in older adults with co-morbid insomnia and osteoarthritis. J Clin Sleep Med. 2009;5(4):355–62.
128. Firestein GS. Etiology and Pathogenesis of Rheumatoid Arthritis. In: Firestein GS, Budd RC, Gabriel SE, McInnes IB, O'Dell JR, editors. Kelley's textbook of rheumatology. 9th ed. Philadelphia: Elsevier Saunders; 2013. p. P1059–95.
129. Kunz M, Ibrahi S. Cytokines and cytokine profiles in human autoimmune diseases and animal models of autoimmunity. Mediators Inflamm. 2009;2009: 979258.
130. Wang F, Xu L, Feng X, Guo D, Tan W, Zhang M. Interleukin-29 modulates proinflammatory cytokine production in synovial inflammation of rheumatoid arthritis. Arthritis Res Ther. 2012;14(5):R228.
131. Arend WP, Gabay C. Cytokines in the rheumatic diseases. Rheum Dis Clin North Am. 2004;30:41–67.
132. Wedderburn L, Nistala K. Etiology and pathogenesis of juvenile idiopathic arthritis. In: Firestein GS, Budd RC, Gabriel SE, McInnes IB, O'Dell JR, editors. Kelley's textbook of rheumatology. 9th ed. Philadelphia: Elsevier Saunders; 2013. p. 1741–51.
133. Yu D, Lories R, Inman R. Pathogenesis of ankylosing spondylitis and reactive arthritis. In: Firestein GS, Budd RC, Gabriel SE, McInnes IB, O'Dell JR, editors. Kelley's textbook of rheumatology. 9th ed. Philadelphia: Elsevier Saunders; 2013. p. 1193–201.
134. Fitzgerald O. Psoriatic Arthritis. In: Firestein GS, Budd RC, Gabriel SE, McInnes IB, O'Dell JR, editors. Kelley's textbook of rheumatology. 9th ed. Philadelphia: Elsevier Saunders; 2013. p. 1243–5.

135. St. Clair EW. Sjogren's syndrome. In: Firestein GS, Budd RC, Gabriel SE, McInnes IB, O'Dell JR, editors. Kelley's textbook of rheumatology. 9th ed. Philadelphia: Elsevier Saunders; 2013. p. 1169–89.
136. Varga J. Etiology and pathogenesis of scleroderma. In: Firestein GS, Budd RC, Gabriel SE, McInnes IB, O'Dell JR, editors. Kelley's textbook of rheumatology. 9th ed. Philadelphia: Elsevier Saunders; 2013. p. 1343–65.
137. Kaufman WS, Mcnamara EK, Jorizzo JL. Behcet's disease. In: Firestein GS, Budd RC, Gabriel SE, McInnes IB, O'Dell JR, editors. Kelley's textbook of rheumatology. 9th ed. Philadelphia: Elsevier Saunders; 2013. p. 1525–32.
138. Miller A, Ranatunga S. Immunotherapy in rheumatologic disorders. Med Clin North Am. 2012;96: 475–96.
139. Kytarris V. Kinase inhibitors: a new class of antirheumatic drugs. Drug Des Devel Ther. 2012;6: 245–50.
140. Otten MH, Anink J, Spronk S, van Suijlekom-Smit LW. Efficacy of biological agents in juvenile idiopathic arthritis: a systematic review using indirect comparisons. Ann Rheum Dis. 2012. [Epub ahead of print]

Sleep Deprivation and Pain

13

Akiko Okifuji and Bradford D. Hare

Introduction

Sleep is an activity that is critical for maintaining our health and well-being. Unfortunately, however, sleep-related problems are one of the most common health problems in our society. Up to 40 % of adults report at least one symptom of insomnia annually [1]. Approximately 75 % of Americans report disturbed sleep in any given week [2]. Disturbance in sleep typically results in a range of physical and mental impairments, including alteration in the nervous, metabolic, endocrine, and immune systems, dermal changes, impaired sensory responses, and deterioration in mood and cognition [3].

It has been well established that disturbed sleep is very prevalent in the chronic pain populations. Clinically significant insomnia has been reported by 53 % of chronic pain patients attending pain clinics compared to 3 % of gender- and age-matched healthy people [4]. Approximately 89 % of chronic pain patients seeking treatments present at least one sleep-related complaint [5]. In people with temporomandibular disorder (TMD), the polysomnographic analyses showed that both insomnia and sleep apnea are common [6]. In fibromyalgia, sleep disturbance is ubiquitous, with the reported prevalence of up to 99 % [7].

A. Okifuji, Ph.D. (✉) • B.D. Hare, M.D., Ph.D.
Pain Research Center, Pain Management Center, Department of Anesthesiology, University of Utah, Salt Lake City, UT, USA
e-mail: akiko.okifuji@hsc.utah.edu

The close relationship between pain and sleep can also be seen in people with a primary presentation of insomnia. A large epidemiological study with 47,000 people [8] found that the presence of insomnia is associated with increased prevalence of pain conditions. Over 40 % of people with insomnia complain of at least one chronic pain problem [9].

In general, the relationship between pain and poor sleep is considered to be bidirectional [10]. That is, having pain disrupts the initiation and maintenance of sleep, whereas sleep disruption also worsens pain. In this chapter, we will review the experimental, clinical, and epidemiological research evaluating the effects of poor sleep on pain. We will also review how sleep may be altered by opioid analgesic use.

Poor Sleep and Hyperalgesia

Reported Poor Sleep and Pain Response to Noxious Stimulation

In general, people exhibit increased pain response to experimentally induced noxious stimulation following poor sleep. Patients with rheumatoid arthritis showed a significant relationship between self-rated poor sleep and lower pressure pain thresholds both in joint and non-joint sites [11]. Similarly, TMD patients with primary insomnia have been shown to exhibit reduced pain thresholds to mechanical stimulations in the affected and distal areas [6].

M.T. Bianchi (ed.), *Sleep Deprivation and Disease: Effects on the Body, Brain and Behavior*,
DOI 10.1007/978-1-4614-9087-6_13, © Springer Science+Business Media New York 2014

In a recent laboratory study by Campbell et al. [12], 28 healthy people were tested under two conditions; the heat-capsaicin nociceptive test and the same test with distracting game playing. The subjects who reported chronically short sleep duration (<6.5 h per night on average) exhibited greater secondary hyperalgesia to the heat-capsaicin test. Secondary hyperalgesia in this case is expressed as increased pain sensitivity to mechanical stimulation in the surrounding, but not including, region of the capsaicin-treated skin. Since secondary hyperalgesia implicates hyperexcitability of dorsal horn interneurons [13], the results suggest the possibility that sleep deprivation has adverse nociceptive effects at the spinal level. They also showed significantly attenuated analgesic benefit from distraction with game playing, even though the groups did not differ in the degree of attention to and focus on the game playing task. Reduced benefit from distraction also suggests a possibility that sleep-deprived people may have trouble disengaging themselves from pain.

Past research has implicated that distraction analgesia may result from the activation of the endogenous opioid system [14]. Attenuated distraction analgesia in people with poor sleep suggests that poor sleep may interfere with this activation thereby reducing the analgesic benefit from the distraction technique. As we review in the next section, animal research also suggests that sleep deprivation interferes with opioid-mediated analgesia. Based upon these results, we may speculate that disordered sleep may attenuate the analgesic effects of certain behavioral coping strategies (e.g., distraction) via compromised endogenous opioid activation and effect. As noted, poor sleep is prevalent in chronic pain patients. Clinicians may need to be aware of the possibility of adverse effects of insomnia on distraction-based techniques.

Effects of Sleep Deprivation on Pain Response to Noxious Stimulation

In general, pain response to noxious stimulation seems to increase following poor sleep.

Animal Data: Effects of REM Deprivation on Pain Behavior

Because of the methodological constraints of animal model (i.e., no self-report data), poor sleep has to be experimentally defined by manipulating the quantity of sleep. Most commonly, the deprivation of rapid eye movement (REM) sleep is used in animals as a sleep measure of poor sleep and behavioral indication of response to noxious stimulations as an outcome. REM deprivation is typically achieved by utilizing a platform placed in shallow water, and when muscle atonia occurs in REM, the animal's limb or entire body falls into the water and it awakens. As reviewed extensively in Kundermann et al. [15], the animal studies showed consistent hypersensitivity with REM deprivation using a range of noxious stimulation modalities. A recent study [16], using the thermal preference apparatus, showed that REM deprivation may impact differentially on the nociceptive sensitivity to different types of noxious stimuli. When the animals had a choice of either staying on the hot plate or cold plate, their occupancy time did not differ between the two plates following a non-deprived sleep, whereas following the REM-deprived night, they stayed significantly longer on the hot plate than the cold plate. Although one often assumes the thermal pain of cold-hot sensations to be on one spectrum, evidence suggests that they do employ somewhat different processes [17]. Mechanisms underlying cold hyperalgesia/allodynia are not very well understood at this time, but likely involve multiple pathways. The results suggest that REM deprivation may more greatly augment sensitivity to cold and heat pain should further be studied to examine whether sleep deprivation differentially affects various thermal pain afferent pathways.

Animal Data: Effects of REM Deprivation on Analgesics

There are a few studies that suggest the possibility of REM deprivation interfering with the antinociceptive efficacy of pharmacologic interventions. Rats undergoing REM deprivation showed attenuated analgesia with morphine administration (2.5, 5 mg/kg) in response to the hot-plate test unless the dosage was very high (10 mg/kg) compared to control rats [18]. Recently, Skinner et al. [19] replicated the results with an interesting supposition that the slowing of paw withdrawal response to heat at the high-dose morphine (10 mg/kg) may not reflect the analgesic effects of opioids but rather it is due to decreased locomotor activity from the high-dose opioid.

It has been suggested [10] that sleep deprivation may reduce opioid binding and/or inhibit opioid protein synthesis, thereby reducing opioid analgesic effects on noxious stimulation. However, the autoradiographical analyses of receptor binding in the aforementioned study [18] showed no difference in the binding of [3H] DAMGO, a highly selective ligand for μ-opiate receptors, to mu receptors in REM-deprived rats compared to control rats. Thus, it is reasonable to assume that attenuated opioid analgesia in sleep-deprived animals do not result from the reduced affinity of mu receptor, although we cannot rule out the involvement of other opioid systems.

Damasceno et al. [20] tested the effects of REM deprivation on analgesic response with tricyclics. They divided rats into two groups: one group underwent REM deprivation whereas the other did not have any restriction of sleep. In each group, rats were given either saline or one of three dose levels of amitriptyline (3, 10 and 30 mg/kg) for 11 days prior to the testing. The REM-deprived rats consistently showed higher sensitivity to nociceptive testing with all doses; the difference was greatest at the highest amitriptyline dose (30 mg/kg) where the control rats showed significant analgesia while such effects were blunted in the REM-deprived rats.

Wei et al. [21] intrathecally administered specific 5-HT receptor subtype antagonists to REM-deprived rats and non-sleep-deprived rats. Compared to non-sleep-deprived rats, REM-deprived rats showed significantly increased pain responses to noxious mechanical stimuli. The effects of spinal 5-HT receptor antagonists are harder to interpret, as there was no effects of 5-HT(3) receptor antagonists, whereas 5-HT(1A) and 5-HT(2C) receptor antagonists had comparable analgesic effects for both REM-deprived and control animals. The results suggest that although some spinally administrated 5-HT receptor antagonists have analgesic effects in general, the effects do not interact with sleep deprivation. This seems at variance with the amitriptyline trial on REM-deprived rats [20] that showed analgesia only for their control subjects. Further studies are needed to clarity the interactive effects between the serotonergic system and sleep deprivation on pain.

Human Data

Experimental deprivation of sleep in humans involves several targets. It may simply reduce the duration of sleep or selectively target three areas: REM deprivation, total sleep deprivation (i.e., subject stays up all night), or deprivation of slow wave sleep (N3 sleep).

Reduced Sleep Duration

Tiede et al. [22] tested heat pain sensitivity in healthy volunteers twice, once after undergoing normal sleep and once after 4 h sleep regimens. The subjects showed significantly increased pain sensitivity to heat stimuli following the deprivation compared to normal sleep. The sleep duration for each phase was confirmed by the use of actigraph; however, how the sleep reduction altered the durations and proportions of each sleep stage could not be ascertained using actigraphy. Interestingly, the study also found that the pain-related-evoked potentials in response to the stimuli were reduced following sleep deprivation. The results appear contradictory; however, the authors argue that this dissociation may present a key to understand the sleep–pain connection in that it reflects an intracortical amplification process, resulting from reduced top-down control of the pain processing accompanied by reduced attentional resource allocation.

Deprivation of Total Sleep or Selective Sleep Stages

In the early uncontrolled study by Moldofsky et al. [23], six healthy young males underwent three consecutive nights of stage IV sleep deprivation. During the deprivation period, their pain sensitivity to pressure stimulation was significantly elevated. Acoustic disruption of N3 sleep without decreasing sleep duration also reduced pressure pain thresholds by 24 % in middle age, sedentary healthy females on next day [24]. However, not all studies found the pain altering effects of selective N3 sleep deprivation. In the study by Older et al. [25], 13 healthy people underwent 3 nights of selective N3 sleep disturbance. Their pressure pain thresholds were unchanged as a function of the N3 sleep disturbance. Similar results were obtained by Arima et al. [26] who found that ten healthy men did not show changes in pressure pain thresholds following 3 nights of N3 sleep disruption. The variance of the results is difficult to explain. Differences in the methods, sample characteristics, and the levels of interruptions may contribute to the inconsistent results. Additionally, it is possible that hyperalgesic response may not occur as a function of N3 sleep deprivation alone, but as a result of interaction between N3 sleep deprivation and other factors. Further studies are warranted to clarify this point.

Other studies have shown that the effects of sleep disturbance on pain may not be limited to N3 sleep deprivation. Onen et al. [27] tested the pain tolerance following three types of sleep deprivation: Total sleep deprivation, REM deprivation, and N3 sleep deprivation. All three types of deprivation produced decreases in pain tolerance to mechanical stimuli with the total sleep deprivation showing the greatest effect. The level of pain tolerance was restored following recovery sleep. Similarly Roehrs et al. [28] demonstrated that healthy people showed significantly greater pain response following REM deprivation or reduction in sleep duration (4 h). In her editorial comment, Baghdoyan [29] speculates that the modulation of acetylcholine release in the reticular formation (RF) may play an important role in the relationship between REM deprivation and pain, given the demonstrated linear relations between release of acetylcholine in the RF and duration of REM sleep. However, not all studies showed the hyperalgesic effects of REM deprivation. Moldofsky et al. [30] failed to demonstrate changes in pain sensitivity after 3 nights of REM deprivation. Similarly, a recent study [31] showed significant increase in pain sensitivity after 2 nights of total sleep deprivation, but pain sensitivity was unchanged after 4 nights of REM deprivation in healthy males.

Kundermann et al. [32] assigned 24 healthy people either to 2 nights of total sleep deprivation (i.e., no sleep) with a recovery sleep night in between, or control condition (no sleep deprivation). The subjects who had been sleep-deprived showed significant decreases in heat pain thresholds that were normalized after the restored sleep. On the other hand, 1 night of total deprivation in healthy people did not alter pain threshold or tolerance to mechanical and thermal stimuli [33]. Similarly, 1 night total sleep deprivation (about 39 h continuous waking) in patients with chronic pain of unknown origin resulted in increased clinical pain report but not alteration in pain thresholds in heat, cold, and pressure stimuli [34].

To summarize, research evaluating the effects of various types of sleep deprivation on pain response shows inconsistent results. The discrepancy is difficult to explain. Many of the studies are well controlled; selective deprivation studies typically show the polysomnographic data to ascertain the effects of deprivation (i.e., deprivation was selectively conducted). It is possible that the relationship between sleep deprivation and pain is not linear and other moderators and mediators are at work to make the effects variable. Human pain perception is known to be influenced by a range of cognitive, emotional, behavioral, and environmental factors [35]. For example, experimental studies have shown that pain-related self-efficacy is associated with greater pain sensitivity in response to noxious stimulation [36–38]. Improvement in self-efficacy reduces pain sensitivity but the effects may be attenuated by a use of naloxone [39], suggesting the involvement of endogenous opioid system in the self-efficacy belief. Other cognitive factors, such as belief that there is nothing one can do to reduce pain, has shown to lead greater neural activation in the pain-perception areas of the brain [40]. Some of those factors may override the adverse hyperalgesic effects of sleep deprivation. Identification of such factors will be helpful in treatment planning for those whose insomnia is particularly recalcitrant.

Another important point to keep in mind is the possibility that acute deprivation of sleep in a laboratory setting can be quite different from chronic insomnia chronic pain patients typically present. We will now review the effects of poor sleep on pain reports. However, it should be noted that unfortunately, research evaluating the effect of chronic insomnia on pain sensitivity is scarce and not well understood.

Cross-Sectional Associations Between Poor Sleep and Clinical Pain

A significant relationship between self-reported poor sleep and pain severity has been reported in people with a range of pain/medical conditions including advanced cancer [41], burn injuries [42], and rheumatoid arthritis [43]. For migraine patients, self-reported poor sleep is associated with the severity of allodynia [44]. O'Brien and colleagues [45] examined 292 patients with chronic facial pain, back pain, and fibromyalgia and found a significant relationship between poor sleep and pain, although emotional distress may also have mediated the relationship. In pediatric patients with headache, severe migraine headaches were associated with more severe sleep disturbance compared to milder headaches [46].

Research provides overwhelming support for the cross-sectional association between self-reported poor sleep and pain. Conditions with high likelihood of sleep disturbance and pain tend to show significant relationship between the two. Similarly, chronic pain patients who report high pain levels also report high degree of sleep disturbance. However, the cross-sectional nature of these studies does not allow us to make an inference for any causal relationship between sleep disturbance and pain.

Furthermore, when sleep is measured objectively, the relationship may become more tenuous. In our recent study [47], self-reported poor sleep (number of times awake during night and how refreshed patients felt upon wakening) was significantly correlated to reported pain severity, whereas the relationship was not present for the objective (actigraphically obtained) sleep measures.

Several studies investigated the possibility that disturbances in specific sleep architecture are related to pain conditions. In the aforementioned study with migrainous children [46], subjects with severe headaches had significantly lowered percents of N3 sleep and REM sleep. Earlier studies [48–50] suggested that fibromyalgia may be associated with greater alpha intrusion to sleep relative to healthy people. However, alpha intrusion does not seem to be present in all fibromyalgia patients and its relationship to symptoms is unclear [51]. Furthermore, a recent study [52] showed that the sleep architecture did not differ between fibromyalgia patients and healthy controls. In contrast, in another study [53], fibromyalgia patients exhibited shorter duration of Stage II, not N3 sleep, than did the matched healthy subjects, with an inverse relationship between daily pain scores and duration of Stage II.

The Relationship Between Poor Sleep and Pain Complaints

Nonclinical Samples

Increased pain complaints seem to follow nights of poor sleep even for healthy individuals, who are typically free of pain problems. In Haack's study [54], 40 healthy adults were asked either to reduce sleep to 50 % of their normal duration or to maintain their normal sleep for 12 consecutive nights. Those with sleep restriction reported greater pain complaints, generalized body pain, back pain, and stomach pain, across days. Other research suggests that not just insomnia but also hypersomnia may result in greater pain. Daily assessment of sleep and pain in a large sample of individuals in the general population showed that shorter (<6 h) or longer (>9 h) sleep duration was followed by increased pain in the next day [55].

Clinical Samples

The sequential relationship seems to hold in the clinical pain populations as well. Affleck et al. [56] followed fibromyalgia patients for 30 days using the temporally sequential analyses of sleep and pain and found that greater pain followed poorer sleep. Similarly, sequential analyses of sleep and pain over 10 days in adolescents with chronic pain [57] revealed that longer sleep duration and higher sleep interruption predicted the pain level in the next day. In a comprehensive study evaluating the two-way relationship between sleep and pain, Tang et al. [58] assessed sleep, pain, mood, and presleep arousal in 119 patients with various chronic pain conditions for 1 week. The results overall showed that no consistent relationship between sleep quality and pain. Presleep pain level was not a reliable predictor of sleep quality, whereas presleep cognitive and physiological arousal level did relate to the quality of sleep that night. Sleep quality seemed to have modest relation to pain next day although the effects are short-lived; the relationship only holds with pain reports taken in the earlier part of the day.

The sequential relationship seems less obvious when the objective measures of sleep are employed. In a recent report, 22 women with chronic pain underwent a 2-week assessment of pain and sleep, both self-report and actigraphic monitoring. Subjectively reported poor sleep, but not the actigraphically obtained sleep measures, was related to increased pain in the next day [59]. Another study using actigraphy [60] compared sleep patterns from ten consecutive nights between 61 teens with chronic pain and 60 healthy controls. Although the two groups were comparable in the sleep patterns of night time sleep, chronic pain teens had significantly greater daytime sleep, which was associated with greater functional limitation.

Sequential analyses between sleep and next day pain generally demonstrate that subjectively determined poor sleep, either insomnia or hypersomnia, seems to adversely impact pain at the later time. However, as in the cross-sectional analyses, the relationship may not hold when the quantity and quality of sleep are measured objectively.

The mismatch between subjectively reported and objectively measured sleep does not represent a pain-specific condition and is fairly common. Such discrepancy has been found in people with sleep disorders [61], depressed patients [62, 63], and community sample [64]. In our study of chronic pain patients whose sleep was measured seven consecutive nights, the average discrepancy between subjective and objective sleep was ±73 min per night, with greater discrepancy associated with restless sleep [47]. At this time, mechanisms underlying the discrepancy are not understood. The results raises an interesting question as to whether some of these discrepancies may reflect a form of sleep misperception ("paradoxical insomnia") in which a person complains of insomnia without any objective signs of sleep deprivation [65]. The misperception can go either direction, under-, or overestimation of the duration of sleep [66]. Future research needs to delineate how the discrepancy may be associated with various aspects of pain and wellness in general.

Effects of Poor Sleep on the Development of Chronic Pain

Research with prospective follow-up evaluation typically suggests that sleep disturbance is one of the contributors to the development of chronic pain. A study that followed 112 children with neck pain showed poor sleep and mood predicted the development of widespread body pain 1 year later [67]. Similarly, a study followed 394 high school students found that sleep disturbance and fatigue are significant predictors for the presence of weekly neck pain at age 22–25 [22–25, 68].

Sleep also seems to predict the development of chronic pain in adults. In a population study with 3,171 people, Gupta et al. [69] found that 324 people developed a new chronic widespread pain (CWP) 15 months later. Poor sleep at the baseline was a significant predictor, with an adjusted odds ratio of 2.7. Kaila-Kangas et al. [70] followed 902 metal workers for 28 years and found that the baseline sleep disturbance was a significant predictor for later hospitalization for back-related problems. Even when the workers with chronic or recurrent back pain at the baseline were excluded, the hazard ratio was 2.1 for those reported with the sleep latency disturbance and 2.9 for those with the latency problem and the multiple wakening. Sleep may also be a factor for facilitating the development of chronic pain in people with a history of severe injury. Castillo et al. [71] found that for those who had severe lower extremity injuries with sleep disturbance at the 3 months post-discharge are more likely to report chronic pain 7 years later.

The development of chronic pain is complex and multifactorial. Research consistently shows that sleep is a significant predictor, albeit the reported ORs suggest modest predictive power. It is reasonable to assume that sleep disturbance is just one of the contributors to the onset of chronic pain. A number of variables, including the pain parameters at onset, disease/injury severity, and other psychological variables, are likely to contribute to the development of chronic pain. However, it is clear although those with a history of pain or injuries are clearly high risk for later development of chronic pain, sleep disturbance seems to further facilitate such development. Assessment and therapy addressing sleep problems may be critical for the secondary prevention of chronic pain for those who are vulnerable.

Effects of Opioid Analgesics on Sleep

We have thus far reviewed the effects of poor sleep on pain. We would like to shift the direction here to discuss how opioid medications may influence sleep. Opioid medications are one of the most commonly prescribed medications [72]. Based upon a population survey [73], it is estimated that over 43 million adult Americans regularly use opioid medications.

Acute administration of opioid to opioid naïve subjects has a significant disrupting impact on sleep architecture. For example, acute administration of 5 mg methadone or 15 mg sustained-release morphine sulfate by month to opioid naïve, healthy people decreased N3 sleep and increased the duration of Stage II [74]. The same results were obtained with an acute administration of IV morphine (0.1 mg/kg) compared to saline IV in healthy individuals. Cronin et al. [75] compared the effects of two types of intraoperative and postoperative epidural analgesia (fentanyl vs. bupivacaine) on sleep in women undergoing a surgery requiring a low abdominal incision. Only the fentanyl group showed significantly reduced N3 sleep percent in the early postoperative phase.

Research is relatively scarce in the investigation of the relationship between chronic opioid therapy and sleep architecture. As reviewed by Wang and Teichtahl [76], the effects of opioids on sleep differ as a function of opioid phasing: Initiation, maintenance, acute abstinence, and prolonged abstinence. In an early study with six healthy men in a federal prison, Martin et al. [77] examined the effects of methadone at these four phases on sleep. They observed an increase in the total sleep duration during the ascending and stabilization weeks; there was a significantly increased duration of N3 sleep and REM 10 weeks after terminating the opioids. On the other hand, the comparisons between methadone maintenance patients (for opioid addiction, not for pain: 2–10 years of therapy) and healthy people showed that the patient group had significantly shorter N3 sleep, less wake after sleep onset, and fewer arousals during sleep than did the healthy controls [78]. Another study [79] also showed that methadone maintenance patients showed longer Stage II and shorter REM durations.

The implications of these studies are difficult to apply to clinical pain populations. It is likely that pain patients may experience significant sleep disturbance with the initiation of opioid treatment, as the studies of acute opioid administration to naïve subjects would imply. Less clear, however, is how chronic opioid therapy would influence sleep architecture in patients with chronic pain. Paradoxical results of both analgesia and pro-nociceptive effects via sleep disturbance may be co-present with prolonged opioid use. Anecdotally, we have observed that some of our patients with short acting opioids complain of waking at night with pain and unable to fall back asleep. The problem tends to resolve when the medication is switched to a long acting one. It is possible that these with short acting treatment may be experiencing nightly micro-withdrawal, thereby disturbing sleep. Further research in this area is urgently needed.

Another important consequence of opioid use is sleep-disordered breathing. Research evaluating the acute administration of opioids is limited to healthy subjects. The results are variable; one study shows decreased ventilatory response to hypoxia [80], whereas others decreased ventilatory response to hyperoxia, or no alteration in respiration during sleep [76, 81]. In contrast, growing evidence suggests that chronic opioid use increases the risk of central sleep apnea. The comparison between methadone maintenance patients and healthy controls [82] revealed significantly reduced hypercapnic ventilatory response and increased hypoxic ventilatory response in methadone maintenance patients relative to healthy controls. Thirty percent of the methadone maintenance patients had the central apnea index of greater than 5, whereas the highest index for the healthy controls was 1. No group difference was found on the obstructive sleep apnea index.

Similarly, an observational investigation of 140 chronic pain patients on chronic opioids [83] revealed that sleep apnea is common in these patients, with 39 % with obstructive sleep apnea and 24 % with the central sleep apnea. The daily doses of methadone and benzodiazepines were linearly related to central apnea index. In a study with people referred for a sleep study [84], patients taking chronic opioids exhibited significantly greater central apnea index than those without opioid medications, although the group did not differ on the obstructive sleep apnea index. The results are replicated by a recent multicenter study with a group of chronic pain patients on chronic opioids ($n=61$), chronic pain patients without opioids ($n=187$), and pain-free control ($n=170$) [85], showing the significantly greater central sleep apnea index in those with chronic opioids compared to the others. The risk of central sleep apnea seems to be related to opioid dose. The regressive analysis estimated 2.8 central apnea events increase per hour, per 100 mg morphine equivalent opioids.

Overall, research suggests that people using chronic opioids are at higher risk of developing central sleep apnea. Given the increasing trend of opioid-related mortality [86], better understanding of the nature of the relationship between central sleep apnea and chronic opioid use is essential. Recently, the use of adaptive servo-ventilation, a form of closed-loop mechanical ventilation, has been shown to improve central apnea related to chronic opioid use [87]. Another important point to keep in mind is that those who are using chronic opioids also tend to use other centrally depressive drugs, such as benzodiazepine which potentiate the ventilatory changes with opioids [88]. How the polypharmacy contributes to mortality, and the extent to which this risk is attributable to the sleep effects, remains to be elucidated.

Effects of Improved Sleep on Pain

An epidemiological follow-up study by Davies et al. [89] suggests that good sleeping habits may be critical in later resolution of chronic pain. In this study, the investigators followed 679 people in the general population with CWP of at least 3-month duration and reassessed 15 months later. Approximately 44 % reported the resolution of their CWP at follow-up. Three parameters of sleep quality at the baseline, short sleep latency, absence of early wakening, and restorative quality of sleep, predicted the resolution of CWP at the follow-up assessment [89].

As noted, disturbed breathing during sleep is common in chronic pain [83]. Resolution of this problem may have an important therapeutic effect. A recent small, randomized controlled trial [90] treated elderly patients with obstructive sleep apnea either with low (4 cmH_2O pressure) or high (5–10 cmH_2O pressure auto-adjusted) capacity continuous positive airway pressure (CPAP) therapy. Although both groups showed improved respiratory functions, only those in the high CPAP group showed significantly increased tolerance to electric stimulation, a return of pain threshold towards normal.

Unfortunately, many trials testing the efficacy of treatments for managing chronic pain tend to focus on pain as a primary outcome and often do not include sleep measures. However, clinical trials on fibromyalgia tend to include sleep as one of the outcomes probably because the adverse impact of poor sleep on the disorder is well recognized. A review of treatment efficacy for fibromyalgia suggests that both the use of amitriptyline and multimodal therapy approaches seems to help sleep and pain, although whether the sleep improvements are correlated with pain reduction is not known [91]. Application of cognitive-behavioral therapy for insomnia to fibromyalgia patients shows strong evidence for improvement in sleep but relatively small effects for pain reduction [92, 93]. In one study [92], however, the post-hoc analyses showed a moderate, though significant, correlation between the improvement in reported pain scores and the improvement in sleep quality (total waking time during night).

The lack of strong effect of better sleep influencing pain with the cognitive-behavioral approach is somewhat surprising as cognitive-behavioral therapy is typically shown to be efficacious for treating fibromyalgia [91]. Both studies, however, provided fairly brief intervention time (6 weeks). Given that the approach requires patients to learn the skills and practice, a longer duration may be needed to significantly impact pain severity. Furthermore, patients in the cognitive-behavioral treatment studies typically take multiple medications, unlike those in the pharmacotherapy trials. The potential confounding effects of those drugs may need to be considered. Having said that, however, this presents an interesting, yet familiar, dilemma. Washing out all the medications is needed to achieve an optimal level of internal validity for the study. On the other hand, the clinical reality is that many chronic pain patients have been taking multiple medications to address not just pain, but also sleep, mood, and function. How to apply the results from a well-controlled study to the actual patient population (that is, external validity) has always been a challenge in pain medicine.

A recent large multicenter, phase III clinical study with the randomized, double-blind, placebo-controlled design evaluated the efficacy of sodium oxybate in fibromyalgia patients [94]. Sodium oxybate is FDA-approved to treat narcolepsy, but the application for the use to treat fibromyalgia was rejected in 2010 for the safety concerns, mostly on the potential misuse and abuse potential of the drug. An earlier, open trial [95] showed that the use of sodium oxybate could normalize N3 sleep disturbance in fibromyalgia. In the multicenter study, 548 highly selected patients were randomized into placebo, sodium oxybate 4.5 or 6 g a day. The study had a high attrition (39 %), with the majority of dropouts being resulted from side effects and lack of efficacy. The series of intent-to-treat analyses revealed that the two sodium oxybate groups showed significant improvement in self-reported sleep quality and pain, as well as, to the lesser degree, tender point sensitivity.

Although clinical studies typically show the correlation of sleep improvement and pain reduction in chronic pain patients, it is still difficult to interpret the causal-effect relationship. Future research should evaluate the relationships; whether decreased pain improves sleep; whether improved sleep reduces pain; or whether other factors affect both sleep and pain.

Conclusion

We have reviewed several areas of research investigating the relationship between poor sleep and pain. Although there is some inconsistency in the results, overall, evidence seems to point to the relationship where poor sleep increases pan sensitivity to experimentally produced stimuli and is related to higher clinical pain report. Furthermore, the animal data suggests the potential interfering effects of poor sleep on the efficacy of analgesic pharmacotherapy. Similarly, the human data suggests that poor sleep may also attenuate the benefit of the behavioral approach to pain management.

In order to provide the other perspectives on the topic, we have reviewed the literature suggesting the possible adverse effects of opioid use on sleep. The area is fairly new but the accumulating evidence certainly suggests the importance of better understanding of how sleep is impacted by opioid analgesics, particularly chronic use, and how sleep disturbance from the opioid use, one of the most widely used pain treatment, may adversely impact the pain condition as a whole.

Treatment of sleep problems in chronic pain is not an easy task, given the likely bidirectional relationship between sleep and pain and its complicated relation to mood and function. Nonetheless, available evidence suggests that sleep is an important treatment target in chronic pain management. Improvement of sleep is essential, if not necessary, for recovery from pain and disability. Thus, better understanding of the sleep–pain relationship is imperative for developing effective sleep management for pain patients.

References

1. Johnson EO, Roth T, Schultz L, Breslau N. Epidemiology of DSM-IV insomnia in adolescence: lifetime prevalence, chronicity, and an emergent gender difference. Pediatrics. 2006;117(2):e247–56.
2. National Sleep Foundation. Summary of findings: sleep in America poll. Washington, DC: National Sleep Foundation; 2005.
3. Orzel-Gryglewska J. Consequences of sleep deprivation. Int J Occup Med Environ Health. 2010; 23(1):95–114.
4. Tang NK, Wright KJ, Salkovskis PM. Prevalence and correlates of clinical insomnia co-occurring with chronic back pain. J Sleep Res. 2007;16(1):85–95.
5. McCracken LM, Iverson GL. Disrupted sleep patterns and daily functioning in patients with chronic pain. Pain Res Manag. 2002;7(2):75–9.
6. Smith MT, Wickwire EM, Grace EG, et al. Sleep disorders and their association with laboratory pain sensitivity in temporomandibular joint disorder. Sleep. 2009;32(6):779–90.
7. Theadom A, Cropley M, Humphrey KL. Exploring the role of sleep and coping in quality of life in fibromyalgia. J Psychosom Res. 2007;62(2):145–51.
8. Sivertsen B, Krokstad S, Overland S, Mykletun A. The epidemiology of insomnia: associations with physical and mental health. The HUNT-2 study. J Psychosom Res. 2009;67(2):109–16.
9. Ohayon MM. Relationship between chronic painful physical condition and insomnia. J Psychiatr Res. 2005;39(2):151–9.
10. Lautenbacher S, Kundermann B, Krieg JC. Sleep deprivation and pain perception. Sleep Med Rev. 2006;10(5):357–69.
11. Lee YC, Chibnik LB, Lu B, et al. The relationship between disease activity, sleep, psychiatric distress and pain sensitivity in rheumatoid arthritis: a cross-sectional study. Arthritis Res Ther. 2009;11(5):R160.
12. Campbell CM, Bounds SC, Simango MB, et al. Self-reported sleep duration associated with distraction analgesia, hyperemia, and secondary hyperalgesia in the heat-capsaicin nociceptive model. Eur J Pain. 2011;15(6):561–7.
13. Westlund KN. Chapter 9 The dorsal horn and hyperalgesia. Handb Clin Neurol. 2006;81:103–25.
14. Tracey I, Ploghaus A, Gati JS, et al. Imaging attentional modulation of pain in the periaqueductal gray in humans. J Neurosci. 2002;22(7):2748–52.
15. Kundermann B, Krieg JC, Schreiber W, Lautenbacher S. The effect of sleep deprivation on pain. Pain Res Manag. 2004;9(1):25–32.
16. Harvey MT, Kline IV RH, May ME, et al. Parametric analysis of thermal preference following sleep deprivation in the rat. Neurosci Lett. 2010;485(2):98–101.
17. Schepers RJ, Ringkamp M. Thermoreceptors and thermosensitive afferents. Neurosci Biobehav Rev. 2010;34(2):177–84.
18. Nascimento DC, Andersen ML, Hipolide DC, Nobrega JN, Tufik S. Pain hypersensitivity induced by paradoxical sleep deprivation is not due to altered binding to brain mu-opioid receptors. Behav Brain Res. 2007;178(2):216–20.
19. Skinner GO, Damasceno F, Gomes A, de Almeida OM. Increased pain perception and attenuated opioid antinociception in paradoxical sleep-deprived rats are associated with reduced tyrosine hydroxylase staining in the periaqueductal gray matter and are reversed by L-dopa. Pharmacol Biochem Behav. 2011;99(1):94–9.
20. Damasceno F, Skinner GO, Gomes A, Araujo PC, de Almeida OM. Systemic amitriptyline administration does not prevent the increased thermal response induced by paradoxical sleep deprivation. Pharmacol Biochem Behav. 2009;94(1):51–5.
21. Wei H, Ma A, Wang YX, Pertovaara A. Role of spinal 5-HT receptors in cutaneous hypersensitivity induced by REM sleep deprivation. Pharmacol Res. 2008;57(6):469–75.
22. Tiede W, Magerl W, Baumgartner U, Durrer B, Ehlert U, Treede RD. Sleep restriction attenuates amplitudes and attentional modulation of pain-related evoked potentials, but augments pain ratings in healthy volunteers. Pain. 2010;148(1):36–42.
23. Moldofsky H, Scarisbrick P, England R, Smythe H. Musculosketal symptoms and non-REM sleep disturbance in patients with "fibrositis syndrome" and healthy subjects. Psychosom Med. 1975;37(4):341–51.
24. Lentz MJ, Landis CA, Rothermel J, Shaver JL. Effects of selective slow wave sleep disruption on musculoskeletal pain and fatigue in middle aged women. J Rheumatol. 1999;26(7):1586–92.
25. Older SA, Battafarano DF, Danning CL, et al. The effects of delta wave sleep interruption on pain thresholds and fibromyalgia-like symptoms in healthy subjects; correlations with insulin-like growth factor I. J Rheumatol. 1998;25(6):1180–6.
26. Arima T, Svensson P, Rasmussen C, Nielsen KD, Drewes AM, Arendt-Nielsen L. The relationship between selective sleep deprivation, nocturnal jaw-muscle activity and pain in healthy men. J Oral Rehabil. 2001;28(2):140–8.

27. Onen SH, Alloui A, Gross A, Eschallier A, Dubray C. The effects of total sleep deprivation, selective sleep interruption and sleep recovery on pain tolerance thresholds in healthy subjects. J Sleep Res. 2001; 10(1):35–42.
28. Roehrs T, Hyde M, Blaisdell B, Greenwald M, Roth T. Sleep loss and REM sleep loss are hyperalgesic. Sleep. 2006;29(2):145–51.
29. Baghdoyan HA. Hyperalgesia induced by REM sleep loss: a phenomenon in search of a mechanism. Sleep. 2006;29(2):137–9.
30. Moldofsky H, Scarisbrick P. Induction of neurasthenic musculoskeletal pain syndrome by selective sleep stage deprivation. Psychosom Med. 1976; 38(1):35–44.
31. Azevedo E, Manzano GM, Silva A, Martins R, Andersen ML, Tufik S. The effects of total and REM sleep deprivation on laser-evoked potential threshold and pain perception. Pain. 2011;152(9):2052–8.
32. Kundermann B, Spernal J, Huber MT, Krieg JC, Lautenbacher S. Sleep deprivation affects thermal pain thresholds but not somatosensory thresholds in healthy volunteers. Psychosom Med. 2004;66(6):932–7.
33. Drewes AM, Rossel P, Arendt-Nielsen L, et al. Sleepiness does not modulate experimental joint pain in healthy volunteers. Scand J Rheumatol. 1997; 26(5):399–400.
34. Busch V, Haas J, Cronlein T, et al. Sleep deprivation in chronic somatoform pain-effects on mood and pain regulation. Psychiatry Res. 2012;195(3):134–43.
35. Okifuji A, Turk DC. The influence of the psychosocial environment in pain comorbidities. In: Giamberadino MA, Jensen TS, editors. Pain comorbidities: understanding and treating the complex patient. Seattle, WA: IASP Press; 2012. p. 157–76.
36. Bandura A. Self-efficacy: toward a unifying theory of behavioral change. Psychol Rev. 1977;84(2):191–215.
37. Dolce JJ, Doleys DM, Raczynski JM, Lossie J, Poole L, Smith M. The role of self-efficacy expectancies in the prediction of pain tolerance. Pain. 1986;27(2): 261–72.
38. Keefe FJ, Lefebvre JC, Maixner W, Salley Jr AN, Caldwell DS. Self-efficacy for arthritis pain: relationship to perception of thermal laboratory pain stimuli. Arthritis Care Res. 1997;10(3):177–84.
39. Bandura A, O'Leary A, Taylor CB, Gauthier J, Gossard D. Perceived self-efficacy and pain control: opioid and nonopioid mechanisms. J Pers Soc Psychol. 1987;53(3):563–71.
40. Salomons TV, Johnstone T, Backonja MM, Davidson RJ. Perceived controllability modulates the neural response to pain. J Neurosci. 2004;24(32):7199–203.
41. Delgado-Guay M, Yennurajalingam S, Parsons H, Palmer JL, Bruera E. Association between self-reported sleep disturbance and other symptoms in patients with advanced cancer. J Pain Symptom Manage. 2011;41(5):819–27.
42. Raymond I, Nielsen TA, Lavigne G, Manzini C, Choiniere M. Quality of sleep and its daily relationship to pain intensity in hospitalized adult burn patients. Pain. 2001;92(3):381–8.
43. Luyster FS, Chasens ER, Wasko MC, Dunbar-Jacob J. Sleep quality and functional disability in patients with rheumatoid arthritis. J Clin Sleep Med. 2011; 7(1):49–55.
44. Lovati C, D'Amico D, Bertora P, et al. Correlation between presence of allodynia and sleep quality in migraineurs. Neurol Sci. 2010;31 Suppl 1:S155–8.
45. O'Brien EM, Waxenberg LB, Atchison JW, et al. Negative mood mediates the effect of poor sleep on pain among chronic pain patients. Clin J Pain. 2010;26(4):310–9.
46. Vendrame M, Kaleyias J, Valencia I, Legido A, Kothare SV. Polysomnographic findings in children with headaches. Pediatr Neurol. 2008;39(1):6–11.
47. Okifuji A, Hare BD. Nightly analyses of subjective and objective (actigraphy) measures of sleep in fibromyalgia syndrome: what accounts for the discrepancy? Clin J Pain. 2011;27(4):289–96.
48. Branco J, Atalaia A, Paiva T. Sleep cycles and alpha-delta sleep in fibromyalgia syndrome. J Rheumatol. 1994;21(6):1113–7.
49. Drewes AM, Nielsen KD, Taagholt SJ, Bjerregard K, Svendsen L, Gade J. Sleep intensity in fibromyalgia: focus on the microstructure of the sleep process. Br J Rheumatol. 1995;34(7):629–35.
50. Roizenblatt S, Tufik S, Goldenberg J, Pinto LR, Hilario MO, Feldman D. Juvenile fibromyalgia: clinical and polysomnographic aspects. J Rheumatol. 1997;24(3):579–85.
51. Carette S, Oakson G, Guimont C, Steriade M. Sleep electroencephalography and the clinical response to amitriptyline in patients with fibromyalgia. Arthritis Rheum. 1995;38(9):1211–7.
52. Chervin RD, Teodorescu M, Kushwaha R, et al. Objective measures of disordered sleep in fibromyalgia. J Rheumatol. 2009;36(9):2009–16.
53. Burns JW, Crofford LJ, Chervin RD. Sleep stage dynamics in fibromyalgia patients and controls. Sleep Med. 2008;9(6):689–96.
54. Haack M, Mullington JM. Sustained sleep restriction reduces emotional and physical well-being. Pain. 2005;119(1–3):56–64.
55. Edwards RR, Almeida DM, Klick B, Haythornthwaite JA, Smith MT. Duration of sleep contributes to next-day pain report in the general population. Pain. 2008;137(1):202–7.
56. Affleck G, Urrows S, Tennen H, Higgins P, Abeles M. Sequential daily relations of sleep, pain intensity, and attention to pain among women with fibromyalgia. Pain. 1996;68(2–3):363–8.
57. Lewandowski AS, Palermo TM, De la Motte S, Fu R. Temporal daily associations between pain and sleep in adolescents with chronic pain versus healthy adolescents. Pain. 2010;151(1):220–5.

58. Tang NK, Goodchild CE, Sanborn AN, Howard J, Salkovskis PM. Deciphering the temporal link between pain and sleep in a heterogeneous chronic pain patient sample: a multilevel daily process study. Sleep. 2012;35(5):675–87A.
59. O'Brien EM, Waxenberg LB, Atchison JW, et al. Intraindividual variability in daily sleep and pain ratings among chronic pain patients: bidirectional association and the role of negative mood. Clin J Pain. 2011;27(5):425–33.
60. Law EF, Dufton L, Palermo TM. Daytime and nighttime sleep patterns in adolescents with and without chronic pain. Health Psychol. 2012;31(6):830–3.
61. Vanable PA, Aikens JE, Tadimeti L, Caruana-Montaldo B, Mendelson WB. Sleep latency and duration estimates among sleep disorder patients: variability as a function of sleep disorder diagnosis, sleep history, and psychological characteristics. Sleep. 2000;23(1):71–9.
62. Tsuchiyama K, Nagayama H, Kudo K, Kojima K, Yamada K. Discrepancy between subjective and objective sleep in patients with depression. Psychiatry Clin Neurosci. 2003;57(3):259–64.
63. Rotenberg VS, Indursky P, Kayumov L, Sirota P, Melamed Y. The relationship between subjective sleep estimation and objective sleep variables in depressed patients. Int J Psychophysiol. 2000;37(3): 291–7.
64. Jackowska M, Dockray S, Hendrickx H, Steptoe A. Psychosocial factors and sleep efficiency: discrepancies between subjective and objective evaluations of sleep. Psychosom Med. 2011;73(9):810–6.
65. McCall WV, Edinger JD. Subjective total insomnia: an example of sleep state misperception. Sleep. 1992;15(1):71–3.
66. Trajanovic NN, Radivojevic V, Kaushansky Y, Shapiro CM. Positive sleep state misperception—a new concept of sleep misperception. Sleep Med. 2007;8(2):111–8.
67. Mikkelsson M, Sourander A, Salminen JJ, Kautiainen H, Piha J. Widespread pain and neck pain in schoolchildren. A prospective one-year follow-up study. Acta Paediatr. 1999;88(10):1119–24.
68. Siivola SM, Levoska S, Latvala K, Hoskio E, Vanharanta H, Keinanen-Kiukaanniemi S. Predictive factors for neck and shoulder pain: a longitudinal study in young adults. Spine (Phila Pa 1976). 2004; 29(15):1662–9.
69. Gupta A, Silman AJ, Ray D, et al. The role of psychosocial factors in predicting the onset of chronic widespread pain: results from a prospective population-based study. Rheumatology (Oxford). 2007;46(4):666–71.
70. Kaila-Kangas L, Kivimaki M, Harma M, et al. Sleep disturbances as predictors of hospitalization for back disorders—a 28-year follow-up of industrial employees. Spine (Phila Pa 1976). 2006;31(1):51–6.
71. Castillo RC, MacKenzie EJ, Wegener ST, Bosse MJ. Prevalence of chronic pain seven years following limb threatening lower extremity trauma. Pain. 2006; 124(3):321–9.
72. Kuehn BM. Opioid prescriptions soar: increase in legitimate use as well as abuse. JAMA. 2007;297(3):249–51.
73. Parsells Kelly J, Cook SF, Kaufman DW, Anderson T, Rosenberg L, Mitchell AA. Prevalence and characteristics of opioid use in the US adult population. Pain. 2008;138(3):507–13.
74. Dimsdale JE, Norman D, DeJardin D, Wallace MS. The effect of opioids on sleep architecture. J Clin Sleep Med. 2007;3(1):33–6.
75. Cronin AJ, Keifer JC, Davies MF, King TS, Bixler EO. Postoperative sleep disturbance: influences of opioids and pain in humans. Sleep. 2001;24(1):39–44.
76. Wang D, Teichtahl H. Opioids, sleep architecture and sleep-disordered breathing. Sleep Med Rev. 2007;11(1):35–46.
77. Martin WR, Jasinski DR, Haertzen CA, et al. Methadone—a reevaluation. Arch Gen Psychiatry. 1973;28(2):286–95.
78. Xiao L, Tang YL, Smith AK, et al. Nocturnal sleep architecture disturbances in early methadone treatment patients. Psychiatry Res. 2010;179(1):91–5.
79. Wang D, Teichtahl H, Goodman C, Drummer O, Grunstein RR, Kronborg I. Subjective daytime sleepiness and daytime function in patients on stable methadone maintenance treatment: possible mechanisms. J Clin Sleep Med. 2008;4(6):557–62.
80. Bailey PL, Lu JK, Pace NL, et al. Effects of intrathecal morphine on the ventilatory response to hypoxia. N Engl J Med. 2000;343(17):1228–34.
81. Shaw IR, Lavigne G, Mayer P, Choiniere M. Acute intravenous administration of morphine perturbs sleep architecture in healthy pain-free young adults: a preliminary study. Sleep. 2005;28(6):677–82.
82. Teichtahl H, Wang D, Cunnington D, et al. Ventilatory responses to hypoxia and hypercapnia in stable methadone maintenance treatment patients. Chest. 2005; 128(3):1339–47.
83. Webster LR, Choi Y, Desai H, Webster L, Grant BJ. Sleep-disordered breathing and chronic opioid therapy. Pain Med. 2008;9(4):425–32.
84. Walker JM, Farney RJ, Rhondeau SM, et al. Chronic opioid use is a risk factor for the development of central sleep apnea and ataxic breathing. J Clin Sleep Med. 2007;3(5):455–61.
85. Jungquist CR, Flannery M, Perlis ML, Grace JT. Relationship of chronic pain and opioid use with respiratory disturbance during sleep. Pain Manag Nurs. 2012;13(2):70–9.
86. Fingerhut LO. Increases in poisoning and methadone-related deaths: United States, 1999–2005. NCHS Health E-Stat CDC, ed. Washington, DC; 2008.
87. Ramar K, Ramar P, Morgenthaler TI. Adaptive servoventilation in patients with central or complex sleep apnea related to chronic opioid use and congestive heart failure. J Clin Sleep Med. 2012;8(5):569–76.
88. Bailey PL, Pace NL, Ashburn MA, Moll JW, East KA, Stanley TH. Frequent hypoxemia and apnea after sedation with midazolam and fentanyl. Anesthesiology. 1990;73(5):826–30.

89. Davies KA, Macfarlane GJ, Nicholl BI, et al. Restorative sleep predicts the resolution of chronic widespread pain: results from the EPIFUND study. Rheumatology (Oxford). 2008;47(12):1809–13.
90. Onen SH, Onen F, Albrand G, Decullier E, Chapuis F, Dubray C. Pain tolerance and obstructive sleep apnea in the elderly. J Am Med Dir Assoc. 2010; 11(9):612–6.
91. Okifuji A, Ashburn M. Fibromyalgia syndrome: toward an integration of the literature. Crit Rev Phys Rehabil Med. 2001;13(1):27–54.
92. Edinger JD, Wohlgemuth WK, Krystal AD, Rice JR. Behavioral insomnia therapy for fibromyalgia patients: a randomized clinical trial. Arch Intern Med. 2005;165(21):2527–35.
93. Miro E, Lupianez J, Martinez MP, et al. Cognitive-behavioral therapy for insomnia improves attentional function in fibromyalgia syndrome: a pilot, randomized controlled trial. J Health Psychol. 2011; 16(5):770–82.
94. Russell IJ, Holman AJ, Swick TJ, Alvarez-Horine S, Wang YG, Guinta D. Sodium oxybate reduces pain, fatigue, and sleep disturbance and improves functionality in fibromyalgia: results from a 14-week, randomized, double-blind, placebo-controlled study. Pain. 2011;152(5):1007–17.
95. Scharf MB, Baumann M, Berkowitz DV. The effects of sodium oxybate on clinical symptoms and sleep patterns in patients with fibromyalgia. J Rheumatol. 2003;30(5):1070–4.

Sleep Loss in Older Adults: Effects on Waking Performance and Sleep-Dependent Memory Consolidation with Healthy Aging and Insomnia

14

Edward F. Pace-Schott and Rebecca M.C. Spencer

Introduction

The effects of acute sleep deprivation on waking cognitive processes such as vigilant attention may be buffered in older adults, in comparison to younger adults, by normal changes in homeostatic and circadian regulation of sleep propensity [1]. These processes may confer a lesser need for total sleep in general, and slow wave sleep (SWS) in particular, in comparison to younger adults [1–3]. Although lowered sleep need may allow older adults a degree of cognitive protection against sleep loss, the sleep-wake regulatory systems in older adults are fragile and vulnerable to disruption. The risk of such disruption increases with aging not only due to a wide variety of medical conditions [4, 5], but also due to psychiatric disorders such as depression, anxiety disorders [6], and especially insomnia, the risk for which increases with aging [7]. Moreover, forms of memory consolidation that are dependent upon neural processes that occur during sleep may become degraded by normal declines in sleep duration and quality. Such changes may then be exacerbated by any further reduction in sleep quantity or quality when insomnia and anxiety are present in older individuals.

E.F. Pace-Schott, Ph.D. (✉)
Department of Psychiatry, Harvard Medical School, Massachusetts General Hospital, Charlestown, MA, USA
e-mail: epace-schott@partners.org

Rebecca M.C. Spencer, Ph.D.
Department of Psychology and Neuroscience and Behavior Program, University of Massachusetts, Amherst, Amherst, MA, USA

Changes in Sleep Quality and Architecture with Aging

Changes in sleep quality and polysomnographic (PSG) architecture as well as in the homeostatic and circadian control of sleep propensity accompany healthy aging (for reviews, see [4, 5, 8–12]. Studies using PSG (e.g., [13, 14]), actigraphy (e.g.,[15]) and subjective measures of sleep (e.g., [14]) reveal changes in sleep quality with aging that include decreased total sleep time (TST), increased wake time after sleep onset (WASO), and decreased sleep efficiency (for review, see ref. [8]). Nocturnal awakenings, especially in the early morning, increase in frequency and duration with aging [4, 5] and PSG studies show that older adults awaken more often from non-rapid eye movement sleep (NREM) vs. rapid eye movement sleep (REM) [16, 17].[1] This latter feature may render older adults more vulnerable to sleep inertia—reduced performance and alertness due to sleep-state carry over following awakening [18]. Studies comparing young-old to old-old individuals further suggest that deterioration of

[1] Cited studies that differentiate REM and NREM or substages of NREM (e.g., slow wave sleep) or that report phasic features of sleep (e.g., sleep spindles) or EEG spectral power (e.g., slow wave activity) all employ PSG.

M.T. Bianchi (ed.), *Sleep Deprivation and Disease: Effects on the Body, Brain and Behavior*,
DOI 10.1007/978-1-4614-9087-6_14,

sleep quality in aging becomes especially prominent with advanced age. For example, a combined PSG and diary study showed that "young-old" individuals (aged 60–74 years) showed few changes in sleep quality over 3 years of longitudinal monitoring, whereas "old-old" individuals (75–87 years) showed increasing WASO and sleep onset latency (SOL) over this same duration [19, 20].

Behavioral factors may further degrade sleep quality with aging. Most prominent of these behavioral factors is a changed frequency of daytime napping [21]. The frequency of diurnal naps increases markedly with aging and this increase continues from "young-old" into "old-old" age [22]. Changes in social patterns may also decrease natural light exposure [23] and reduce exposure to other naturally occurring time cues (zeitgebers) [12]. Circadian disruption may be further exacerbated by the normative circadian phase advance that accompanies healthy aging [12].

Sleep is additionally disrupted by medical conditions common in older adults such as arthritic pain, gastroesophageal reflux, nocturia, and polypharmacy [4, 5, 24]. Much greater disruption of sleep ensues with serious medical conditions such as obstructive sleep apnea (OSA) [25], heart failure [26], and neurodegenerative illnesses [27].

Reduced polysomnographically scored SWS as well as reduced Slow Wave Activity (SWA), defined as spectral power in the delta (0.5–4.5 Hz) frequency range, are the most prominent changes in sleep architecture that accompany healthy aging [2, 3, 28, 29]. Decreasing SWA reflects decline in both the amplitude and frequency of slow waves [2, 30, 31] and is also accompanied by reductions in the slow (<1 Hz) oscillation [28]. For example, in a carefully controlled study, Dijk et al. [3] demonstrated reduction in SWS in middle-aged (40–55 years) and older (66–83 years) adults compared to young (20–30 years) adults with the greatest change observed between the young and middle-aged groups. These age-related declines in SWA are most prominent in frontal brain regions [32]. Unlike in young adults for whom SWS is concentrated in the first one or two NREM-REM cycles of the night, SWS is distributed more evenly across the night in older adults [32, 33]. Carrier et al. [30] have shown that such changes relative to young adults are present at a mean age of 51 ± 4.6 years. They also showed that, by this age, slow waves are reduced in density and their morphology has changed such that the positive component of such waves has a reduced slope and increased duration. SWS declines less with aging in females vs. males [34] and older females better maintain the characteristic morphology of slow waves [30].

The total amount and percentage of REM sleep declines only slightly with aging [29, 35]. However, REM density, the number of rapid eye movements per unit time, is more prominently decreased [36]. With the decline in SWS and REM, lighter NREM sleep (N1 and N2) is increased proportionately. However, N2 sleep spindles are reduced in number, density, and amplitude [2, 37–42] as are the frequency and amplitude of N2 K-complexes [37, 43].

Experimental Sleep Loss and Cognition in Healthy Aging

Harrison and colleagues [44] have suggested that total sleep deprivation (TSD) in young adults may model the cognitive changes typical of normally rested, healthy older adults. However, paradoxically, waking performance is *less* disrupted in older vs. younger adults following TSD [45–49], reviewed in [1]. Moreover, performance of older adults is superior to young adults after sleep restriction [50, 51] and sleep fragmentation [52].

In an early study, the effects of 64 h TSD were compared between healthy young males (18–28 years) and older males (55–71 years) with and without insomnia [53]. Using a verbal memory and a reaction time (RT) test, individuals in these three groups were tested at bedtime, following three nocturnal awakenings by study staff, and upon morning awakening on baseline and recovery nights as well as at the corresponding times across 64 h (2 nights) of TSD [53]. Whereas performance on both the memory and RT task deteriorated across 2 night's TSD in young males, it remained near baseline values in both the healthy and insomniac older males. In another study, during 26 h of constant routine conditions (continuous waking in a semi-recumbent position under dim light with regularly spaced caloric intake), performance on the psychomotor vigilance test (PVT) did not differ between young and older adults during the hours that they were normally awake. However, during hours that they were normally asleep, performance in older subjects was less impaired as indicated by both faster RTs and fewer lapses (RT>500 ms) in performance [47]. Very similar results were seen in another study using TSD with a constant routine protocol in which a baseline slower RT on the PVT in older (mean 65 years) vs. younger (mean 25 years) adults disappeared during the hours normally occupied by sleep [48]. Similarly, in a sleep-laboratory study that employed repeated PVT testing over 40 h TSD, young males (mean 25.2 years) compared to older males (mean 66.4 years) displayed greater slowing of RT, more PVT lapses, and greater RT variability beginning after the 16 h of normal wake had elapsed [46]. This greater impact of TSD on young participants became highly pronounced by the time of the circadian nadir (the 24-h core temperature minimum occurring around 4 a.m.) and continued into the subsequent day. In a similar study, using a within-subject crossover design, young males (mean 22.5 years) showed a significant increase in number of lapses on a simple RT task following 24 h TSD compared to a night of normal sleep [49]. Older males (mean 58.2 years), on the other hand, showed no change in lapses with TSD. Along with a lesser performance deficit, older adults in some [46] but not all [49] studies report less subjective sleepiness during prolonged TSD. Older adults also display less increase, during TSD, in objective measures of sleepiness such as the multiple sleep latency test or MSLT [54].

These findings support earlier studies reporting less sleep deprivation-related decrement in older vs. younger individuals on a choice reaction time task [55] as well as on a vigilance task in old-old individuals (80 years) compared to young adults (20 years) [56]. In more ecologically realistic settings, cognitive resistance to sleep deprivation may buffer older-adult performance in some situations such as in a driving simulator [57] but not in others, such as maintaining postural control [58]. The latter effect of sleep deprivation has significant health and safety implications with regard to the risk of falling in older adults.

Older adults also show lesser cognitive sequela of sleep loss under conditions of partial sleep deprivation. For example, Bliese et al. [50] showed that 7 days of sleep restriction to 5 or 3 h time-in-bed (TIB) resulted in deterioration of PVT performance compared to performance following sufficient sleep (7 and 9 h TIB). Notably, however, this reduction in performance under partial sleep deprivation was negatively related to increasing age.

Similarly, although older adults are less able than younger adults to adapt their sleep schedules to shifted circadian phase [16, 59], they have been shown to display less subjective sleepiness as well as better-maintained vigilance performance during extended exposure to experimentally altered circadian phase [14, 60]. In one such study, older (mean 64 years) and younger (mean 24 years) adults underwent 18 days of a forced desynchrony protocol—an experimental procedure whereby circadian and homeostatic influences (see below) can be dissociated by imposing day–night schedules outside the range that can entrain the intrinsic human circadian clock—in this case consisting of 20-h days [60]. Across this extended disruption of circadian rhythmicity, unlike the younger adults, older adults showed neither an increase in subjective sleepiness nor an increase in RT on the PVT.

Changes in Circadian and Homeostatic Sleep Regulation with Aging

The Two-Process Model [61] postulates that sleep propensity results from the interaction of a homeostatic process (Process S) by which sleep propensity increases with increased duration of prior waking and a circadian process (Process C) by which intrinsic drive to sleep or waking varies predictably across a 24-h period. The interaction of these two processes allows for a consolidated bout of nocturnal sleep in healthy adults [62]. Both homeostatic and circadian processes are believed to be damped in older adults [2, 3, 12] and changes in the homeostatic regulation of sleep may be of particular importance to the above-noted cognitive resistance to sleep deprivation with aging.

Circadian Changes in Sleep Patterns with Aging

The master circadian signal from the suprachiasmatic nucleus (SCN) of the anterior hypothalamus is believed to weaken with age [63, 64]. Biological changes in the human SCN with aging include decreases in cell number and neuroendocrine activity [12, 63]. These changes result in a decreased amplitude of circadian rhythms of both objective and subjective sleepiness [13] as well as of core body temperature, melatonin and cortisol, the amplitude of which may be 20–30 % lower in older compared to younger adults [11, 12, 63–66]. In older adults, the circadian rhythms of core body temperature, melatonin, and cortisol are phase advanced by approximately 1 h relative to younger adults [11, 12, 65, 67]. Nonetheless, the circadian period remains approximately 24.2 h across the lifespan [68].

The sensitivity of the SCN to photic entrainment appears also to diminish with age [64]. Nonetheless, bright light can reset the circadian clock in both young and older adults [69, 70]. The weakening of the circadian signal with aging may be exacerbated by behavioral and environmental factors such as increased time indoors away from natural light cues [71], degenerative changes in the eye [72], or reduced exposure to zeitgebers such as social stimuli [73] (see ref.[12] for a review). Older adults have more difficulty with sleep maintenance when attempting sleep at an unfavorable circadian phase as occurs with jet lag [16, 59]. Similarly, older adults may suffer greater sleep inertia because of their tendency both to awaken at an earlier circadian phase and to more frequently awaken from NREM relative to REM sleep in comparison to younger adults [18]. In addition to effects on cognition brought about by age-related effects on the circadian timing of sleep, age may also influence cognition-related circadian oscillators in the brain independently of the effects of such oscillators on sleep itself [64].

Homeostatic Changes in Sleep Patterns in Healthy Aging

The increase in SWS and SWA following sleep loss (discussed above) constitutes a sensitive measure of sleep homeostatic recovery [74]. Because of the increase in nocturnal awakenings and decrease in subjective and objective daytime sleepiness with aging, it has been suggested that concurrent reductions in SWS and SWA indicate a decrease in the degree to which sleep homeostatic pressure increases over prolonged wakefulness [1–3]. For example, in a large-scale study, Dijk et al. [3] used acoustic disruption of SWS in young, middle-aged, and older adults to examine age-related differences in homeostatic rebound of SWS. Compared to age-matched controls who were allowed undisturbed sleep, disruption of SWS produced a rebound of SWS as well as increased objective (MSLT) and subjective daytime sleepiness in all three age groups. This responsivity to curtailment of SWS in older adults indicated that their ability to homeostatically compensate for loss of SWS relative to their baseline remained intact. Dijk et al. [3] therefore concluded that the observed age-related baseline differences in SWS and SWA reflect a lesser buildup of homeostatic sleep pressure during normal waking rather than a putative inability to compensate for sleep loss that would lead to chronic sleep debt. As further evidence of lesser sleep need in aging, a smaller additional amount of TST was achieved by older compared to younger adults when an extended 16-h sleep opportunity was provided [75].

Nonetheless, other investigators have found differences in the way in which the sleep EEG responds to sleep loss in older vs. younger adults. For example, following 40 h TSD under constant routine conditions, young adults (mean 25 years) showed a distinct frontal predominance of SWA during recovery sleep, whereas older adults (mean 65 years) had SWA more evenly distributed between frontal and posterior derivations as well as a slower decline in overall delta power across the remainder of recovery sleep [32]. However, as in Dijk et al. [3], a significant increase in SWS on the recovery vs. baseline night was present in both older and younger groups, a finding also replicated in middle-aged (40–60 years) adults [76]. Age differences in the response to the *lowering* of homeostatic sleep pressure using daytime naps have also been reported in some, but not all studies. For example, Campbell and Feinberg [77] report a nearly identical reduction in delta power relative to baseline following daytime naps in young (mean 22 years) and old (mean 71 years) adults. Similarly, Munch et al. (2007) showed that, following the lowering of sleep pressure using a constant routine procedure with extended naps, a reduction of delta power during the first sleep cycle occurred in both young (20–31 years) and older (57–74 years) adults. In contrast, however, in the young adults, this reduction persisted longer into recovery night sleep and showed a more posterior scalp-EEG topography. Nonetheless, there is a clear consensus that, despite such small differences, a functional homeostatic response to sleep and SWS loss persists into later adulthood [3, 32, 76, 78].

Recent findings suggest that the age-related increase in resistance to sleep deprivation-induced deficits in vigilance and subjective sleepiness may result from changes in adenosinergic systems underlying the buildup of homeostatic sleep pressure [1]. Desensitization of adenosine receptors with age is suggested by a positron emission tomography (PET) study showing reduced binding of an adenosine A1 receptor ligand in older vs. younger adults [79]. Vigilance in young adults who show high sensitivity to caffeine, a non-specific adenosine A1 and A2A receptor antagonist, is impacted more by sleep deprivation than in those with lower sensitivity, and such sensitivity is mediated by a polymorphism in the adenosine A2A receptor gene [1]. In both younger and older adults, sleep deprivation increased and caffeine decreased two indices of elevated homeostatic sleep pressure, namely, increased theta activity at frontal relative to posterior sites in the waking EEG and performance impairment on the psychomotor vigilance task (PVT). However, attenuated responses of these indices in older adults resembled more those of caffeine-insensitive vs. caffeine-sensitive young adults leading Landolt and colleagues (2012) to suggest possible reduction in adenosine A2A receptor function with aging.

Whereas in older adults vigilance and other forms of attention may suffer less from acute sleep loss compared to younger adults, normal changes in sleep quality and architecture may impact neural processes that take place during sleep itself. The best known of these processes is sleep-dependent memory consolidation [80, 81] and changes in this process with healthy aging are considered next.

Changes in Sleep-Dependent Cognition with Healthy Aging

Declarative memory recall is greater following an intersession interval containing sleep compared to when the intersession interval contains wake in young adults (e.g., [82]). Such facilitation has been demonstrated for intervals containing overnight sleep as well as daytime naps [83], thus ruling out circadian explanations for such effects. Offline changes in learning over sleep are thought to reflect consolidation of the memory, a process by which memory storage and retrieval become more efficient. Whereas memory consolidation takes place during both sleep and wake, a major component of consolidation takes place during sleep (e.g., [84], likely as a means to prevent consolidation processes from interfering with encoding of new material and vice versa [80]).

Studies using neural recordings in rat hippocampus suggest that sleep-dependent memory consolidation stems from neural replay. Wilson and colleagues [85] recorded hippocampal place cell activity during active exploration and sleep. During exploration, place cells are active when the animal is in particular areas of an environment such that, collectively, place cells code a map of space. Interestingly, sequences of neural firing recorded during subsequent sleep mimicked patterns observed during waking exploration. Neuroimaging in humans suggests a similar neural process. Using PET imaging, Peigneux and colleagues [86] demonstrated hippocampal activation during learning that predicted subsequent reactivation during sleep. Moreover, the amount of hippocampal activity during sleep predicted performance improvements in the maze navigation task.

Given the drastic changes in sleep that occur with aging, one might expect sleep-dependent memory consolidation to be reduced in older adults. Indeed, performance changes over sleep relative to wake are reduced for procedural learning tasks even when participants are screened for sleep disorders, medication use, and other confounds. For instance, when young adults (mean 20.8 years) and older adults (mean 59 years) learned a ten-item sequence of finger movements, initial learning did not differ for the two groups [87]. When tested 12-h later, young adults demonstrated performance improvements of approximately 5 % if the interval contained wake and 18 % if the interval contained sleep. However, performance of older adults improved by only 2–5 % regardless of whether the interval contained wake or sleep. In other words, the performance benefits sleep exerted on this procedural task for young adults were absent in the older adult group. This result was subsequently replicated by the same group [88] and others [89, 90].

Likewise, Peters and colleagues [91] reported reduced sleep-related performance changes on a pursuit rotor learning task in a group of older adults (mean 69.8 years) relative to young adults (mean 20.1 years). Pursuit rotor learning requires participants to use a stylus to track a moving target. In this particular study, the target moved in a predictable fashion, thus the task requires learning of the stable movement pattern and prediction of the target's velocity, both forms of procedural learning. Performance improvements on this task 1 week later were associated with sleep spindles in NREM stage 2 in the young adults but not older adult participants.

While benefits to procedural learning from sleep are reduced or absent in older adults, (but see ref. [92]), declarative memory consolidation may be preserved. We directly contrasted over-sleep changes in performance on a declarative word-pair learning task and a procedural motor sequence learning task in young (20–34 years), middle-aged (35–50 years), and older (51–70 years) adults [88]. While changes in motor sequence learning over sleep relative to wake were greater in the young adults (and nearly absent in middle-age and older adults), sleep's benefit on word-pair learning was spared. In fact, using a sleep benefit score which subtracts the change in performance over wake from changes over sleep (i.e., yielding a positive value indicating that the intersession interval with sleep was better than wake), we found no difference in sleep's benefit on word-pair learning across the three age groups. Likewise, older adults have been shown to have greater recall of personal events and standardized narratives (WMS-III Logic Memory stories) following sleep compared to wake [93], although the effect on memory for personal events was reduced relative to young adults. Differences in the amount of declarative memory consolidation achieved within the older adult group may be related to the quality of sleep. For instance, older women (61–74 years) with high spindle density had better performance on the Rey-Osterrieth Complex Figure Test, a measure of declarative memory, than women with low spindle density [94].

While it may be tempting to conclude that sleep-dependent consolidation is reduced for procedural but not declarative memories in older adults, the picture is not yet entirely clear. For instance, one recent study [95], using a similar word-pair learning task as [88], reported that older adults (mean 70.7 years) failed to consolidate declarative memory over sleep while the young adult group (mean 19.7 years) in this study showed a significant improvement. Notably, this improvement over sleep in young adults was associated with the percent of TST spent in SWS. Notably, these older adults had significantly reduced SWS relative to the young adults. In fact, performance changes over sleep for older adults were on par with that of the younger adults who happened to have similar amounts of SWS [95]. This is consistent with a study by Backhaus and colleagues [96] who reported that middle-aged adults benefitted similarly from sleep on a declarative learning task when SWS time was equated.

Although healthy aging is, therefore, associated with a degree of preservation of sleep-dependent memory consolidation, further changes in sleep quality and architecture that accompany the increased risk of medical, neurological, and psychiatric illness with aging are likely to seriously impact this function of sleep in a large percentage of older adults. Indeed sleep-dependent memory consolidation has been shown to be diminished due to mild cognitive impairment [97, 98] and even more so with the onset of Alzheimer's disease [99]. Similarly, sleep disorders can impair sleep-dependent memory consolidation (for a review, see ref. [100]). For example, even the sleep fragmentation associated with mild OSA has been shown to diminish sleep-dependent memory consolidation in young to middle-aged (mean 30 years) adults [101] as has moderate OSA in middle-aged (mean 47 years) adults [102]. In the next sections, we examine associations of anxiety and insomnia—conditions that may affect a large percentage of otherwise healthy older adults—and consider whether resultant sleep disruption might also impact sleep-dependent memory consolidation.

Interactions of Anxiety and Insomnia in Aging

Incidence of sleep disorders greatly increases with advancing age [5, 103, 104]. Complaints of insomnia symptoms, including difficulty with sleep maintenance, early-morning awakening, and daytime fatigue and sleepiness, all become more prevalent with aging [5, 105, 106]. Indeed, aging itself constitutes the greatest independent risk factor for insomnia [7]. Difficulty sleeping is an increasing problem as aging advances [107] and may constitute the primary somatic complaint in old-old individuals [108].

An intriguing potential trigger for insomnia complaints in the elderly was suggested by Dijk et al. [3] who note that a normatively reduced sleep propensity might be interpreted as abnormal sleep loss by older individuals who believe that longer or more consolidated sleep is required for good health. Since maladaptive cognitions focused on sleep can themselves become initiating or perpetuating factors for chronic insomnia [109], misinterpretation of reduced sleep need as a health problem can lead to a positive feedback cycle that results in worsening symptoms of insomnia. For example, an individual may nap excessively during the day in the belief that it is necessary to compensate for shorter nocturnal sleep [110]. As such, they may unintentionally exacerbate sleep onset or maintenance problems by reducing homeostatic sleep pressure prior to their nocturnal sleep bout. Similarly, long-term use of hypnotic drugs can lead to a worsening rather than the intended improvement of sleep difficulties over time in older adults [111]. A common source of anxiety among older adults is concern regarding physical and, especially, mental decline particularly in the domain of memory. Such concerns during presleep rumination can exacerbate insomnia in much the same way as described above [110]. However, despite this potential for misattribution with regard to normal changes in sleep, self-reported poor sleep [112] and excessive daytime sleepiness [113, 114] have indeed both been found to be significantly associated with cognitive decline.

Anxiety disorders are highly comorbid with sleep disturbance in older adults [108, 110] with even subclinical levels of anxiety contributing significantly to sleep disturbance [115, 116]. Although overall prevalence of anxiety disorders is less in older compared to younger adults [6], they remain common in this population. Up to 10 % of older adults suffer from anxiety disorders [117] that can persist for many years [118]. Even in those of an advanced age (85–103 years), a 2.3 % prevalence of anxiety disorders has been reported [119]. Moreover, even greater numbers of older adults report significant anxiety symptoms that do not fully meet diagnostic criteria for an anxiety disorder [110]. Poor sleep and anxiety have been found to constitute major risk factors for one another in older adults with the above-noted concerns about physical health and cognitive integrity being a major contributor to both conditions [110]. For example, in a large prospective study of adults in Norway that included older cohorts, persistent insomnia was shown to be a significant risk factor for later development of an anxiety disorder [120]. Thus, poor sleep may represent an independent risk factor for anxiety disorders in older adults, of the same order of magnitude as other risk factors such as severe stressors and neuroticism [121].

Large prospective epidemiological studies in older adults have clearly shown that sleep difficulties also constitute significant risk factors for both physical and cognitive decline. In a large cohort of non-frail men aged 67, poor sleep has been identified as a major risk factor for the onset of frailty (following the definitional criteria of Fried et al. [122]) at 3–4 year follow-up [123, 124]. Similar findings have been reported in a large sample of elderly women [125]. In the cognitive domain, a longitudinal study of 1,664 cognitively unimpaired older adults aged 65–95 showed that elevated Pittsburgh Sleep Quality Index (PSQI) scores and habitual sleep duration predicted Mini-Mental Statues Exam scores within the range of cognitive impairment at 12-month follow-up [126]. Similarly, sleep duration shorter than 6.5 h per night and excessive daytime sleepiness in older (median 75 years) adults at baseline were found to predict cognitive decline at 10-year follow-up [127]. Indicators of disrupted circadian rhythmicity such as delay in activity peak [128] and damped amplitude of circadian rhythms [129] have also been shown to predict cognitive decline. Therefore, buffering of the cognitive impact of sleep loss in older adults appears to be somewhat fragile and easily overcome by other factors that severely perturb sleep.

One such factor that is of great public health importance due to its ubiquity is insomnia, a disorder that, in turn, is clearly comorbid with and, in many cases the result of, subclinical anxiety and anxiety disorders [110, 115]. It is important to note that insomnia and sleep disturbances accompanying mood disorders may also have great impact on cognition in the elderly [130, 131] and mood disorders may bear a similar reciprocal etiological risk with insomnia as do anxiety disorders [110, 132].

Interaction of Sleep-Dependent Memory Consolidation with Insomnia

A small number of studies have begun to suggest that sleep-dependent memory consolidation can be impaired by insomnia. For example, middle-aged individuals (mean 41 years) with primary insomnia have been shown to have diminished consolidation of declarative memory (word pairs) relative to controls while, at the same time, showing preserved sleep-dependent consolidation of procedural (mirror-tracing) learning [133]. In contrast, in middle-aged (mean 46 years) subjects, those with primary insomnia who slept vs. those who remained awake failed to show greater percent improvement on the mirror-tracing task or enhanced retention of declarative learning on the visual verbal task (VVT) that were apparent in good-sleeping controls [134]. Both studies, however, demonstrate that primary insomnia can negatively impact sleep-dependent memory consolidation in otherwise healthy middle-aged adults. Similarly, psychiatric disorders that are associated with insomnia such as depression may impair sleep-dependent memory consolidation [135, 136] as may disorders such as schizophrenia that alter specific aspects of sleep such as sleep spindles [137–139].

Conclusions and Clinical Implications

In the future, it will be important to determine if sleep disruption associated with subclinical anxiety disorders and associated mild or situational insomnia can also impact the memory consolidation function of sleep in older adults. If this proves to be the case, anxiety, insomnia, and cognitive impairment might constitute mutually reinforcing conditions that lead to increasing severity in symptoms of each. Hence, even cognitively intact older adults may find themselves experiencing daytime memory problems that lead to increased nocturnal rumination and, in turn increased sleep difficulties [3, 110]. Bearing in mind the actual epidemiological associations of sleep difficulties and neurodegenerative disease described above, sleep clinicians and mental health providers who treat older adults may benefit from considering such complex interactions of normal worry, memory, and sleep when advising and treating patients. In such patients, if more severe illnesses can be ruled out, cognitive-behavioral therapy for insomnia [140] may prove especially helpful and reduce the need for or the duration of treatment with hypnotic drugs.

References

1. Landolt HP, Retey JV, Adam M. Reduced neurobehavioral impairment from sleep deprivation in older adults: contribution of adenosinergic mechanisms. Front Neurol. 2012;3:62. Epub 2012/05/05.
2. Carrier J, Land S, Buysse DJ, Kupfer DJ, Monk TH. The effects of age and gender on sleep EEG power spectral density in the middle years of life (ages 20–60 years old). Psychophysiology. 2001;38(2):232–42.
3. Dijk DJ, Groeger JA, Stanley N, Deacon S. Age-related reduction in daytime sleep propensity and nocturnal slow wave sleep. Sleep. 2010;33(2):211–23.
4. Vitiello MV. Sleep in normal aging. Sleep Med Clin. 2006;1:171–6.
5. Crowley K. Sleep and sleep disorders in older adults. Neuropsychol Rev. 2011;21(1):41–53. Epub 2011/01/13.
6. Wolitzky-Taylor KB, Castriotta N, Lenze EJ, Stanley MA, Craske MG. Anxiety disorders in older adults: a comprehensive review. Depress Anxiety. 2010;27(2):190–211.
7. Foley D, Ancoli-Israel S, Britz P, Walsh J. Sleep disturbances and chronic disease in older adults: results of the 2003 National Sleep Foundation Sleep in America Survey. J Psychosom Res. 2004;56(5):497–502.
8. Bliwise D. Normal aging. In: Kryger MH, Roth T, Dement WC, editors. Principles and practice of sleep medicine. 5th ed. Philadelphia: Elsevier; 2011.
9. Pace-Schott EF, Spencer RM. Age-related changes in the cognitive function of sleep. Prog Brain Res. 2011;191:75–89.
10. Colrain IM. Sleep and the brain. Neuropsychol Rev. 2011;21(1):1–4. Epub 2011/01/25.
11. Dijk DJ, Duffy JF, Czeisler CA. Contribution of circadian physiology and sleep homeostasis to age-related changes in human sleep. Chronobiol Int. 2000;17(3):285–311.
12. Naylor E, Zee PC. Circadian rhythm alterations with aging. Sleep Med Clin. 2006;1:187–96.
13. Buysse DJ, Monk TH, Carrier J, Begley A. Circadian patterns of sleep, sleepiness, and performance in older and younger adults. Sleep. 2005;28(11):1365–76.
14. O'Donnell D, Silva EJ, Munch M, Ronda JM, Wang W, Duffy JF. Comparison of subjective and objective assessments of sleep in healthy older subjects without sleep complaints. J Sleep Res. 2009;18(2):254–63.
15. Huang YL, Liu RY, Wang QS, Van Someren EJ, Xu H, Zhou JN. Age-associated difference in circadian sleep-wake and rest-activity rhythms. Physiol Behav. 2002;76(4–5):597–603.
16. Dijk DJ, Duffy JF, Czeisler CA. Age-related increase in awakenings: impaired consolidation of nonREM sleep at all circadian phases. Sleep. 2001;24(5):565–77.
17. Salzarulo P, Fagioli I, Lombardo P, Gori S, Gneri C, Chiaramonti R, et al. Sleep stages preceding spontaneous awakenings in the elderly. Sleep Res Online. 1999;2(3):73–7.
18. Silva EJ, Duffy JF. Sleep inertia varies with circadian phase and sleep stage in older adults. Behav Neurosci. 2008;122(4):928–35.
19. Hoch CC, Dew MA, Reynolds III CF, Buysse DJ, Nowell PD, Monk TH, et al. Longitudinal changes in diary- and laboratory-based sleep measures in healthy "old old" and "young old" subjects: a three-year follow-up. Sleep. 1997;20(3):192–202.
20. Hoch CC, Dew MA, Reynolds III CF, Monk TH, Buysse DJ, Houck PR, et al. A longitudinal study of laboratory- and diary-based sleep measures in healthy "old old" and "young old" volunteers. Sleep. 1994;17(6):489–96.
21. Carskadon MA, Brown ED, Dement WC. Sleep fragmentation in the elderly: relationship to daytime sleep tendency. Neurobiol Aging. 1982;3(4):321–7.
22. Martin JL, Ancoli Israel S. Napping in older adults. Sleep Med Clin. 2006;1:177–86.
23. Campbell SS, Kripke DF, Gillin JC, Hrubovcak JC. Exposure to light in healthy elderly subjects and Alzheimer's patients. Physiol Behav. 1988;42(2):141–4. Epub 1988/01/01.
24. Asplund R, Aberg H. Nocturnal micturition, sleep and well-being in women of ages 40–64 years. Maturitas. 1996;24(1–2):73–81.
25. Ancoli-Israel S, DuHamel ER, Stepnowsky C, Engler R, Cohen-Zion M, Marler M. The relationship between congestive heart failure, sleep apnea,

and mortality in older men. Chest. 2003;124(4):1400–5.
26. Riegel B, Weaver TE. Poor sleep and impaired self-care: towards a comprehensive model linking sleep, cognition, and heart failure outcomes. Eur J Cardiovasc Nurs. 2009;8(5):337–44.
27. Petit D, Gagnon JF, Fantini ML, Ferini-Strambi L, Montplaisir J. Sleep and quantitative EEG in neurodegenerative disorders. J Psychosom Res. 2004; 56(5):487–96. Epub 2004/06/03.
28. Cajochen C, Munch M, Knoblauch V, Blatter K, Wirz-Justice A. Age-related changes in the circadian and homeostatic regulation of human sleep. Chronobiol Int. 2006;23(1–2):461–74.
29. Ohayon MM, Carskadon MA, Guilleminault C, Vitiello MV. Meta-analysis of quantitative sleep parameters from childhood to old age in healthy individuals: developing normative sleep values across the human lifespan. Sleep. 2004;27(7):1255–73.
30. Carrier J, Viens I, Poirier G, Robillard R, Lafortune M, Vandewalle G, et al. Sleep slow wave changes during the middle years of life. Eur J Neurosci. 2011;33(4):758–66. Epub 2011/01/14.
31. Darchia N, Campbell IG, Tan X, Feinberg I. Kinetics of NREM delta EEG power density across NREM periods depend on age and on delta-band designation. Sleep. 2007;30(1):71–9. Epub 2007/02/22.
32. Munch M, Knoblauch V, Blatter K, Schroder C, Schnitzler C, Krauchi K, et al. The frontal predominance in human EEG delta activity after sleep loss decreases with age. Eur J Neurosci. 2004;20(5):1402–10.
33. Lombardo P, Formicola G, Gori S, Gneri C, Massetani R, Murri L, et al. Slow wave sleep (SWS) distribution across night sleep episode in the elderly. Aging (Milano). 1998;10(6):445–8.
34. Fukuda N, Honma H, Kohsaka M, Kobayashi R, Sakakibara S, Kohsaka S, et al. Gender difference of slow wave sleep in middle aged and elderly subjects. Psychiatry Clin Neurosci. 1999;53(2):151–3.
35. Floyd JA, Janisse JJ, Jenuwine ES, Ager JW. Changes in REM-sleep percentage over the adult lifespan. Sleep. 2007;30(7):829–36.
36. Darchia N, Campbell IG, Feinberg I. Rapid eye movement density is reduced in the normal elderly. Sleep. 2003;26(8):973–7.
37. Crowley K, Trinder J, Kim Y, Carrington M, Colrain IM. The effects of normal aging on sleep spindle and K-complex production. Clin Neurophysiol. 2002; 113(10):1615–22.
38. Landolt HP, Dijk DJ, Achermann P, Borbely AA. Effect of age on the sleep EEG: slow-wave activity and spindle frequency activity in young and middle-aged men. Brain Res. 1996;738(2):205–12.
39. Wei HG, Riel E, Czeisler CA, Dijk DJ. Attenuated amplitude of circadian and sleep-dependent modulation of electroencephalographic sleep spindle characteristics in elderly human subjects. Neurosci Lett. 1999;260(1):29–32.
40. Guazzelli M, Feinberg I, Aminoff M, Fein G, Floyd TC, Maggini C. Sleep spindles in normal elderly: comparison with young adult patterns and relation to nocturnal awakening, cognitive function and brain atrophy. Electroencephalogr Clin Neurophysiol. 1986;63(6):526–39. Epub 1986/06/01.
41. Nicolas A, Petit D, Rompre S, Montplaisir J. Sleep spindle characteristics in healthy subjects of different age groups. Clin Neurophysiol. 2001;112(3):521–7. Epub 2001/02/27.
42. Wauquier A. Aging and changes in phasic events during sleep. Physiol Behav. 1993;54(4):803–6. Epub 1993/10/01.
43. Crowley K, Trinder J, Colrain IM. An examination of evoked K-complex amplitude and frequency of occurrence in the elderly. J Sleep Res. 2002;11(2):129–40.
44. Harrison Y, Horne JA, Rothwell A. Prefrontal neuropsychological effects of sleep deprivation in young adults—a model for healthy aging? Sleep. 2000; 23(8):1067–73.
45. Bonnet MH, Arand DL. Sleep loss in aging. Clin Geriatr Med. 1989;5(2):405–20.
46. Adam M, Retey JV, Khatami R, Landolt HP. Age-related changes in the time course of vigilant attention during 40 hours without sleep in men. Sleep. 2006;29(1):55–7.
47. Duffy JF, Willson HJ, Wang W, Czeisler CA. Healthy older adults better tolerate sleep deprivation than young adults. J Am Geriatr Soc. 2009;57(7):1245–51.
48. Blatter K, Graw P, Munch M, Knoblauch V, Wirz-Justice A, Cajochen C. Gender and age differences in psychomotor vigilance performance under differential sleep pressure conditions. Behav Brain Res. 2006;168(2):312–7.
49. Philip P, Taillard J, Sagaspe P, Valtat C, Sanchez-Ortuno M, Moore N, et al. Age, performance and sleep deprivation. J Sleep Res. 2004;13(2):105–10.
50. Bliese PD, Wesensten NJ, Balkin TJ. Age and individual variability in performance during sleep restriction. J Sleep Res. 2006;15(4):376–85.
51. Stenuit P, Kerkhofs M. Age modulates the effects of sleep restriction in women. Sleep. 2005;28(10):1283–8.
52. Bonnet MH. The effect of sleep fragmentation on sleep and performance in younger and older subjects. Neurobiol Aging. 1989;10(1):21–5.
53. Bonnet MH, Rosa RR. Sleep and performance in young adults and older normals and insomniacs during acute sleep loss and recovery. Biol Psychol. 1987;25(2):153–72.
54. Carskadon MA, Dement WC. Sleep loss in elderly volunteers. Sleep. 1985;8(3):207–21.
55. Smulders FT, Kenemans JL, Jonkman LM, Kok A. The effects of sleep loss on task performance and the electroencephalogram in young and elderly subjects. Biol Psychol. 1997;45(1–3):217–39. Epub 1997/03/21.

56. Brendel DH, Reynolds III CF, Jennings JR, Hoch CC, Monk TH, Berman SR, et al. Sleep stage physiology, mood, and vigilance responses to total sleep deprivation in healthy 80-year-olds and 20-year-olds. Psychophysiology. 1990;27(6):677–85. Epub 1990/11/01.
57. Roge J, Pebayle T, El Hannachi S, Muzet A. Effect of sleep deprivation and driving duration on the useful visual field in younger and older subjects during simulator driving. Vision Res. 2003;43(13):1465–72. Epub 2003/05/28.
58. Robillard R, Prince F, Filipini D, Carrier J. Aging worsens the effects of sleep deprivation on postural control. PLoS One. 2011;6(12):e28731. Epub 2011/12/14.
59. Dijk DJ, Duffy JF, Riel E, Shanahan TL, Czeisler CA. Ageing and the circadian and homeostatic regulation of human sleep during forced desynchrony of rest, melatonin and temperature rhythms. J Physiol. 1999;516(Pt 2):611–27.
60. Silva EJ, Wang W, Ronda JM, Wyatt JK, Duffy JF. Circadian and wake-dependent influences on subjective sleepiness, cognitive throughput, and reaction time performance in older and young adults. Sleep. 2010;33(4):481–90.
61. Borbely AA. A two process model of sleep regulation. Hum Neurobiol. 1982;1(3):195–204.
62. Dijk DJ, Czeisler CA. Paradoxical timing of the circadian rhythm of sleep propensity serves to consolidate sleep and wakefulness in humans. Neurosci Lett. 1994;166(1):63–8.
63. Hofman MA, Swaab DF. Living by the clock: the circadian pacemaker in older people. Ageing Res Rev. 2006;5(1):33–51.
64. Kondratova AA, Kondratov RV. The circadian clock and pathology of the ageing brain. Nat Rev Neurosci. 2012;13(5):325–35. Epub 2012/03/08.
65. Monk TH. Aging human circadian rhythms: conventional wisdom may not always be right. J Biol Rhythms. 2005;20(4):366–74.
66. Skene DJ, Swaab DF. Melatonin rhythmicity: effect of age and Alzheimer's disease. Exp Gerontol. 2003;38(1–2):199–206. Epub 2003/01/25.
67. Duffy JF, Dijk DJ, Klerman EB, Czeisler CA. Later endogenous circadian temperature nadir relative to an earlier wake time in older people. Am J Physiol. 1998;275(5 Pt 2):R1478–87.
68. Czeisler CA, Duffy JF, Shanahan TL, Brown EN, Mitchell JF, Rimmer DW, et al. Stability, precision, and near-24-hour period of the human circadian pacemaker. Science. 1999;284(5423):2177–81.
69. Benloucif S, Green K, L'Hermite-Baleriaux M, Weintraub S, Wolfe LF, Zee PC. Responsiveness of the aging circadian clock to light. Neurobiol Aging. 2006;27(12):1870–9.
70. Van Someren EJ, Riemersma RF, Swaab DF. Functional plasticity of the circadian timing system in old age: light exposure. Prog Brain Res. 2002;138:205–31.
71. Van Someren EJ. Circadian and sleep disturbances in the elderly. Exp Gerontol. 2000;35(9–10):1229–37.
72. Bliwise DL. Normal aging. In: Kryger MH, Roth T, Dement WC, editors. Principles and practice of sleep medicine. 4th ed. Philadelphia: Elsevier; 2005. p. 24–38.
73. Ohayon MM, Zulley J, Guilleminault C, Smirne S, Priest RG. How age and daytime activities are related to insomnia in the general population: consequences for older people. J Am Geriatr Soc. 2001;49(4):360–6. Epub 2001/05/12.
74. Achermann P, Dijk DJ, Brunner DP, Borbely AA. A model of human sleep homeostasis based on EEG slow-wave activity: quantitative comparison of data and simulations. Brain Res Bull. 1993;31(1–2):97–113. Epub 1993/01/01.
75. Klerman EB, Dijk DJ. Age-related reduction in the maximal capacity for sleep—implications for insomnia. Curr Biol. 2008;18(15):1118–23. Epub 2008/07/29.
76. Gaudreau H, Morettini J, Lavoie HB, Carrier J. Effects of a 25-h sleep deprivation on daytime sleep in the middle-aged. Neurobiol Aging. 2001;22(3):461–8.
77. Campbell IG, Feinberg I. Homeostatic sleep response to naps is similar in normal elderly and young adults. Neurobiol. Aging 2005;26(1):135–44.
78. Munch M, Knoblauch V, Blatter K, Wirz-Justice A, Cajochen C. Is homeostatic sleep regulation under low sleep pressure modified by age? Sleep. 2007;30(6):781–92.
79. Meyer PT, Elmenhorst D, Boy C, Winz O, Matusch A, Zilles K, et al. Effect of aging on cerebral A1 adenosine receptors: a [18F]CPFPX PET study in humans. Neurobiol Aging. 2007;28(12):1914–24. Epub 2006/09/26.
80. Diekelmann S, Born J. The memory function of sleep. Nat Rev Neurosci. 2010;11(2):114–26.
81. Stickgold R. Sleep-dependent memory consolidation. Nature. 2005;437(7063):1272–8.
82. Donohue K, Spencer RMC. Continuous re-exposure to environmental sound cues during sleep does not improve memory for semantically unrelated word pairs. J Cognit Educ Psychol. 2011;10(2):167–77.
83. Tucker MA, Hirota Y, Wamsley EJ, Lau H, Chaklader A, Fishbein W. A daytime nap containing solely non-REM sleep enhances declarative but not procedural memory. Neurobiol Learn Mem. 2006;86(2):241–7.
84. Stickgold R, Walker MP. Sleep-dependent memory consolidation and reconsolidation. Sleep Med. 2007;8(4):331–43.
85. Ji D, Wilson MA. Coordinated memory replay in the visual cortex and hippocampus during sleep. Nat Neurosci. 2007;10(1):100–7.
86. Peigneux P, Laureys S, Fuchs S, Collette F, Perrin F, Reggers J, et al. Are spatial memories strengthened in the human hippocampus during slow wave sleep? Neuron. 2004;44(3):535–45.

87. Spencer RM, Gouw AM, Ivry RB. Age-related decline of sleep-dependent consolidation. Learn Mem. 2007;14(7):480–4.
88. Wilson JK, Baran B, Pace-Schott EF, Ivry RB, Spencer RM. Sleep modulates word-pair learning but not motor sequence learning in healthy older adults. Neurobiol Aging. 2012;33(5):991–1000. Epub 2012/01/17.
89. Siengsukon CF, Boyd LA. Sleep enhances implicit motor skill learning in individuals poststroke. Top Stroke Rehabil. 2008;15(1):1–12.
90. Siengsukon C, Boyd LA. Sleep enhances off-line spatial and temporal motor learning after stroke. Neurorehabil Neural Repair. 2009;23(4):327–35.
91. Peters KR, Ray L, Smith V, Smith C. Changes in the density of stage 2 sleep spindles following motor learning in young and older adults. J Sleep Res. 2008;17(1):23–33.
92. Tucker M, McKinley S, Stickgold R. Sleep optimizes motor skill in older adults. J Am Geriatr Soc. 2011;59(4):603–9. Epub 2011/03/18.
93. Aly M, Moscovitch M. The effects of sleep on episodic memory in older and younger adults. Memory. 2010;18(3):327–34.
94. Seeck-Hirschner M, Baier PC, Weinhold SL, Dittmar M, Heiermann S, Aldenhoff JB, et al. Declarative memory performance is associated with the number of sleep spindles in elderly women. Am J Geriatr Psychiatry. 2012;20(9):782–8. Epub 2011/10/15.
95. Scullin MK. Sleep, memory, and aging: the link between slow-wave sleep and episodic memory changes from younger to older adults. Psychol Aging. 2013;28(1):105–14. Epub 2012/06/20.
96. Backhaus J, Born J, Hoeckesfeld R, Fokuhl S, Hohagen F, Junghanns K. Midlife decline in declarative memory consolidation is correlated with a decline in slow wave sleep. Learn Mem. 2007;14(5):336–41.
97. Westerberg CE, Lundgren EM, Florczak SM, Mesulam MM, Weintraub S, Zee PC, et al. Sleep influences the severity of memory disruption in amnestic mild cognitive impairment: results from sleep self-assessment and continuous activity monitoring. Alzheimer Dis Assoc Disord. 2010;24:325–33. Epub 2010/07/02.
98. Westerberg CE, Mander BA, Florczak SM, Weintraub S, Mesulam MM, Zee PC, et al. Concurrent impairments in sleep and memory in amnestic mild cognitive impairment. J Int Neuropsychol Soc. 2012;18(3):490–500. Epub 2012/02/04.
99. Rauchs G, Schabus M, Parapatics S, Bertran F, Clochon P, Hot P, et al. Is there a link between sleep changes and memory in Alzheimer's disease? Neuroreport. 2008;19(11):1159–62.
100. Cipolli C, Mazzetti M, Plazzi G. Sleep-dependent memory consolidation in patients with sleep disorders. Sleep Med Rev. 2013;17(2):91–103. Epub 2012/04/07.
101. Djonlagic I, Saboisky J, Carusona A, Stickgold R, Malhotra A. Increased sleep fragmentation leads to impaired off-line consolidation of motor memories in humans. PLoS One. 2012;7(3):e34106. Epub 2012/04/04.
102. Kloepfer C, Riemann D, Nofzinger EA, Feige B, Unterrainer J, O'Hara R, et al. Memory before and after sleep in patients with moderate obstructive sleep apnea. J Clin Sleep Med. 2009;5(6):540–8.
103. Ancoli-Israel S, Ayalon L, Salzman C. Sleep in the elderly: normal variations and common sleep disorders. Harv Rev Psychiatry. 2008;16(5):279–86.
104. Neikrug AB, Ancoli-Israel S. Sleep disorders in the older adult—a mini-review. Gerontology. 2010;56(2):181–9.
105. Morphy H, Dunn KM, Lewis M, Boardman HF, Croft PR. Epidemiology of insomnia: a longitudinal study in a UK population. Sleep. 2007;30(3):274–80. Epub 2007/04/12.
106. Foley DJ, Monjan AA, Brown SL, Simonsick EM, Wallace RB, Blazer DG. Sleep complaints among elderly persons: an epidemiologic study of three communities. Sleep. 1995;18(6):425–32. Epub 1995/07/01.
107. Giron MS, Forsell Y, Bernsten C, Thorslund M, Winblad B, Fastbom J. Sleep problems in a very old population: drug use and clinical correlates. J Gerontol A Biol Sci Med Sci. 2002;57(4):M236–40. Epub 2002/03/23.
108. Spira AP, Friedman L, Flint A, Sheikh JI. Interaction of sleep disturbances and anxiety in later life: perspectives and recommendations for future research. J Geriatr Psychiatry Neurol. 2005;18(2):109–15. Epub 2005/05/25.
109. Bootzin RR, Epstein DR. Understanding and treating insomnia. Annu Rev Clin Psychol. 2011;7:435–58. Epub 2007/08/25.
110. Magee JC, Carmin CN. The relationship between sleep and anxiety in older adults. Curr Psychiatry Rep. 2010;12(1):13–9. Epub 2010/04/29.
111. Beland SG, Preville M, Dubois MF, Lorrain D, Voyer P, Bosse C, et al. The association between length of benzodiazepine use and sleep quality in older population. Int J Geriatr Psychiatry. 2011;26(9):908–15. Epub 2010/10/22.
112. Bruce AS, Aloia M. Sleep and cognition in older adults. Sleep Med Clin. 2006;1:207–20.
113. Whitney CW, Enright PL, Newman AB, Bonekat W, Foley D, Quan SF. Correlates of daytime sleepiness in 4578 elderly persons: the Cardiovascular Health Study. Sleep. 1998;21(1):27–36. Epub 1998/03/05.
114. Ohayon MM, Vecchierini MF. Daytime sleepiness and cognitive impairment in the elderly population. Arch Intern Med. 2002;162(2):201–8. Epub 2002/02/13.
115. Spira AP, Friedman L, Aulakh JS, Lee T, Sheikh JI, Yesavage JA. Subclinical anxiety symptoms, sleep, and daytime dysfunction in older adults with primary insomnia. J Geriatr Psychiatry Neurol. 2008;21(2):149–53. Epub 2008/05/14.
116. Spira AP, Stone K, Beaudreau SA, Ancoli-Israel S, Yaffe K. Anxiety symptoms and objectively measured

sleep quality in older women. Am J Geriatr Psychiatry. 2009;17(2):136–43. Epub 2009/01/22.
117. Beekman AT, Bremmer MA, Deeg DJ, van Balkom AJ, Smit JH, de Beurs E, et al. Anxiety disorders in later life: a report from the Longitudinal Aging Study Amsterdam. Int J Geriatr Psychiatry. 1998;13(10):717–26. Epub 1998/11/18.
118. Schuurmans J, Comijs HC, Beekman AT, de Beurs E, Deeg DJ, Emmelkamp PM, et al. The outcome of anxiety disorders in older people at 6-year follow-up: results from the Longitudinal Aging Study Amsterdam. Acta Psychiatr Scand. 2005;111(6):420–8. Epub 2005/05/10.
119. Schaub RT, Linden M. Anxiety and anxiety disorders in the old and very old—results from the Berlin Aging Study (BASE). Compr Psychiatry. 2000;41(2 Suppl 1):48–54. Epub 2000/04/04.
120. Neckelmann D, Mykletun A, Dahl AA. Chronic insomnia as a risk factor for developing anxiety and depression. Sleep. 2007;30(7):873–80. Epub 2007/08/09.
121. de Beurs E, Beekman AT, Deeg DJ, Van Dyck R, van Tilburg W. Predictors of change in anxiety symptoms of older persons: results from the Longitudinal Aging Study Amsterdam. Psychol Med. 2000;30(3):515–27. Epub 2000/07/07.
122. Fried LP, Tangen CM, Walston J, Newman AB, Hirsch C, Gottdiener J, et al. Frailty in older adults: evidence for a phenotype. J Gerontol A Biol Sci Med Sci. 2001;56(3):M146–56. Epub 2001/03/17.
123. Ensrud KE, Blackwell TL, Ancoli-Israel S, Redline S, Cawthon PM, Paudel ML, et al. Sleep disturbances and risk of frailty and mortality in older men. Sleep Med. 2012;13(10):1217–25. Epub 2012/06/19.
124. Ensrud KE, Blackwell TL, Redline S, Ancoli-Israel S, Paudel ML, Cawthon PM, et al. Sleep disturbances and frailty status in older community-dwelling men. J Am Geriatr Soc. 2009;57(11):2085–93. Epub 2009/10/02.
125. Spira AP, Covinsky K, Rebok GW, Punjabi NM, Stone KL, Hillier TA, et al. Poor sleep quality and functional decline in older women. J Am Geriatr Soc. 2012;60(6):1092–8. Epub 2012/06/14.
126. Potvin O, Lorrain D, Forget H, Dube M, Grenier S, Preville M, et al. Sleep quality and 1-year incident cognitive impairment in community-dwelling older adults. Sleep. 2012;35(4):491–9. Epub 2012/04/03.
127. Keage HA, Banks S, Yang KL, Morgan K, Brayne C, Matthews FE. What sleep characteristics predict cognitive decline in the elderly? Sleep Med. 2012;13(7):886–92. Epub 2012/05/09.
128. Cochrane A, Robertson IH, Coogan AN. Association between circadian rhythms, sleep and cognitive impairment in healthy older adults: an actigraphic study. J Neural Transm. 2012;119(10):1233–9. Epub 2012/04/11.
129. Tranah GJ, Blackwell T, Stone KL, Ancoli-Israel S, Paudel ML, Ensrud KE, et al. Circadian activity rhythms and risk of incident dementia and mild cognitive impairment in older women. Ann Neurol. 2011;70(5):722–32. Epub 2011/12/14.
130. Naismith SL, Norrie L, Lewis SJ, Rogers NL, Scott EM, Hickie IB. Does sleep disturbance mediate neuropsychological functioning in older people with depression? J Affect Disord. 2009;116(1–2):139–43. Epub 2009/01/09.
131. Mallon L, Broman J-E, Hetta J. Sleeping difficulties in relation to depression and anxiety in elderly adults. Nord J Psychiatry. 2000;54:355–60.
132. Perlis ML, Smith LJ, Lyness JM, Matteson SR, Pigeon WR, Jungquist CR, et al. Insomnia as a risk factor for onset of depression in the elderly. Behav Sleep Med. 2006;4(2):104–13.
133. Backhaus J, Junghanns K, Born J, Hohaus K, Faasch F, Hohagen F. Impaired declarative memory consolidation during sleep in patients with primary insomnia: Influence of sleep architecture and nocturnal cortisol release. Biol Psychiatry. 2006;60(12):1324–30. Epub 2006/08/01.
134. Nissen C, Kloepfer C, Nofzinger EA, Feige B, Voderholzer U, Riemann D. Impaired sleep-related memory consolidation in primary insomnia—a pilot study. Sleep. 2006;29(8):1068–73.
135. Genzel L, Ali E, Dresler M, Steiger A, Tesfaye M. Sleep-dependent memory consolidation of a new task is inhibited in psychiatric patients. J Psychiatr Res. 2011;45(4):555–60. Epub 2010/09/28.
136. Dresler M, Kluge M, Genzel L, Schussler P, Steiger A. Impaired off-line memory consolidation in depression. Eur Neuropsychopharmacol. 2010;20(8):553–61. Epub 2010/03/05.
137. Manoach DS, Cain MS, Vangel MG, Khurana A, Goff DC, Stickgold R. A failure of sleep-dependent procedural learning in chronic, medicated schizophrenia. Biol Psychiatry. 2004;56(12):951–6.
138. Manoach DS, Thakkar KN, Stroynowski E, Ely A, McKinley SK, Wamsley E, et al. Reduced overnight consolidation of procedural learning in chronic medicated schizophrenia is related to specific sleep stages. J Psychiatr Res. 2010;44(2):112–20.
139. Wamsley EJ, Tucker MA, Shinn AK, Ono KE, McKinley SK, Ely AV, et al. Reduced sleep spindles and spindle coherence in schizophrenia: mechanisms of impaired memory consolidation? Biol Psychiatry. 2012;71(2):154–61. Epub 2011/10/05.
140. Schutte-Rodin S, Broch L, Buysse D, Dorsey C, Sateia M. Clinical guideline for the evaluation and management of chronic insomnia in adults. J Clin Sleep Med. 2008;4(5):487–504. Epub 2008/10/16.

Part V

Performance, Economics, and Operational Topics

Noise-Induced Sleep Deprivation: Toward Sleeping Soundly on Noisy Nights

15

Jeffrey M. Ellenbogen

Introduction

"In space, no one can hear you scream." With that terrifying tagline, the 1979 sci-fi blockbuster, "Alien," reminded us that sounds are pressure waves that require a medium to travel. Interstellar space is so sparse that it simply cannot transmit sound. But our Earth's atmosphere is replete with molecules—gases, liquids, and solids—and these relay a host of vibrations generated by wiggling objects. When those wiggles occur with enough energy, and in frequencies of the audible range (20–20,000 Hz), our ear can translate those mechanical movements into electrical and chemical languages of neurons. Enter the brain, a complex, biological machine that can perceive, comprehend, and react to a host of complex sounds.

Clearly this is a wonderful thing. Sounds allow us to communicate through language; sounds warn us of danger; they delight us with music. But there is a cost to acoustic perception, a cost that can be summed up in a single word: noise. And while the laws of physics make no distinction between noise and sound, our minds certainly do. A cardiac alarm is an important sound to a doctor, but it's an aggravating hassle to a nearby, sleeping patient.

J.M. Ellenbogen, M.M.Sc., M.D. (✉)
Department of Neurology, Johns Hopkins University, Baltimore, MD, USA
e-mail: jme@jhu.edu

Fortunately, our brains evolved mechanisms to protect sleep from noise. Though the secrets of that process are yet to be fully revealed, the phenomenon is certainly familiar to our experience: if I were awake, people could gain my attention with a whisper; when asleep, they would need to shout.

How does sleep achieve this substantial shift in the brain's response to audible signals? This difference might provide essential clues into sleep physiology, and it might also reveal key information regarding the fundamental mechanisms of perception. Knowing this combined information could enable us to harness the brain's natural abilities, could we then use the brain itself to reduce sound perception during sleep—reducing the likelihood of noise-induced sleep disruption? Perhaps we could make adjustments to these cerebral activities—guided by the needs of the situation confronting the sleeper. In theory, this could be immediately useful for people with sleep impairments; or those living in challenging environments, such as noisy urban neighborhoods; or they could help people trying to sleep in military environments, hospitals or nursing homes, airplanes, etc.

Biases and Caveats

Before proceeding, it is important for me to disclose my potential bias: sleep is essential for health and well-being. Though this assertion itself is the source of spirited debate, it is beyond

M.T. Bianchi (ed.), *Sleep Deprivation and Disease: Effects on the Body, Brain and Behavior*,
DOI 10.1007/978-1-4614-9087-6_15, © Springer Science+Business Media New York 2014

my ability to adequately address this broad topic in a brief chapter (a reader motivated by an in-depth discussion of the purpose of sleep might consider reading articles dedicated to this topic, including [1]). Further, it is commonly claimed that disruption of sleep will jeopardize the myriad of biological functions that rely on it. I will take this complex topic for granted, for the purpose of this chapter, as it is addressed by various other chapters of this book and elsewhere.

In short, for the purpose of this chapter, I will focus exclusively on noise-induced sleep disruption, without discussion of the essence of sleep or the implications of its disruption. The reader interested in learning about personal-health and public-health consequences of noise-induced sleep disruption might choose to become familiar with a myriad of topics, including important issues surrounding impairments in cognitive performance, e.g., [2], and I also encourage inspection of less well-worn paths in our emerging understanding about sleep disruption, including heart rate elevation [3–5], blood sugar intolerance [6], memory consolidation, and other topics of ongoing investigation in the emerging sciences of sleep medicine.

Finally, there are many worthy subtopics and important articles on a myriad of issues pertaining to noise-induced sleep disruption, including examination of the interface between sleep and noises from aircraft, trains, automobiles [3, 5]. In order to keep this article within reasonable length and focus, I will largely examine noise-induced sleep disruption in hospital settings, and on brain-based sciences related therein. Hopefully these concepts convey a set of principles that generalize to other areas pertinent to noise and sleep.

Noise Sources: Help or Harm

Heuristically, the sources of sounds can be organized by their source's location. Outside the building (e.g., airplanes), inside the building (e.g., elevator shaft), or inside the room itself (e.g., snoring bed partner). They can be further organized by natural or synthetic noises, and through many other practical categories.

No matter how you organize your thinking, what is readily apparent is that noises are all around us. Urban environments are filled with synthetic sounds that cause nocturnal noises: apartment-building neighbors play loud music; nearby airports roar with the takeoff and landing of planes; train stations rumble with combusting engines and shriek with metal brakes; car motors grumble; police, ambulances, and fire trucks siren with alarms. The list goes on and on. Rural environments face more a combination of synthetic and natural noises: bull elks bugle in mating season; crickets chirp in droves; roosters crow at all hours; tractor engines fire up early in the morning.

One important distinction between types of sounds might include whether the sound is intended or not, and whether it serves a good purpose. For example, most people would not complain about a smoke alarm waking them up at night. The alerting signal can be lifesaving, and so the cost of disrupted sleep is trivial. On the other hand, what if the neighbor's alarm sirens? Were you in position to help, you might feel one way; were you not able to help, you might feel another.

An ambulance is an even more provocative example. Its alarm benefits some and irritates others—often at the same time. An ambulance gets the patient to the hospital more expeditiously, because the warning signals (sounds and lights) tell other cars and trucks to get out of the way; a clear benefit. The sirens also warn potential pedestrians to watch out, as the truck wisps through red lights at speeds too fast to abruptly stop. Another benefit. But what about the child living in an apartment building along a road near a hospital? He is frequently awoken by the ambulances' alarms, but he is neither in position to provide medical assistance, nor is he able to help speed things along on the road, nor is he a pedestrian in danger of being hit. The same sound can serve a benefit to some and detriment to others, simultaneously.

Sleep in Hospitals

Ironically, hospitals are notorious for providing patients inadequate opportunity to sleep [7], even though, presumably, sleep is important for health and well-being. The hospital is replete with scenarios where sounds are ambiguously helpful and harmful. No doubt, there are unwanted noises that are byproducts of providing medical treatment. No one would argue that the familiar thud-thud-thud noise of a helicopter landing on the hospital's roof benefits none. As a society, we tolerate that noise since we wish to provide the service of an air ambulance. But try explaining that to a patient in a hospital bed near the helicopter landing pad.

The hospital setting has even more ambiguous scenarios. Take an intravenous (IV) pump, infusing antibiotics all night long to a patient with a bacterial infection of his leg. If the tubing kinks—and it frequently does—the pump will alarm. This alerts the nurse or doctor that the medication infusion is inadequate, so that it can be fixed. In that sense, the alarm clearly benefits the patient. But the patient himself is not in position to fix the pump. So to him, the alarm becomes a noise source that frequently disrupts his needed sleep (never mind the further nuisance that his alarming IV pump causes his sleeping roommate). In this example, the sound both benefits and harms the same person; it is further needed for some and not for others.

It is no wonder that patients rate noise in and around their hospital room as one of the key areas in need of improvement for hospitalized patients [8]. Yet hospitals are getting noisier and noisier. A major urban hospital reported steadily increasing nighttime noise levels over a 45-year period, from sound-pressure levels (SPLs) averaging 45 dBA to more than 55 dBA in 2005 [9], which is 5–10 dBA higher than that at sustained levels in the emergency department [10].

Keep in mind that *sound-pressure level* (SPL, or sound level, for short) is a unit of measure from an instrument. It is recorded on a log scale, decibels (dB). Ten points higher on this scale is ten times the power. *Loudness*, on the other hand, is a term referring to a person's perception of sound. As a crude rule of thumb, a 10-point increase in sound level yields the psychological sensation of hearing something twice as loud. While a SPL of 50 dBA is that of conversation, 70 dBA is a vacuum cleaner just a few feet away.

Seeking to examine the sleep among patients in the intensive care unit, one study demonstrated poor sleep quality and quantity, employing conventional, polysomnographic sleep measures across numerous patients [11]. The same study also demonstrated high SPLs throughout the entire night. When weighting the recorded sounds to those that the human ear is most sensitive—so-called A weighting of decibels, or dBA—this recent study showed the mean SPL to be >50 dBA across the night in these patient areas. While the study did not attempt to control for light exposure, or medical interventions at night, or medications, or medical disorders—all events that would likely contribute to poor sleep—it seems reasonable to assume that an average sound level of that degree would represent severe impediment to sleep. Also, it is important to remember that the average SPL overnight is only one broad metric. One could easily imagine pulses of very brief, very loud noises, with relative quiet in between. This would register as a reasonably low average SPL, but would likely be very disruptive to sleep nonetheless.

Taking hospital-based sounds to the sleep laboratory, another study attempted to isolate the effects of noises on sleep, examining sound level, sound type, and sleep stage [4]. The investigators first made sound recordings from a local hospital. They took the 14 most commonly encountered sounds—IV alarms, overhead pages, snoring, etc.—and then brought those recordings into a sleep laboratory at a nearby hotel. The sleep room was designed to mimic the soundscape of a hospital, including surrounding the bed with speakers and playing the hospital sounds while healthy volunteers attempted to sleep. Surround-sound allowed for three-dimensional movement of sounds: planes flew across the room, for example. The SPL for any given sound played to a sleeping subject was adjusted based on real-time analysis of the human electroencephalogram (EEG).

Researchers first determined that the participant was asleep. If so, they cycled randomly through a series of 14 different sounds. Each one was played at a low level first. If that did not awaken the subject, then the sound was played at a more substantial SPL, and higher and higher until the subject was awoken. When sleep was disrupted, the noise was abruptly stopped. The subject was allowed to fall back asleep, and when asleep, another sound was chosen to play.

By employing this step-function technique—where the sleepers were subjected to higher and higher "doses" of noise until they were awoken—the investigators attempted to quantify what sound-pressure levels wake people up. Since brain-wave patterns of sleep were being quantified with EEG alongside the sound presentation, these investigators were also able to control for what sleep stage the subject was sleeping in when awoken. Taken together, the study characterized three variables: sleep stage; SPL; and type of sound that awakens healthy volunteers.

This study had several results worth noting. First, it showed that "deep sleep" (N3, formerly called NREM 3 and NREM 4) is, in fact, deeper sleep than other stages. Comparing the same type of sound at different decibel levels across different stages of sleep, it took higher levels to awaken people from N3 than any other stage of sleep. Further, the effects of sounds differed quite a bit: alarm-like sounds awoken people more readily than voices, etc. This was possibly due to their abrupt sounds, alternating on and off signal, or other acoustic characteristics such as pitch.

Interestingly, however, these distinctions between types of sounds were less apparent in REM sleep. In REM, it appeared that all sounds had similar effects on sleep at similar sound levels. This finding is somewhat unexpected, given prior studies showing that people can more readily respond to their name during REM sleep, compared to hearing another person's name—implying that the brain can distinguish between types of sounds in REM sleep [12]. Interestingly, a follow-up study showed that REM sleep appears to make no distinction between pseudo-words and congruous words, implying that REM sleep fails to distinguish between normal and absurd types of sound presentations [13]. Taken together, it might be that a person's name represents a notable exception, but in the broader context, REM sleep appears to afford little distinction between sound types. The underlying psychobiology remains elusive.

One immediate potential application for this study would be to assist architects putting together building plans for future hospitals that limit noise. In making material decisions about certain types of sounds, they can gauge the degree of need for noise mitigation based on empirical data. Or engineers can focus on smart devices that dampen certain types of sounds at certain sound levels. However, to optimally employ this kind of data for the purpose of a hospital construction, it would ideally be replicated in a population of older people, which would be a more representative sample of hospitalized patients. It is already known, for instance, that advanced age can reduce sleep depth and adjust circadian biology [14]. And young patients in neonatal and pediatric settings also have different sleep and circadian physiology than healthy adults.

Three other variables limit the real-world applicability of this study. First, hospitalized patients are sick. Those illnesses can cause stress and discomfort—each of which might influence sleep for the worse. Next, the illnesses themselves might influence sleep. And finally, the medications used during hospitalization might have effects on sleep.

Indeed, many medications are given to hospitalized patients for their illness, and these can inadvertently influence sleep. While these are often unwanted or incidental effects, some hospitalized patients receive medications taken for the sole purpose of helping them sleep. Yet so-called sleep-specific medications, like all medications, have their risks and side effects [15]. And there is even healthy debate about whether the sleep obtained by these medications represents healthy sleep, or a poor, synthetic replica of natural sleep that does not behave normally [16, 17]. Left unresolved, it seems preferable to reduce the use of sleep medications—ideally by reducing their need. And the recipe for reducing need includes creating an environment that is conducive to sleep—no small challenge for a hospital setting.

With this in mind, investigators sought to reduce sleep medication use by employing a broad set of limitations to hospital routines, including reduced noise [18]. They blinded the medical staff from the fact that sleep-medication use was being recorded. Investigators then implemented a protocol that reduced noise made by staff, including a period of "quiet time" overnight. This lead to an impressive 50 % reduction in the use of sleep medications. The study will need to be repeated to isolate the effect of noise, however, as one of the main interventions was not only noise reduction, but also the reduction in nursing staff disturbing sleeping patients overnight for routine tests and measurements. So it remains unclear what specific contribution the quiet played in reducing the need for sleep medications.

Another recent study examined sound levels in the neonatal intensive care unit [19]. They found levels to be quiet high. Background noise was 56 dBA. And frequent alarms brought levels commonly in the 1980s. But neonates live inside an isolate. And so the investigators measured in and out of the isolate. As expected, this isolate afforded modest reduction of ambient noise from the room (47 dBA, instead of 56 dBA), but not from the noises made inside the isolate. For that, they introduced a sound absorbing panel (SAP) to the walls and ceiling of the isolate itself. This led to substantial reductions of SPLs in the isolate, but still unacceptably high (e.g., 82 dBA brought down to 72 dBA with use of SAP).

Noise Mitigation

The potential for noise-induced sleep disruption raises an important challenge: how can we reduce noises or mitigate their effects, in order to enhance sleep? Generally speaking, these fall into two broad approaches: traditional, acoustic, or electrical engineering approaches; and futuristic, neuro-engineering approaches.

Traditional approaches to noise include three broad categories: passive noise control, active noise control, and sound masking.

Passive noise control deals with either the source of a sound, or its path. The focus is, respectively, either taking efforts to eliminating sound itself, or if not eliminated, disrupting its path such that it is not perceived by the potential listener.

At the source, efforts can be made to reduce the existence of sounds altogether. The simplest form of this approach involves a sign that says "quiet" or "$350 fine for honking after 10 p.m." or "welcome to the concert, please turn your phones off." At the level of public policy, passive noise control that focuses on the source of sounds might refer to laws preventing airplanes from flying at night over populated areas, or a mandated "quiet car" on a train. Though often easy to articulate what the policy might be, this form of passive noise control is challenging to implement, partly because it requires agreement and participation of non-sleeping people. And who wants to whisper without being the direct beneficiary from that limitation?

So beyond the source of the sound, the other part of passive noise control involves the path. That is, once a sound is generated, what can be done to limit its perception by a sleeping person? This technique involves any technique, often a physical material, strategically placed between a sound and sleeping person. At its simplest level, one might insert earplugs into their external auditory canal, between the sound and the tympanic membrane of the ear. One might thicken walls; or hang thick materials such as mass-loaded-vinyl over the windows. More advanced construction materials and techniques exist as well. As a rule, smartly constructed homes, hotels, hospitals, and other sleep environments will seek to reduce SPLs before they reach the potential listener.

But what if sounds reach the listener? Two further approaches can be employed, beyond passive noise control: active noise control and sound masking.

Active noise control derives its name from the fact that a new sound wave is being introduced into the environment to cancel the waveform of the existing, undesirable noise. Active noise control is different from sound masking. With active noise control, a precise physical sound is produced in response to the existence of an unwanted noise, nullifying resulting physical properties and reducing the perception of both sounds altogether. Sound masking, on the other hand, introduces broad-band noise into the environment order to cover up the existing, unwanted noise from being perceived. Think of how much louder you have to talk in order to be heard, if standing next to a large, industrial fan or an airport propeller. In the extreme, you might have to shout just to be heard by the person inches away. More comfortable sound masking should be less apparent, as there is a clear balance between masking the annoying noise source, while avoiding creation of a different annoying noise source to achieve that effect.

Beyond these traditional, active, and passive noise controls, another approach to reducing noise-induced sleep disruption is to consider the brain, and attempt to harness its natural, protective mechanisms. Can these mechanisms be quantified and manipulated in order to maximize their effect?

The thalamus ranks high among the brain structures that might be responsible for mitigating the perception of sounds in the sleeping brain. After all, the thalamus is the gateway of sensory information, a way station for neurons communicating information about the external world, including sound, light, touch, temperature, etc. to the broader cortex of the brain where sounds are mentally perceived. Fortunately, at least part of the activity of the thalamus can be quantified at the surface of the brain, in the form of EEG signals. By placing harmless, sticky electrodes on a person's scalp, we can detect faint electromagnetic signals generated by the brain. If we amplify these signals and display them over time, we get a picture of brain waves that have been measured since the early twentieth century [20]. The EEG has been employed for a century, so there is substantial familiarity with these signals. But the (relatively) recent transition to digital recordings of these sleep brain waves affords the opportunity to employ advanced signal-processing techniques previously unavailable to paper and pen recordings.

Among the markers of activity from the thalamus includes the sleep spindle, a thalamocortical rhythm manifested on the EEG as an 11–15 Hz oscillation, and is thought to be capable of modulating the influence of external stimuli [21]. The rate of occurrence of spindles, while variable across people, appears to be relatively stable across nights for any given person [22, 23]. And interestingly, noise tolerance during sleep [24], like spindle rate [25], diminishes with age.

A recent study leveraged these finding by systematically challenging sleeping people with noises [22]. They demonstrated that healthy, young individuals who generated more sleep spindles during a quiet night of sleep went on to exhibit higher tolerance for noise during a subsequent, noisy night of sleep. This result argues that the sleeping brain's spontaneous activity provides a window onto the sleeper's ability to protect their sleep in the face of noise. This finding further raises fundamental questions about whether augmenting spindle production—with drug or device—one might be able to enhance sleep continuity when confronted with noise.

In the future, perhaps the sleep spindle could serve as a biomarker, predicting an individual's ability to maintain sleep in the face of external sound: those with more abundant spindles are more resistant to sounds during sleep. But even if we were to fully believe this finding, and its relatively small sample size of healthy young adults, it remains to be seen, however, whether this relationship emerges directly from thalamic activity—represented by the sleep spindle—or whether it is due to a yet undetermined biological process. Knowing this information might pave the roads for pursuit of techniques to protect sleep by harnessing the spindle's ability to deflect sensory information.

In a related study, subjects were challenged with noises during sleep [26]. Whereas the spindle study (above) asked whether there are certain traits of sleep overall that predict sound sleep in the face of noise, this study looked at the moments immediately prior to disrupted sleep, to see if the EEG signal offered a signature of moment-to-moment sleep depth. To achieve this, the researchers computed the amount of energy in the alpha band, an 8–13 Hz EEG rhythm prominent over posterior scalp locations, where the visual system of the brain is located, among other functions. Traditionally considered the signature of wakefulness, alpha intensity discloses immediate levels of alertness and dissipates in concert with fading awareness as sleep begins. This alpha brain activity pattern, however, is largely ignored once sleep begins. Yet behind the prominent slow waves and other physical features of sleep, energy in the alpha band subtly waxes and wanes in the background. It is this background signal that was discovered to convey information about sleep depth: for any given stage of sleep, the micro-environment of alpha intensity predicted the ability of the sleeper to maintain sleep when confronted with noises. More alpha activity right before a sound was played meant that it was more likely for sleep to be disturbed by that sound. More alpha waves means more fragile sleep, it seems.

Taken together, it appears that there are numerous biomarkers that might disclose information about the brain's ability to withstand sleep in the face of noises. It's tantalizing to consider these signals to represent targets of intervention. If, for example, sleep spindles could be amplified, or alpha activity reduced, could we boost the brain's natural abilities to maintain sleep in noisy environments? Answers to these questions currently remain out of reach. For one thing, we don't fully understand the sleep spindle. Its source appears to be the reticular nucleus of the thalamus [27, 28], but noninvasive techniques of EEG record brain activity near the surface of the brain, not directly measuring deep structures like the thalamus. Even if a device were to increase spindle activity that we measure, would it actually behave in a biological manner similar to a naturally occurring spindle? More concerning, while spindles correlate with sleep stability, do they play a causal role, or are they merely a marker for another biological function that boosts sleep depth? And as for alpha activity, we know even less about its underlying biological mechanisms.

Though spindles and alpha waves represent interesting biomarkers of stable sleep, the classic signature of deep sleep continues to be represented by the so-called slow oscillation. Ironic to this topic of noise-induced sleep disruption, two recent studies examined the ability to bolster native sleep rhythms by strategically introducing brief pulses of sounds [29, 30]. The slow oscillation was only boosted when the sound was precisely timed to coincide in-phase with the slow oscillation itself. Out of phase presentations of sound were disruptive. These new findings represent exciting areas of early-phase basic science that complement other attempts to bolster slow oscillations. Conversely, other recent studies attempt to selectively reduce certain components of deep sleep by introducing subtle sounds into sleep [6]. The technical limitations and clinical benefits of this group of studies will clearly need to be further examined in this fascinating arena in the coming years.

Limitations abound. But the promise of bolstering sleep through principled alterations in biological activity of the brain represents a new and exciting frontier for tools available to maintain sound sleep on noisy nights. In the meantime, continue to keep your eye out for signs reading "no honking after 10 p.m."

References

1. Cirelli C, Tononi G. Is sleep essential? PLoS Biol. 2008;6:e216.
2. Van Dongen HP, Maislin G, Mullington JM, Dinges DF. The cumulative cost of additional wakefulness: dose-response effects on neurobehavioral functions and sleep physiology from chronic sleep restriction and total sleep deprivation. Sleep. 2003;26:117–26.
3. Basner M, Griefahn B, Berg MVD. Aircraft noise effects on sleep: mechanisms, mitigation and research needs. Noise Health. 2010;12:95–109.
4. Buxton OM, Ellenbogen JM, Wang W, et al. Sleep disruption due to hospital noises: a prospective evaluation. Ann Intern Med. 2012;157:170–9.
5. Basner M, Müller U, Elmenhorst E-M. Single and combined effects of air, road, and rail traffic noise on sleep and recuperation. Sleep. 2011;34:11–23.
6. Tasali E, Leproult R, Ehrmann DA, Van Cauter E. Slow-wave sleep and the risk of type 2 diabetes in humans. Proc Natl Acad Sci U S A. 2008;105:1044–9.
7. Dogan O, Ertekin S, Dogan S. Sleep quality in hospitalized patients. J Clin Nurs. 2005;14:107–13.
8. Jha AK, Orav EJ, Zheng J, Epstein AM. Patients' perception of hospital care in the United States. N Engl J Med. 2008;359:1921–31.

9. Busch-Vishniac IJ, West JE, Barnhill C, Hunter T, Orellana D, Chivukula R. Noise levels in Johns Hopkins Hospital. J Acoust Soc Am. 2005;118:3629–45.
10. Orellana D, Busch-Vishniac IJ, West JE. Noise in the adult emergency department of Johns Hopkins Hospital. J Acoust Soc Am. 2007;121:1996–9.
11. Elliott R, McKinley S, Cistulli P, Fien M. Characterisation of sleep in intensive care using 24 hour polysomnography: an observational study. Crit Care. 2013;17:R46.
12. Perrin F, Garcia-Larrea L, Mauguiere F, Bastuji H. A differential brain response to the subject's own name persists during sleep. Clin Neurophysiol. 1999;110: 2153–64.
13. Perrin F, Bastuji H, Garcia-Larrea L. Detection of verbal discordances during sleep. Neuroreport. 2002;13: 1345–9.
14. Dijk DJ, Duffy JF, Czeisler CA. Contribution of circadian physiology and sleep homeostasis to age-related changes in human sleep. Chronobiol Int. 2000;17: 285–311.
15. Bianchi MT, Thomas RJ, Ellenbogen JM. Hypnotics and mortality risk. J Clin Sleep Med. 2012;8:351–2.
16. Seibt J, Aton SJ, Jha SK, Coleman T, Dumoulin MC, Frank MG. The non-benzodiazepine hypnotic zolpidem impairs sleep-dependent cortical plasticity. Sleep. 2008;31:1381–91.
17. Aton SJ, Seibt J, Dumoulin MC, Coleman T, Shiraishi M, Frank MG. The sedating antidepressant trazodone impairs sleep-dependent cortical plasticity. PLoS One. 2009;4:e6078.
18. Bartick MC, Thai X, Schmidt T, Altaye A, Solet JM. Decrease in as-needed sedative use by limiting nighttime sleep disruptions from hospital staff. J Hosp Med. 2010;5:E20–4.
19. Altuncu E, Akman I, Kulekci S, Akdas F, Bilgen H, Ozek E. Noise levels in neonatal intensive care unit and use of sound absorbing panel in the isolette. Int J Pediatr Otorhinolaryngol. 2009;73:951–3.
20. Berger H. Über das Elektroenkephalogramm des Menschen. Arch Psychiatr Nervenkr. 1929;87:527–70.
21. Steriade M. Alertness, quiet sleep, dreaming. In: Peters A, Jones EJ, editors. Cerebral cortex vol. 9: normal and altered states of function. New York: Plenum Press; 1991. p. 279–357.
22. Dang-Vu TT, Mckinney SM, Buxton OM, Solet JM, Ellenbogen JM. Spontaneous brain rhythms predict sleep stability in the face of noise. Curr Biol. 2010;20:R626–7.
23. Azumi K, Shirakawa S. Characteristics of spindle activity and their use in evaluation of hypnotics. Sleep. 1982;5:95–105.
24. Busby KA, Mercier L, Pivik RT. Ontogenetic variations in auditory arousal threshold during sleep. Psychophysiology. 1994;31:182–8.
25. De Gennaro L, Ferrara M. Sleep spindles: an overview. Sleep Med Rev. 2003;7:423–40.
26. Mckinney SM, Dang-Vu TT, Buxton OM, Solet JM, Ellenbogen JM. Covert waking brain activity reveals instantaneous sleep depth. PLoS One. 2011;6:e17351.
27. Steriade M. Corticothalamic resonance, states of vigilance and mentation. Neuroscience. 2000;101:243–76.
28. Steriade M. The corticothalamic system in sleep. Front Biosci. 2003;8:d878–99.
29. Ngo H-VV, Claussen JC, Born J, Mölle M. Induction of slow oscillations by rhythmic acoustic stimulation. J Sleep Res. 2012;22:22–31.
30. Ngo H-VV, Martinetz T, Born J, Mölle M. Auditory closed-loop stimulation of the sleep slow oscillation enhances memory. Neuron. 2013;78(3):545–53.

Sleep Deprivation and Cognitive Performance

16

William D.S. Killgore and Mareen Weber

Introduction

Over the past half century, people living in Westernized societies have been showing a steady decline in their nightly sleep. While in the 1960s, most Americans were sleeping between 8 and 9 h per night [1], by the mid 1990s, this level had dropped to about 7 h nightly [2]. Recent epidemiologic data actually suggest that about one in three workers currently report sleeping less than 6 h most nights [3]. At present, the impact of sleep loss on cognitive and emotional functioning is only modestly understood. With more people getting less sleep, it is vital that science advances our understanding of the effects that sleep loss can have on cognitive and emotional functioning.

While a comprehensive review of the effects of sleep deprivation on cognitive performance is beyond the scope of this volume, we will provide a concise and selective review that focuses on several of the major cognitive domains that may be affected when sleep is restricted or completely prevented for a period of 24 h or more. From a simplistic perspective, neuropsychological capacities generally function in a hierarchical fashion, with more complex higher order capacities (e.g., decision-making) building upon more elementary ones (e.g., attention; memory) [4]. Accordingly, the present chapter will follow an ordered discussion of the effects of sleep loss on cognitive capacities, beginning with elementary ones such as simple alertness, vigilance, and attention, which generally form the foundation for more complex cognitive abilities. This will be followed by the effects of sleep deprivation on sensory perception, emotion, and long-term memory, followed by its effects on higher order cognitive processes, including mental flexibility, planning and sequencing, abstract concept formation, and decision-making.

Alertness, Vigilance, and Simple Attention

In order to engage in most forms of complex cognitive processing, an individual must first be conscious, alert, and able to focus attentional resources for a sufficient period of time to solve the problem at hand. It is at this basic level that sleep loss appears to have its most consistent and profound effects on cognition [5, 6]. For a healthy well-rested person, general alertness only fluctuates in a subtle manner throughout the day, generally corresponding to the normal circadian cycle, with slight dips that are often most noticeable in the early afternoon hours. However, after about

W.D.S. Killgore (✉)
Center for Depression, Anxiety, and Stress Research, McLean Hospital, Harvard Medical School, Belmont, MA, USA

M. Weber
McLean Hospital, Harvard Medical School, Belmont, MA, USA

M.T. Bianchi (ed.), *Sleep Deprivation and Disease: Effects on the Body, Brain and Behavior*, DOI 10.1007/978-1-4614-9087-6_16, © Springer Science+Business Media New York 2014

16 h of continuous wakefulness, the ability to sustain alertness and vigilant attention begins to wane dramatically for most people. This is particularly notable on specialized tests designed to repeatedly measure reaction time over a period of several minutes [7].

Psychomotor Vigilance

One of the most common measures of alertness and vigilance is known as the psychomotor vigilance test (PVT), a computerized test of reaction time that requires the respondent to press a key every time a stimulus appears on the screen [8]. In the most widely used version of the test, stimuli are presented at pseudorandom intervals for a total duration of 10 min. Though simple in design and presentation, the PVT is exquisitely sensitive to total sleep deprivation [9] and chronic partial sleep restriction [10]. One of the primary effects of sleep deprivation on this task is slowing of simple reaction time. Figure 16.1 shows the effects of 82 h of sleep deprivation on psychomotor vigilance speed (i.e., 1/Reaction Time × 1,000) in ten healthy participants [11]. As evident in the figure, speed of responding on the PVT remains close to 100 % of baseline throughout most of the first day, but shows remarkable slowing after about 23:00 h and continues to decline until 08:00 the next morning, at which time the performance decline is reversed temporarily, due to the circadian phase. This pattern is even more pronounced during the second and third nights without sleep. A useful rule of thumb that has been proposed for operational settings suggests that response times on the PVT and other similar tasks can be expected to slow by about 25 % for each night without sleep [12]. While total sleep deprivation can bring about rapid and dramatic declines in psychomotor vigilance, degraded performance can also emerge more insidiously during periods of chronic partial sleep restriction over several nights. One study showed that when total sleep time was limited to only 6 h per night for two consecutive weeks, PVT performance declined to a level similar to that of individuals who had undergone 2 nights of total sleep deprivation [13] (Fig. 16.1).

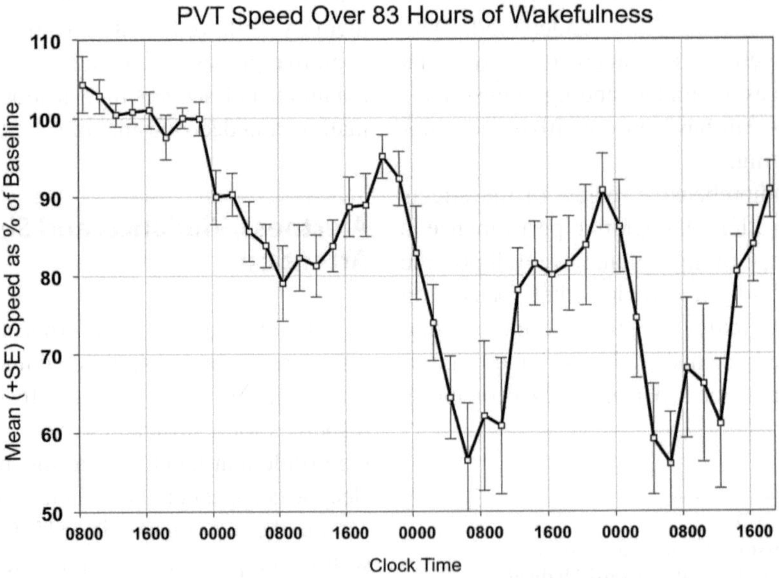

Fig. 16.1 Psychomotor vigilance speed (1/RT × 1,000) over 83 h of sleep deprivation (n=10) shows the combined effects of accumulating homeostatic sleep pressure (*downward* trend of the data) and the circadian rhythm of alertness (*sinusoidal* trend across days). Speed performance is normalized to each participant's own baseline and presented as a percentage of that baseline (Data from Wesensten et al. [11])

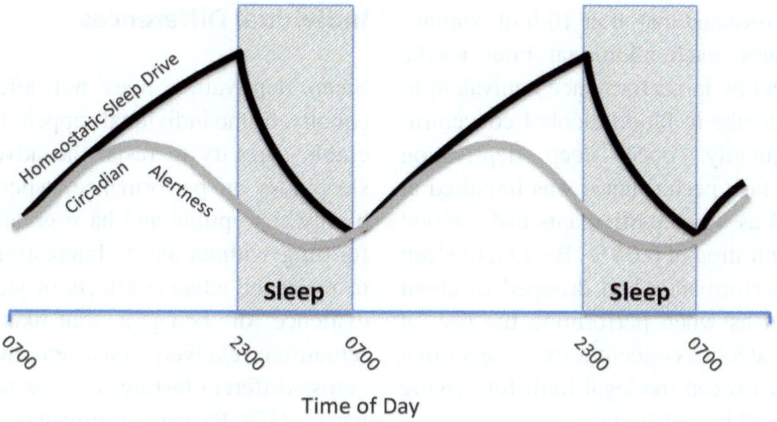

Fig. 16.2 The two-process model of sleep homeostasis [14]. The propensity to sleep is dependent upon two interacting processes, (1) a homeostatic drive for sleep, which increases the longer an individual goes without sleep, and is dissipated rapidly with sleep, and (2) an oscillating circadian pattern of alertness that is lowest in the early morning and highest in early evening. At any particular time of day, these two processes combine to influence an individual's level of alertness and propensity to sleep

Not only does sleep deprivation lead to slowing of response times, it also increases the duration and frequency of momentary "lapses" in attention (i.e., periods of nonresponsiveness lasting a half second or longer). While lapses are rare occurrences among well-rested individuals, they become quite common during periods of prolonged wakefulness. Two interacting biological processes govern the probability of a lapse [14]. First, extended periods of wakefulness lead to increased homeostatic sleep pressure (i.e., the biological drive for sleep). The longer an individual is awake, the stronger is the drive to fall asleep. Second, alertness is also influenced by the circadian phase (i.e., the time of day), which tends to affect the level of alertness in a sinusoidal pattern that rises and falls throughout the day. Figure 16.2 shows the hypothesized interaction of these two processes over a 2-day period. An individual's level of alertness and vigilance at any particular moment emerges from the combined product of these interacting processes. The effects of accumulated homeostatic sleep pressure may be only minimal and hard to detect when the circadian rhythm is at its peak, but when the circadian rhythm is at its nadir (i.e., usually in the early morning), the impairing effects of sleep deprivation on alertness and vigilance performance can be dramatic, leading to significant slowing of response time and increased probability of momentary lapses [15] (Fig. 16.2).

Attention and Motor Tracking

Sleep deprivation can affect simple attention and motor tracking capacities in a manner that closely parallels alcohol intoxication. In a compelling and practically relevant study, investigators equated the hour-by-hour effects of continuous wakefulness with the drink-by-drink effects of blood alcohol concentration during a visual-motor tracking task [16]. During 28 h of sleep deprivation, participants were tested repeatedly on a simple test of hand-eye tracking and coordination. The researchers found, as expected, that performance showed a linear decline with longer sleep deprivation. On a different day, the same subjects returned to the lab and completed the same motor tracking task when well-rested. The interesting twist to this study was that while the rested subjects completed the motor tracking task they also slowly consumed alcoholic beverages to the point of intoxication. A comparison between the sleep-deprived and alcohol-intoxicated performances revealed that after 10 h of continuous wakefulness, each additional hour awake produced a decline in performance equivalent to a 0.004 % increase in blood alcohol concentration. Consequently, once sleep deprivation reached 17 h, task performance was impaired at the same level as when participants had a blood alcohol concentration of 0.05 %. By 24 h of sleep deprivation, performance had dropped to about the same level as when performing the task at 0.10 % blood alcohol concentration, a level that would meet or exceed the legal limit for driving while intoxicated in all US states.

Wake State Instability

One of the most consistent findings from the research on the effects of sleep deprivation on psychomotor vigilance is that sleep-deprived performance is unstable. Compared to rested wakefulness, the performance of a sleep-deprived person is variable and prone to unexpected lapses. At one moment, a sleep-deprived person may appear to be relatively alert and responsive, only to be followed by a momentary slowing of performance or even an unexpected failure to respond altogether. This phenomenon has been described as "wake state instability" which suggests that the hallmark of sleep loss is *variability* in the ability to sustain wakefulness and resulting *inconsistency* of performance [9]. This instability is believed to be the net output from the interaction of reciprocally inhibiting neurobiologic systems, one pressuring the individual to fall asleep and the other struggling to sustain wakefulness [7]. Instability in wakefulness is most reliably observed in performance lapses (i.e., PVT response times exceeding 500 ms), which occur with greater frequency and last for longer durations with progressively greater time spent awake [9]. At the extreme, lapses in attention can become so prolonged (e.g., 30 s or longer) that they are more accurately described as "functional sleep attacks" [5].

Individual Differences

Sleep deprivation does not affect all people equally. Some individuals appear to have considerable capacity to resist the adverse effects of sleep loss on performance, whereas others are highly susceptible and have great difficulty performing without sleep. Interestingly, the ability to resist the adverse effects of sleep loss shows evidence of being a trait-like phenomenon, remaining relatively consistent and reproducible across different testing sessions within the same person [17]. By some estimates, systematic individual differences may explain up to 67.5 % of variability in PVT performance, and more than 90 % of variability in subjective sleepiness ratings, suggesting that such resistance may indeed reflect a trait-like capacity [17]. Interestingly, this capacity appears to confer resistance in a variety of sleep loss situations. For example, one recent study showed that total sleep deprivation (63 h) and prolonged sleep restriction (7 nights of 3 h time in bed) yielded very similar effects on cognitive performance and mood within the same individuals, suggesting that vulnerability to one also involves vulnerability to the other—regardless of the performance capacity demonstrated at baseline [18].

Can these individual differences in resistance capacity be predicted or identified before sleep deprivation? So far, it has been difficult to identify a reliable marker for this phenomenon. A number of sensible candidate markers, including prior sleep history, baseline cognitive functioning, standard blood and urine laboratory test findings, and psychological traits such as personality have not emerged as reliable predictors of resistance or vulnerability to sleep loss [19]. Some recent studies have reported such relationships for some personality traits or sensory capacities [20–22], but these findings will require further replication to determine their reliability and the degree to which they are affected by external or environmental factors [23]. Interestingly, the ability to identify odors (an

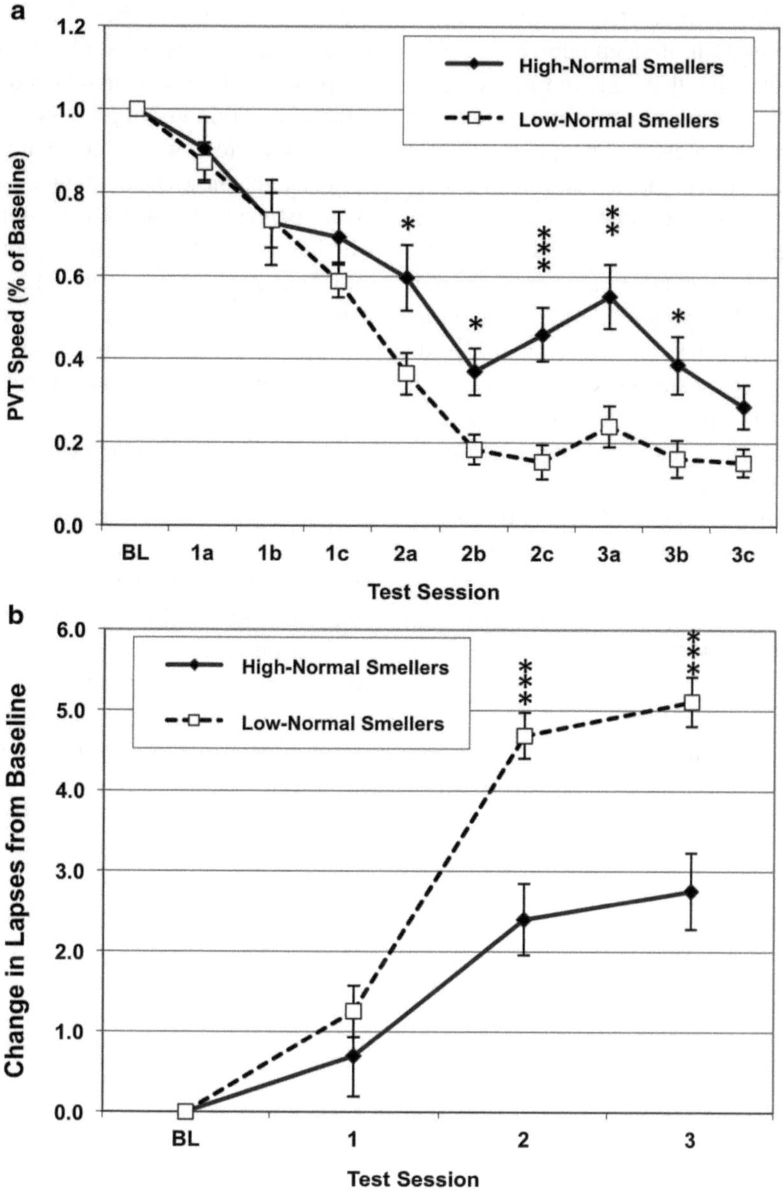

Fig. 16.3 Differences in "high-normal" and "low-normal" performers on the smell identification test discriminate the magnitude of degradation of psychomotor vigilance over a 3-day sleep deprivation study [21]. (**a**) Psychomotor vigilance speed (1/RT × 1,000) declines to a greater extent among "low-normal" smellers (*dashed line*) compared to "high-normal" smellers (*solid line*). Each 9-h night is subdivided into thirds (i.e., *a*, *b*, *c*). (**b**) The number of attentional lapses (i.e., non-responses >500 ms) on the PVT was significantly greater among "low-normal" smellers compared to "high-normal" smellers. $*p<0.05$, $**p<0.01$, $***p<0.005$ (Reprinted with permission from Killgore et al. [21])

ability that involves the orbitofrontal cortex) when well-rested was highly effective at discriminating between more and less resistant individuals in one study (see Fig. 16.3), raising the possibility that baseline orbitofrontal integrity may confer some resistance to sleep loss [21]. Individual differences might also arise from baseline brain activation during rested wakefulness. For example, greater activation of the ventrolateral prefrontal cortex (VLPFC) during rested wakefulness predicted greater signal change following 31 h of sleep deprivation on a working memory task that required participants to decide whether an on-screen stimulus was the same as the stimulus presented one, two, or three trials before the current presentation [24]. This means that the more this area was involved in task performance when tested at rested baseline, the greater was the reduction in brain activation following sleep deprivation. Perhaps the most promising avenue toward identifying the basis for the ability to resist sleep loss will come from genetic research. There is some evidence that there may be a several candidate gene polymorphisms that contribute to individual differences in sensitivity to the effects of sleep loss, sleep pressure, and circadian influences [25–27].

Sensory Perception

Building upon the neurobiological foundation of alertness, vigilance, and attention, the next section briefly summarizes the effects of sleep deprivation on the sensory and perceptual systems.

Visuospatial Perception

Vision is arguably the most highly studied and well mapped of the sensory-perceptual systems. However, there have been only a relatively small number of studies that have specifically tested the effects of sleep deprivation on visual perception. One recent study showed that a single night of sleep loss was sufficient to degrade perceptual sensitivity on a computerized visual perception task and was associated with more conservative perceptual decisions [28]. Functional neuroimaging data also suggest that the visual system may be particularly affected by sleep loss [29]. For example, Chee and colleagues found that sleep deprivation induced a significant decline in visual task-related activation within the occipital cortex. Moreover, these reductions in visual cortex activity were most prominent when an individual was experiencing a lapse in attention [29], suggesting that a sleep-deprived person may actually experience moments where they fail to "see" a visual stimulus. In a follow-on study by the same group, sleep deprivation was associated with reduced activation within visual processing regions of the occipital cortex, which correlated with poorer performance on a visual memory and a matched visual-perceptual task [30]. It remains uncertain whether these effects are due to a primary deficit in visual processing or whether the observed deficits may actually reflect impairments in attentional allocation. Some evidence seems to support the latter position [31], but more research is necessary.

In addition to simple visual object processing, the visual system is also heavily involved in spatial perception. For instance, most healthy normal individuals show a visual-perceptual bias to overestimate the length of the left half of bisected horizontal lines. This relatively stable finding has been attributed to a right-hemispheric dominance for attention and spatial processing, leading normal healthy individuals to assign greater perceptual weight to the left side of stimuli [32, 33]. Manly and colleagues [34] examined this bias in sleep-deprived participants and found that sleep deprivation induced a rightward shift in attention, negating the normal leftward bias seen when rested. The authors suggest that sleep loss may particularly impair the right hemisphere, leading to a shift in normal visuospatial biases away from the contralateral left hemi-space and toward the right side of space. Thus, these findings seem to suggest that sleep deprivation may tend to adversely affect right-hemispheric spatial attention systems to a greater extent than the left.

Some studies, however, have failed to find lateralized visual perception effects. For example, Kendall and colleagues [35] presented small light flashes at locations around a 150° horizontal visual arc during a divided attention paradigm before and after a night of sleep deprivation. However, other than a general decline in responsiveness across the entire visual field, there was no evidence of lateralized deficits in visual perception. Similarly, another visual perception study failed to show any significant effects of sleep deprivation on the ability to perceive line angles [36], although the task that was studied was relatively brief, suggesting that participants were able to perform normally at least for a short time period. Thus, visual sensory perception may be affected by sleep loss, but subtle spatial biases have been less consistently replicated.

Auditory Perception

Few studies have examined the effect of sleep deprivation on auditory perception. Overall, sleep deprivation appears to be associated with a general decline in auditory response latency, but it is possible that these findings are simply due to reduced attention and vigilance, rather than degradation of primary auditory sensation [37]. There is some evidence, however, that sleep deprivation may affect auditory temporal resolution, which involves the ability to discriminate the order of presentation of two successive stimuli [38]. A single night of sleep deprivation resulted in a 28 % decline in auditory temporal resolution on this task [38]. Such findings could have particular relevance in operational settings where verbal communication is critical, such as for air traffic control or military radio communications. A single night of sleep deprivation has also been found to significantly impair the ability to identify dichotically presented sounds (i.e., presented separately to the left and right ears) [39]. However, similar to impairments in temporal resolution of auditory stimuli following sleep deprivation, it remains to be shown whether and to what extent this effect is influenced by the previously described degrading effect of sleep deprivation on alertness and attention. One practically important area that has been minimally explored involves the effects of sleep deprivation on auditory comprehension. One preliminary study in a very small sample demonstrated that a single night of sleep deprivation was associated with deficits in allocation of auditory attention and possible deterioration of lexical search and selection processes within the brain [40].

Tactile Perception/Pain

This is also an area that has been understudied. Some evidence suggests that sleep deprivation has no significant effect on sensing hot and cold temperatures, but that it does reduce pain tolerance when exposed to extremes of temperature [41]. Sleep-deprived individuals also show increased ratings of general body pains such as complaints of physical discomfort, stomach pain, headache, muscle pain, and body pain [42].

Taste Perception

There has been very little research on actual taste perception during sleep deprivation. Limited evidence suggests that sleep-deprived individuals show lower sensory thresholds for detecting sour tastes, but not for sweet or salty tastes [43], but as with many of the sensory studies, it is difficult to rule out the effects of simple alertness or attention on these findings.

Olfactory Perception

Some evidence suggests that sleep deprivation may adversely affect simple odor recognition. For example, Killgore and McBride administered the smell identification test (SIT), a standardized measure of olfactory discrimination, to a sample of healthy volunteers during 24 h of sleep deprivation [44]. Performance on the SIT declined with sleep loss, despite the fact that several other more complex cognitive capacities remained intact. Essentially the same findings emerged in a second independent sample after 52 h of continuous wakefulness [45]. There have been no studies of odor detection thresholds during sleep deprivation.

Emotional Processing

One of the most rapidly growing areas of sleep deprivation research is focused on the effects of insufficient sleep on emotional processes. Here, we will review some of the major trends in research in this area.

Mood, Frustration Tolerance, and Emotional Control

Degradation of mood is a common finding during even relatively brief periods of sleep deprivation [46, 47], with people generally becoming more irritable and less happy when sleep is curtailed. Sleep loss also alters how people perceive and respond to frustrating and stressful circumstances. Franzen and colleagues recently showed that when sleep-deprived, participants showed greater systolic blood pressure reactivity to a psychological stressor than when rested [48]. The psychological interpretation of a stressful or frustrating situation also appears to be affected by sleep loss. For example, 1 night of sleep deprivation increases subjective stress and anxiety in response to mildly stressful activities, but does not appear to alter normal reactions to highly stressful conditions, suggesting that sleep loss reduces the threshold for becoming stressed but does not increase magnitude of high stress emotional reactions [49]. In another study, participants were shown semi-projective cartoon scenarios depicting a variety of frustrating situations and were asked to write in a verbal response for one of the characters in the scenario. After 2 nights of sleep deprivation, participants showed significantly greater tendencies to blame others for problems and showed reduced willingness to consider mutually beneficial solutions to predicaments [50]. Sleep deprivation also appears to reduce several aspects of proactive coping and emotional intelligence capacities [51]. Declines in coping ability included decreased reliance on positive thinking, reduced behaviorally oriented problem solving, and increased belief in the effectiveness of unrealistic or even magical solutions to problems [51]. Similarly, self-perceived emotional intelligence was reduced following 2 nights of sleep deprivation, a finding that was particularly notable for self-ratings of self-esteem, comprehension of interpersonal situations, impulse control, and capacities for delaying gratification [51].

Evidence also suggests that sleep deprivation and sleep restriction weaken the inhibition of aggressive behaviors. For example, victims of domestic violence report more aggressive behaviors in their partners following nights of poor sleep, and such nights appear also to be of greater frequency in this population compared to non-abused women (see [52] for a review on sleep and aggression). Along the same lines, healthy people show increases on a number of scales measuring various facets of psychopathology following sleep deprivation [53]. In particular, 56 h of sleep deprivation was associated with increased scores on scales measuring the cognitive and affective components of depression, physiological symptoms of anxiety, paranoia and feelings of persecution, and health-related somatic complaints [53]. Overall, the evidence suggests that individuals become more easily frustrated, unforgiving, intolerant, less empathic, and more anxious, depressed, and self-absorbed following a period of sleep deprivation.

Emotional Perception and Experience

In addition to affecting mood and emotional self-ratings, sleep deprivation also has an effect on how individuals perceive and rate external emotionally relevant stimuli. Emerging evidence suggests that this may be due to the effects of sleep deprivation on the functioning of mesolimbic pathways involved in reward processing and altered functional connectivity among key regions involved in regulating the balance of pleasure and punishment [54]. These changes may affect the perception of emotional stimuli, and ultimately, the experience of positive and negative affect.

Sleep loss has a number of effects on emotional perception. Following sleep deprivation, physiological measures of emotional arousal, such as pupillary response, are exaggerated to negative, but not neutral or positive visual stimuli, suggesting that sleep loss enhances the strength of reactions to negative emotional information [55]. In another study [47], participants rated a series of photographs containing pleasant, neutral, and unpleasant content. After either a night of total sleep deprivation in the lab or 1 night of normal sleep at home, participants again rated a similar set of images. Ratings of pleasant and unpleasant images were unaffected by sleep deprivation, but this was not the case for the neutral images, which were rated significantly more negatively without sleep. Selective REM sleep deprivation also leads to enhanced emotional reactivity to threatening stimuli compared to habitual sleep and compared to disrupted sleep containing only non-REM sleep interruptions [56]. This suggests that REM sleep plays a key role in maintaining adequate control over emotional reactivity. This interpretation is bolstered by functional brain activation data collected concurrently. That study showed that compared to the baseline assessment of emotional reactivity, task-relevant brain activation in the VLPFC remained at similar levels in the REM sleep deprivation group, whereas it was reduced in the non-REM sleep interruption group. This suggests that even though the emotional task was performed twice, subjects deprived of REM sleep required additional compensatory supervisory control from the prefrontal cortex during task performance. The role of REM sleep in emotion processing was further supported by research showing that REM sleep is particularly important for sustaining the emotional valence of memories [57].

Sleep deprivation can also affect the perception of humor, a highly complex cognitive capacity. The ability to detect and appreciate humor requires the integration of contextual information with emotional processes. To date, only one study has examined the effects of sleep loss on humor appreciation [58]. In that study, sleep-deprived participants judged which of two stimuli, either cartoons or printed statements with multiple meanings, was funnier. Sleep-deprived subjects scored significantly worse than normative data for normally rested subjects in their ability to identify the more humorous stimuli [58], suggesting that humor appreciation is negatively affected by insufficient sleep.

Lack of sleep can also reduce emotional expression in the voice. McGlinchey and colleagues analyzed vocal expressions of emotion before and after sleep deprivation and found that expressions of positive emotion were decreased following sleep loss [59]. Reduced expression of positive emotion was evident regardless of whether the data were analyzed via human raters, computerized acoustic waveform analysis, or computerized textual analysis. Human raters were also able to detect increased negative emotional expression in the voice following sleep deprivation as well.

Appetite and Motivational Responses to Food Stimuli

Sleep loss also alters the perception of food [60], an effect that may have significant consequences for the current epidemic of obesity. It is well known that people tend to crave carbohydrates and snack more when sleep-deprived [61]. This is due in part to alterations in appetite-regulating hormones [62], but may also be due to changes in cognitive processing related to food and its consumption. Benedict and colleagues showed that when participants were asked to rate food images for their appetizing appeal, normal-weight males rated significantly more images as appetizing following 1 night of sleep deprivation than after 1 night of normal sleep [60]. This was particularly true for images of high-calorie food. Using functional magnetic resonance imaging (MRI), the same authors also reported that total sleep deprivation yielded greater activation in the right anterior cingulate cortex (ACC) to food images independent of calorie content suggesting that sleep loss may impact the human reward circuit in order to regulate food intake in response to the increased energy expenditure during sleep deprivation [63]. Using functional MRI, greater overall brain activation to food images has also been found following chronic partially restricted sleep (4 h time in bed for 6 days) compared to habitual sleep (9 h time in bed) in a sample of males and females [64]. Again, this increase in activation was particularly prominent in structures of the human reward circuit such as putamen, nucleus accumbens, thalamus, insula, and prefrontal cortex. These findings suggest that sleep-deprived individuals are more likely to show increased appetite and be more attracted to unhealthy food choices. Given the gravity of the health problems associated with the current epidemic of obesity, the role of sleep loss in overeating remains an important topic for further research.

Learning and Memory

Sleep appears to be a vital process in learning and memory. Without sufficient sleep prior to learning, the brain appears less able to acquire and encode new information; when sleep is prevented after learning, consolidation of acquired information is hindered [7, 65, 66]. The role that sleep contributes to memory processing represents a large and rapidly growing field of research. Due to space constraints, only a limited overview of the topic is possible here, and the interested reader is referred to several excellent reviews on this topic [65–68]. In brief, there are two primary ways in which sleep is hypothesized to contribute to memory. First, in order to maximize the acquisition of information, an individual needs to be well-rested. A good night of sleep prepares the brain to acquire new information [69]. Second, sleep after exposure to new information appears to facilitate the consolidation (i.e., stabilization) and integration (i.e., assimilation) of new learning into existing memory structures [65, 67]. Thus sleep is critical *before* and *after* learning, but for different reasons.

Pre-learning Sleep Deprivation

Too little sleep hinders subsequent learning. This statement has been supported by extensive research. For example, in one study, 35 h of sleep deprivation significantly reduced verbal learning relative to rested baseline performance [70]. During that same study, sleep deprivation also led to reduced activation within regions of the temporal lobe during the memory task, but this occurred in the context of increased activation of prefrontal and parietal cortex regions. Because this activation correlated with better memory performance, it was interpreted as reflecting compensatory recruitment of parietal regions to sustain performance at near baseline levels despite the impairing effects of insufficient sleep. In another study, healthy participants were deprived of a single night of sleep and then had to memorize a series of scenic images during functional MRI scanning [71]. A matched control group received a normal night of sleep, but underwent the same scene-encoding procedure as those who were sleep-deprived. After both groups slept at home for two additional nights, memory retention for the previously learned images was tested. Interestingly, the brain imaging data showed significantly reduced activation of the posterior hippocampus, a key brain structure involved in memory encoding, in the sleep-deprived relative to the well-rested group [71]. Subsequent work has shown that selective deprivation of only slow wave sleep was sufficient to reduced hippocampal memory encoding [72]. Together, these findings suggest that sleep deprivation adversely affects hippocampal structures involved in the encoding process, as well as other brain regions such as the prefrontal and parietal cortices, which may also be recruited to compensate for deficits brought about by sleep loss.

In addition to the impairments in declarative memory, sleep deprivation also impairs temporal memory, which is the ability to remember when in time a specific event occurred. In one of the few studies of temporal memory in sleep deprivation [73], participants viewed two series of 12 facial photographs separated by a 5-min interval. After viewing all of the images and waiting for an additional 5-min delay, participants were tested for their memory of the previously seen faces. In this case, previously seen faces were intermixed with an equal number of never before seen faces to determine how accurately participants could recognize from which group the faces originated. Overall, sleep-deprived subjects were just as accurate at identifying previously seen faces as the participants who had a normal night of sleep. Interestingly, however, sleep deprivation impaired the ability to determine whether the previously seen faces were from the distant (first) set or the more recent (second) set. The sleep-deprived subjects, surprisingly, were even more confident than the well-rested participants in their incorrect guesses [73].

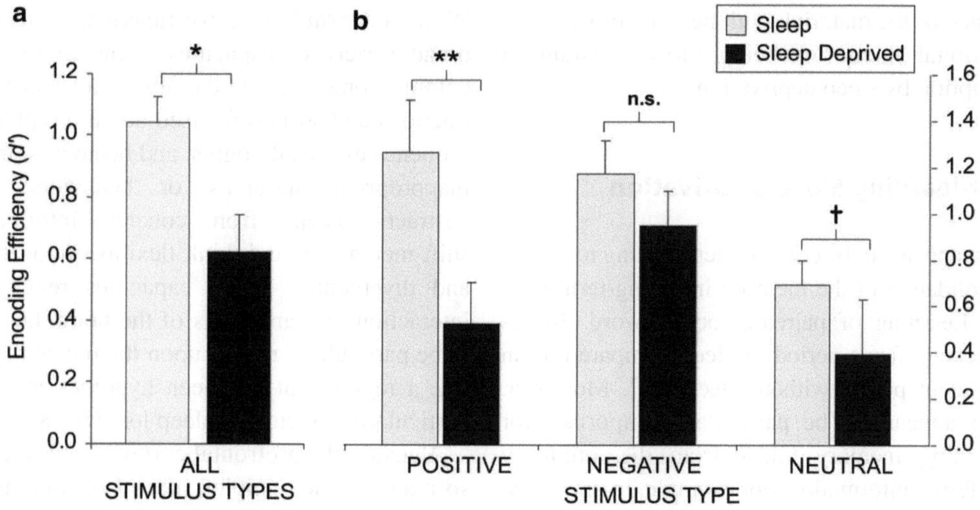

Fig. 16.4 Sleep deprivation and encoding of emotional and nonemotional declarative memory. Effects of 38 h of total sleep deprivation on encoding of human declarative memory (**a**) when combined across all emotional and nonemotional categories, (**b**) when separated by emotional (positive and negative valence) and nonemotional (neutral valence) categories, demonstrating a significant Group (sleep, sleep deprivation) × Emotion Category (positive, negative, neutral) interaction. Post hoc *t*-test comparisons: †$p = 0.08$. *$p = 0.05$. **$p = 0.01$. *n.s.* = not significant; d' = *d*-prime (discrimination index) (Reprinted with permission from Walker and van der Helm [113])

Emerging evidence now suggests that encoding of emotional memories may be particularly susceptible to sleep deprivation. For example, Walker and Stickgold [66] deprived participants of sleep for 36 h and then had them complete an incidental memory-encoding task. A control group slept normally before completing the same task. During the task, participants viewed emotionally positive, negative, or neutral words. After the task, participants slept normally at home for another 2 nights. After being fully rested, performance on a surprise recognition test showed that those who were originally deprived of sleep had a 40 % impairment in recognition scores compared to those who learned the words when well-rested. Moreover, sleep deprivation had a differential effect on memory recognition depending on the emotional category of the words (i.e., positive, negative, neutral). For well-rested subjects, emotional words (positive and negative) were remembered better than neutral words, but for those who were deprived of sleep, memory for both neutral and positive words was significantly impaired (see Fig. 16.4). Interestingly, memory for negative words was not affected by sleep deprivation, suggesting that the encoding of negative memories may be relatively resistant to sleep deprivation compared to other types of emotional memories [66]. This finding could have important implications in understanding the role of insufficient sleep in the development of mood disorders. Recent research suggests that reward expectancy may ameliorate, but not eliminate the effect of sleep deprivation effects on memory recognition [74]. Following sleep deprivation, recognition accuracy was higher for items that were rewarded compared to nonrewarded items. This effect might be related to the upregulation of dopamine following sleep deprivation [75]. Finally, deficits in hippocampal-dependent learning that occur with continuous wakefulness can be prevented and even reversed by a nap [76].

The accumulated evidence strongly suggests that sleep is important for preparing the brain for subsequent learning. Without adequate sleep, functioning of the hippocampus becomes impaired, and new memory formation is hindered. However, the effect of sleep deprivation on emotional material may also depend on the emotional valence of the material, with negatively valenced emotional memories being most resistant to disruption by sleep deprivation.

Post-learning Sleep Deprivation

Sleep appears to be critical after learning to ensure consolidation of the memory into long-term storage. Learning of paired-associate word lists is improved after a period of sleep compared to an equivalent period without sleep [77]. Moreover, sleep appears to be particularly important for protecting memory traces from disruption by interfering information. For example, in one study, participants learned a list of paired-associate words (e.g., brick–shoe), which was followed by a 12-h retention interval, which either included sleep or no sleep. After the 12-h retention period, participants then learned a second list comprised of the previously learned stem words paired with new words (e.g., brick–pen). When asked to recall the original paired-associate words, those without sleep performed significantly worse than those who had slept during the intervening period [77], suggesting that sleep allowed the original memories to be consolidated, conferring resistance to subsequent interference. Evidence suggests that slow wave sleep obtained early in the night may be a critical factor in hippocampal-dependent consolidation, as evidenced by reduced memory recall following selective deprivation of slow wave sleep in the first part of the night after learning [78]. Brain imaging has shown that following spatial learning in humans, there is a replay of hippocampal activity during post-training slow wave sleep, which correlates with next day task performance [79]. Without sleep, hippocampal-dependent memory consolidation is not fully executed and memories remain fragile and prone to interference.

Executive Functions

Executive functions include a variety of higher order capacities involved in the control and coordination of willful action to achieve a goal state [7]. While the term "executive functions" refers to a broad variety of capacities, some of the most common ones include the ability to: ignore distractions and sustain focused attention; plan and sequence events, thoughts, and behaviors; inhibit inappropriate thoughts or behaviors; form abstract concepts from concrete information; shift mental set; and think flexibly, innovatively, and divergently. These capacities require the interaction of many areas of the brain, but seem to be particularly reliant upon the prefrontal cortex, a region that has been hypothesized to be particularly affected by sleep loss [80, 81].

Because the prefrontal cortex is necessary for so many of the complex mental operations that are carried out each day and may become particularly fatigued due to overuse, it has been suggested that the prefrontal cortex may be especially vulnerable to the effects of sleep deprivation [80, 81]. Indeed, the prefrontal cortex shows reduced glucose metabolism following sleep deprivation [82, 83] (see Fig. 16.5), and a number of studies have shown altered prefrontal responses and prefrontal connectivity using functional MRI following sleep loss [84, 85]. Similarly, near-infrared spectroscopy, a technique that measures regional cerebral oxygenation, also demonstrated reduced oxygenation of the bilateral frontal lobes in response to a cognitive task following a night of sleep deprivation [24, 86]. At the behavioral level, however, the prefrontal deficit model has received mixed support. While many studies report deficits in executive functions [87], others have failed to find evidence of such impairments [88, 89]. This suggests that not all aspects of executive functioning may be equally sensitive to sleep loss.

Working Memory

Essentially all executive function tasks rely to some extent on working memory capacity (i.e., maintenance and manipulation of information in immediate memory) [7]. Complex cognition requires the capacity to hold and manipulate information in real time. Such working memory systems in the brain draw extensively upon the

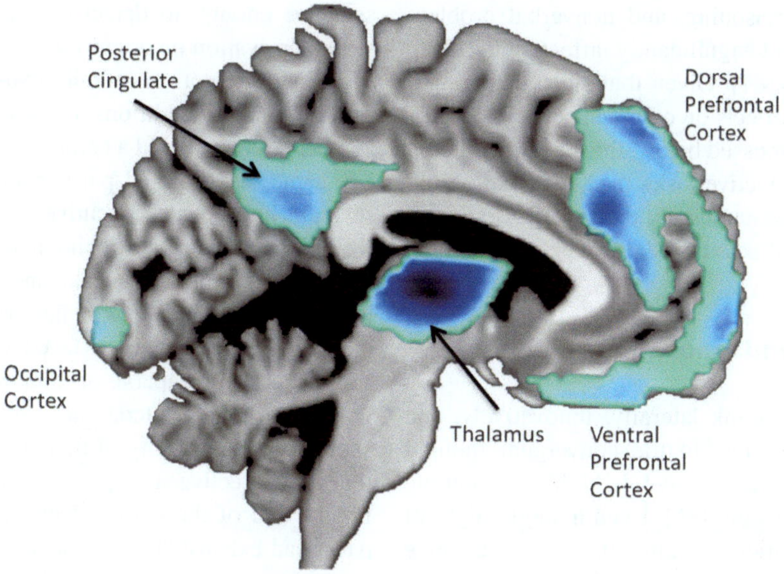

Fig. 16.5 A positron emission tomography (PET) image showing the effects of 24 h of sleep deprivation on regional cerebral glucose metabolism [82] (Courtesy of Maria Thomas, with special thanks to Gregory Belenky of the Walter Reed Army Institute of Research and Henry Halcomb of Johns Hopkins University)

capacities of the dorsolateral prefrontal cortex [90]. Because this region shows significant reductions in metabolic activity during sleep deprivation [82], it would be reasonable to hypothesize that insufficient sleep would be associated with decrements in working memory.

In a recent meta-analysis, Lim and Dinges found that both accuracy and response time during working memory tasks were affected by sleep deprivation [6]. Working memory capacity is not specifically localized to the prefrontal cortex and appears to draw upon multiple regions of the brain, including the parietal cortex. In fact, evidence suggests that the effects of sleep deprivation on parietal functioning may be particularly important in influencing subsequent cognition. For example, the parietal cortex may play an important role in compensating for deficits in other regions that occur during sleep deprivation [70]. Finally, a recent study examined working memory performance during sleep deprivation, and mathematically decomposed "executive" from "non-executive" aspects of this capacity [89]. When parsed in this manner, sleep deprivation only impaired the "non-executive" aspects of the task (i.e., response time), but not the "executive" features of the task such as working memory scanning efficiency and resistance to proactive interference. Their findings raise the possibility that many of the observed deficits in working memory secondary to sleep deprivation may be due simply to degradation of alertness, attention, and psychomotor vigilance rather than in the ability to manipulate information within the immediate memory buffer.

Convergent Thinking and Logical Deduction

There are various ways to arrive at a solution to a problem. Convergent thinking refers to the process of arriving at a solution through logical reasoning and the application of established rules. From this perspective, a problem can be solved by starting with known information and using logical inference to deduce the correct solution. As complex as this process sounds, evidence suggests that convergent thinking is not significantly degraded by sleep deprivation [81]. In fact, most studies examining measures of intellectual functioning, logical deduction, reading comprehension, grammatical reasoning, and nonverbal problem solving are not significantly affected by sleep deprivation [6, 81]. Given that sleep deprivation has profound effects on other aspects of complex thought, as discussed below, this negative finding for logical deductive tasks may eventually help refine our understanding of the specific brain systems that are affected by sleep deprivation.

Divergent and Innovative Thinking

The ability to think laterally, innovatively, and flexibly, in contrast to the convergent thought processes discussed above, is highly susceptible to sleep deprivation [81]. Even a single night of sleep deprivation results in fewer creative responses and greater difficulty shifting away from unsuccessful strategies [91]. Sleep deprivation also reduces the ability to generate lists of novel words, leads to slower and less efficient performance on the Tower of London, a complex task that requires cognitive flexibility, planning, and sequencing abilities. Interestingly, in one study from our lab, performance on the Tower of London test remained below average for sleep-deprived participants, even after administration of a dose of 600 mg of caffeine and restoration of normal reaction times [92]. Another type of divergent thinking, the ability to continuously vocally generate a series of random numbers, was also impaired during sleep deprivation [93]. Without sleep, subjects showed more frequent redundancy and stereotypy of responses and a higher number of rule violations [93]. Consistent with the aforementioned findings from the Tower of London, caffeine was ineffective at restoring the ability to generate random numbers, suggesting that the deficits were unlikely due to degraded alertness or attention. One task that has shown inconsistent findings during sleep loss is the Wisconsin card sorting test (WCST), a clinically based measure of concept formation, mental flexibility, and set shifting [87]. However, most clinically based tasks such as the WCST were originally developed to detect relatively severe brain lesions in a clinical setting and may not be sensitive enough to detect the subtle effects of sleep deprivation on cognition.

In an attempt to mimic real-life decision-making under conditions of sleep deprivation, another study included a complex marketing strategy game that required participants to engage in several high-level executive function tasks, including monitoring ongoing activities, revising strategies in light of new data, and using available information to come up with flexible, creative, and innovative solutions when faced with time pressure [94]. While capable of thinking innovatively when normally rested, the same participants showed greater rigidity of thought and perseveration on ineffective strategies once sleep-deprived. By the end of the game, sleep-deprived participants had exhausted their financial resources and were significantly worse off than they had been when they played the game when rested [94]. The drawback of this type of task is that it is so complex that it is nearly impossible to decipher the underlying cognitive processes that are actually affected by sleep loss, a weakness in many studies that is known as the "task impurity problem" [89, 95]. While such studies do not allow isolation of the specific cognitive systems that may be affected, they do carry some external validity and show the dramatic effects that sleep deprivation can have on "real life" types of problems. Although the evidence suggests that many divergent thinking tasks are impaired during sleep deprivation, additional research will need to clarify the specific component processes affected.

Cognitive Control

A key aspect of executive functioning is the ability to control and modulate mental activity. Cognitive control includes the ability to switch flexibly and rapidly among multiple different rule sets according to situational demands. This capacity is particularly relevant in modern society where "multi-tasking" (e.g., talking on a phone while simultaneously eating breakfast, writing an email, and searching the internet) is often considered to be a necessary or even laudable skill, but which can have devastating effects when combined with the operation of heavy equipment such as motor vehicles. While multi-tasking can degrade overall efficiency even in alert well-rested subjects [96], recent evidence suggests that sleep deprivation appears to further impair the ability to switch efficiently between cognitive tasks [97]. Similar findings appear to be true even for chronic partial sleep restriction [98]. Thus, without sleep, multi-tasking and other cognitive switching tasks are likely to be significantly degraded and the potential for making errors will be increased. Another aspect of cognitive control also involves ignoring irrelevant or distracting information in order to stay focused on the task at hand. This ability is sometimes measured with the Stroop interference paradigm. In its most common form, this paradigm presents a series of words denoting a particular color, but the text is printed in a different color (e.g., the word "red" printed in green ink). The participant is required to state the color of the ink in which each word is printed, effectively ignoring the meaning of the printed word. This is a difficult task for most people, even when fully alert and rested. Interestingly, studies of the Stroop interference effect have not found that it is affected consistently by sleep deprivation. For example, Sagaspe and colleagues [99] found no deficits from 36 h of sleep deprivation for three different Stroop tasks, including the standard color-word, emotional, or sleep content-specific Stroop tasks. It is not entirely clear why deficits are found for task-switching but not for Stroop tasks, but it seems plausible that these two types of tasks may recruit different brain regions and functional networks that are differentially sensitive to sleep deprivation.

Inhibitory Control

One of the hallmark executive capacities is the ability to inhibit inappropriate behavior. The appropriateness of a behavior often depends on the context or circumstances in which it occurs. A highly adaptive behavior in one context may be completely inappropriate in another. A person with intact executive functions is able to accurately assess the immediate context and withhold behavior when appropriate. Inhibitory control is commonly assessed using some form of the "go/no-go" paradigm. In a go/no-go task, a participant learns to respond (i.e., "go") to one stimulus while learning to withhold that response (i.e., "no-go") to another stimulus. Brain imaging studies suggest that the go/no-go paradigm typically recruits the right inferior lateral prefrontal cortex [100]. This same prefrontal region demonstrates reduced metabolic activity following a night of sleep deprivation [82]. Consequently, one would expect that sleep loss would degrade the ability to inhibit inappropriate responses, and in fact, this is what is observed. One study found that inhibitory capacity on a go/no-go task was impaired at 23, 32, and 55 h of sleep deprivation, but returned to normal following recovery sleep [101]. Interestingly, correct "go" responses, which indicate simple attention and response speed, were not affected by sleep deprivation until the 55-h assessment. From these data, it appears that inhibitory control declines rapidly during the first night of sleep deprivation, even when simple attention remains relatively unaffected for a longer period of time. Consequently, simple measures of response time degradation may not be adequate to determine whether a sleep-deprived person is showing deficits in these higher-level inhibitory capacities.

Risk-Taking, Judgment, and Decision-Making

Decision-making is a particularly difficult and complex cognitive process to study because the outcome (i.e., the decision) is the final product of a large number of interacting cognitive processes. Thus, tests of decision-making are often plagued by the "task-impurity problem" described earlier. At a minimum, conscious decision-making requires an individual be awake, attentive, and able to process the relevant sources of information that weigh into a decision. Further, decision-making also usually requires some level of intact sensory processing, sufficient working memory capacity, and reliable access to prior knowledge for comparison. Additionally, various scenarios or models may need to be run to estimate the possible outcomes of a decision. At some point, judgments about the probability of potential outcomes need to be integrated with motivation and emotional factors that determine the subjective value of options to the individual. Of course, each of these complex cognitive processes is also made up of even more elementary processes. Sleep deprivation may impair any combination of these processing stages, potentially leading to different outcomes. Due to these complexities, current knowledge of the effects of sleep loss on decision-making is in its infancy, and most studies have simply focused on fairly crude measures of overall decision outcomes or risk-preferences.

One series of studies in our lab looked at the effects of sleep deprivation on risky decision-making using a gambling task that tends to reveal decision-making deficits among individuals with lesions to the ventromedial prefrontal cortex (vmPFC). On this measure, known as the Iowa gambling task (IGT), patients with damage to the vmPFC show a preference for seeking short-term gains even if such predilections lead ultimately to long-term losses. Killgore and colleagues found that following 49 h of sleep deprivation, healthy normal people begin to show a pattern that is quite similar to (though not as severe as) patients with lesions to the vmPFC [102]. Compared to baseline performance, sleep-deprived individuals became riskier in their choices, preferring to select cards from the decks that led to short-term wins but longer-term losses. This same pattern of disadvantageous decision-making was replicated in a follow-on study that extended the sleep deprivation period out to 75 h [103]. In the second study, longer durations of sleep deprivation were associated with similar risky decision-making in a different sample, a finding that was not reversed by repeated overnight doses of caffeine. In a third sample of participants, Killgore and colleagues again administered the IGT at rested baseline, 23 h of sleep deprivation, again following 46 h of sleep deprivation, and finally after a night of recovery sleep [104]. Consistent with the previous studies, greater sleep deprivation was associated with greater impairment in IGT performance, and sleep-deprived performances were essentially unaffected by acute administration of caffeine (600 mg), dextroamphetamine (20 mg), or modafinil (400 mg). Overall, across all three studies, sleep deprivation led to a focus on short-term gains while devaluing long-term losses, a finding that was unaffected by stimulant medications. Some evidence suggests that sleep deprivation may actually impair rule acquisition on the IGT. For example, when participants were provided a short preview of the IGT that was insufficient for acquiring a full understanding of the underlying rules (i.e., participants were not given sufficient opportunity to learn about the advantageous versus disadvantageous decks and associated gains and potential losses) followed by a delay period of 12 h, better full task performance was observed for those who were able to obtain their habitual sleep during the delay than those who were required to stay awake [105]. Interestingly, the benefit of sleep was greatest among those who initially did not perform well on this task due to limited task understanding. This suggests that task-related benefits of sleep might be more pronounced at earlier stages of learning or rule understanding.

Sleep deprivation may also affect other factors associated with risk-taking. Notably, the willingness to select riskier options during sleep deprivation is also affected by whether the risk is framed as a potential gain or a potential loss. McKenna and colleagues showed that when an outcome was presented in terms of a potential gain, sleep deprivation was associated with an increase in risk-taking compared to rested baseline, whereas if the risk was framed in terms of a potential loss, the same sleep-deprived subjects became risk averse [106]. This may be due to altered brain functioning within brain regions involved in processing of reward. Neuroimaging data suggest that sleep deprivation is associated with increased activation of reward centers when engaged in risky decision-making, but reduced activation of brain regions involved in aversion and punishment when experiencing a loss [107].

These findings suggest that sleep deprivation may alter the normal functional activity within systems of the brain that assess the value of rewards and punishments, altering risk-related judgments. Ultimately, these alterations may lead to overly optimistic expectations of the possibility of future gains and an underestimation of the possibility of losses. Further work is needed to clarify how these various internal and external factors may interact to affect risky behavior.

Insufficient sleep also appears to influence socio-emotional decisions. In one study, sleep-deprived volunteers completed a series of "bargaining" and "trust" games that had tangible financial consequences [108]. Compared to rested baseline, sleep-deprived participants were more likely to engage in aggressive social exchanges with their counterparts. For example, sleep deprivation led to reduced willingness to trust an unknown partner in the game and a greater willingness to reject bargaining offers put forth by their partner when those offers were perceived as "unfair." What was particularly remarkable was that sleep-deprived individuals were more likely to reject these "unfair" offers, even when doing so would incur a financial cost to themselves. This unwillingness to concede or cooperate is consistent with the emotional symptoms discussed in a previous section of this chapter, particularly the findings showing that sleep loss leads to reduced empathy, and elevated symptoms of paranoia, feelings of resentment, and a general perception of being persecuted or unfairly treated. Clearly, sleep deprivation leads to a greater influence of emotions over some aspects of decision-making.

Finally, sleep deprivation alters emotionally guided moral decision-making [109]. Compared to judgments made when well-rested, subjects deprived of sleep for 53 h showed significant slowing of decisions related to highly personal and emotionally charged moral dilemmas. Moreover, sleep deprivation was associated with a greater tendency to make utilitarian type judgments that violated the participant's own moral beliefs when compared to responses provided at baseline [109]. In other words, when lacking sleep, these subjects were more likely to agree with a personally inconsistent moral position than they would have when normally rested. A recent study using the same dilemmas found no significant effect during only a single night of sleep deprivation, suggesting that changes in moral judgments may only be observable after prolonged periods of sleep loss [110]. However, there is evidence that partial sleep restriction to about 2.5 h a night for 5 days during actual military training exercises was enough to significantly impair the ability to engage principle-oriented moral reasoning [111]. That study showed that, when sleep restricted, the moral decisions of military cadets became more rules-focused and self-oriented and less able to engage in principle-oriented moral reasoning than when rested. Notably, the findings were most evident among individuals who relied on principle-oriented moral reasoning the most when well-rested, suggesting that sleep loss impaired the capacity to utilize these types of moral processes. Overall, the evidence suggests that sleep deprivation adversely affects specific executive function systems that involve the ability to integrate emotional information with cognition to guide decisions [112].

Conclusions

Within the context of the laboratory, experimental sleep deprivation has been conducted for extreme durations, sometimes in excess of 70–80 h. While these data provide clues into the role that sleep plays in brain functioning and cognitive performance, such extreme conditions are unlikely to have much generalizability to most "real life" situations where sleep is curtailed by merely a few hours or even when a whole night of sleep is missed. A much more common situation is one of chronic sleep restriction, where an individual repeatedly obtains less than sufficient sleep for many nights in a row. Notably, chronic curtailment of sleep by even a couple of hours per night for up to 2 weeks can produce deficits in psychomotor vigilance that are similar to what is seen after 2 nights of total sleep deprivation. On the whole, findings from studies involving rather short-term sleep deprivation (i.e., 1 or 2 nights) are much more transferable to real-life setting such as shift work or military duty than findings from studies involving extreme sleep loss. Irrespective of difference in study design, however, lack of sleep has a profound effect on several aspects of cognitive functioning. Even a single night of sleep deprivation impairs some of the most elementary aspects of cognitive functioning, including simple alertness, attention, and psychomotor vigilance. The net effect of this impairment is slow and inconsistent responses. There is also some evidence that various sensory systems may be affected by sleep loss, but the extent to which these declines are due simply to reduced alertness and attention remains to be determined. Without sufficient sleep, memory processing is degraded as well, as sleep-deprived individuals have difficulty encoding new information and, if sleep is prevented after learning, consolidation of memories and subsequent recall will also be impaired. Another profound effect of sleep loss is mood and emotional dysregulation. Sleep-deprived individuals tend to be more irritable, prone toward negative mood, less empathic, and more willing to assign blame to others. Emerging evidence from neuroimaging suggests that this may occur because sleep deprivation weakens functional connectivity between prefrontal cortex inhibitory and limbic emotional systems of the brain. Dysregulation of these emotional systems may then shift the affective balance toward negative mood states, which may then influence other aspects of perception, memory, and higher-level judgments and decisions.

References

1. Kripke DF, Simons RN, Garfinkel L, Hammond EC. Short and long sleep and sleeping pills. Is increased mortality associated? Arch Gen Psychiatry. 1979;36:103–16.
2. Gallup Organization. Sleep in America. Princeton, NH: Gallup Organization; 1995.
3. Centers for Disease Control and Prevention. Short sleep duration among workers—United States, 2010. Morb Mortal Wkly Rep. 2012;61(16):281–5.
4. Lezak MD. Neuropsychological assessment. 3rd ed. New York, NY: Oxford University Press; 1995.
5. Lim J, Dinges DF. Sleep deprivation and vigilant attention. Ann N Y Acad Sci. 2008;1129:305–22.
6. Lim J, Dinges DF. A meta-analysis of the impact of short-term sleep deprivation on cognitive variables. Psychol Bull. 2010;136:375–89.
7. Goel N, Rao H, Durmer JS, Dinges DF. Neurocognitive consequences of sleep deprivation. Semin Neurol. 2009;29:320–39.
8. Dinges DF, Powell JW. Microcomputer analyses of performance on a portable, simple, visual RT task during sustained operations. Behav Res Methods Instrum Comput. 1985;17:652–5.
9. Doran SM, Van Dongen HP, Dinges DF. Sustained attention performance during sleep deprivation: evidence of state instability. Arch Ital Biol. 2001;139:253–67.
10. Dinges DF, Pack F, Williams K, et al. Cumulative sleepiness, mood disturbance, and psychomotor vigilance performance decrements during a week of sleep restricted to 4-5 hours per night. Sleep. 1997;20:267–77.
11. Wesensten NJ, Killgore WD, Balkin TJ. Performance and alertness effects of caffeine, dextroamphetamine, and modafinil during sleep deprivation. J Sleep Res. 2005;14:255–66.
12. Belenky G, Penetar D, Thorne D, et al. The effects of sleep deprivation on performance during continuous combat operations. In: Marriott BM, editor. Food components to enhance performance. Washington, DC: National Academy Press; 1994. p. 127–35.
13. Van Dongen HP, Maislin G, Mullington JM, Dinges DF. The cumulative cost of additional wakefulness: dose-response effects on neurobehavioral functions and sleep physiology from chronic sleep restriction and total sleep deprivation. Sleep. 2003;26:117–26.
14. Borbely AA. A two process model of sleep regulation. Hum Neurobiol. 1982;1:195–204.
15. Babkoff H, Caspy T, Mikulincer M, Sing HC. Monotonic and rhythmic influences: a challenge for sleep deprivation research. Psychol Bull. 1991;109:411–28.
16. Dawson D, Reid K. Fatigue, alcohol and performance impairment. Nature. 1997;388:235.
17. Van Dongen HP, Baynard MD, Maislin G, Dinges DF. Systematic interindividual differences in neurobehavioral impairment from sleep loss: evidence of trait-like differential vulnerability. Sleep. 2004;27:423–33.
18. Rupp TL, Wesensten NJ, Balkin TJ. Trait-like vulnerability to total and partial sleep loss. Sleep. 2012;35:1163–72.
19. Van Dongen HP, Belenky G. Individual differences in vulnerability to sleep loss in the work environment. Ind Health. 2009;47:518–26.
20. Killgore WDS, Richards JM, Killgore DB, Kamimori GH, Balkin TJ. The trait of introversion-extraversion predicts vulnerability to sleep deprivation. J Sleep Res. 2007;16:354–63.

21. Killgore WDS, McBride SA, Killgore DB, Balkin TJ, Kamimori GH. Baseline odor identification ability predicts degradation of psychomotor vigilance during 77 hours of sleep deprivation. Int J Neurosci. 2008;118:1207–25.
22. Killgore WDS, Grugle NL, Reichardt RM, Killgore DB, Balkin TJ. Executive functions and the ability to sustain vigilance during sleep loss. Aviat Space Environ Med. 2009;80:81–7.
23. Rupp TL, Killgore WD, Balkin TJ. Socializing by day may affect performance by night: vulnerability to sleep deprivation is differentially mediated by social exposure in extraverts vs introverts. Sleep. 2010;33:1475–85.
24. Lythe KE, Williams SC, Anderson C, Libri V, Mehta MA. Frontal and parietal activity after sleep deprivation is dependent on task difficulty and can be predicted by the fMRI response after normal sleep. Behav Brain Res. 2012;233:62–70.
25. Goel N, Banks S, Mignot E, Dinges DF. PER3 polymorphism predicts cumulative sleep homeostatic but not neurobehavioral changes to chronic partial sleep deprivation. PLoS One. 2009;4:e5874.
26. Groeger JA, Viola AU, Lo JC, von Schantz M, Archer SN, Dijk DJ. Early morning executive functioning during sleep deprivation is compromised by a PERIOD3 polymorphism. Sleep. 2008;31:1159–67.
27. von Schantz M. Phenotypic effects of genetic variability in human clock genes on circadian and sleep parameters. J Genet. 2008;87:513–9.
28. Roge J, Gabaude C. Deterioration of the useful visual field with age and sleep deprivation: insight from signal detection theory. Percept Mot Skills. 2009;109:270–84.
29. Chee MW, Tan JC, Zheng H, et al. Lapsing during sleep deprivation is associated with distributed changes in brain activation. J Neurosci. 2008;28:5519–28.
30. Chuah LY, Chee MW. Cholinergic augmentation modulates visual task performance in sleep-deprived young adults. J Neurosci. 2008;28:11369–77.
31. Chee MW, Tan JC. Lapsing when sleep deprived: neural activation characteristics of resistant and vulnerable individuals. Neuroimage. 2010;51:835–43.
32. Fink GR, Marshall JC, Shah NJ, et al. Line bisection judgments implicate right parietal cortex and cerebellum as assessed by fMRI. Neurology. 2000;54:1324–31.
33. Milner AD, Brechmann M, Pagliarini L. To halve and to halve not: an analysis of line bisection judgements in normal subjects. Neuropsychologia. 1992;30:515–26.
34. Manly T, Dobler VB, Dodds CM, George MA. Rightward shift in spatial awareness with declining alertness. Neuropsychologia. 2005;43:1721–8.
35. Kendall AP, Kautz MA, Russo MB, Killgore WD. Effects of sleep deprivation on lateral visual attention. Int J Neurosci. 2006;116:1125–38.
36. Killgore WDS, Kendall AP, Richards JM, McBride SA. Lack of degradation in visuospatial perception of line orientation after one night of sleep loss. Percept Mot Skills. 2007;105:276–86.
37. Horne JA, Anderson NR, Wilkinson RT. Effects of sleep deprivation on signal detection measures of vigilance: implications for sleep function. Sleep. 1983;6:347–58.
38. Babkoff H, Zukerman G, Fostick L, Ben-Artzi E. Effect of the diurnal rhythm and 24 h of sleep deprivation on dichotic temporal order judgment. J Sleep Res. 2005;14:7–15.
39. Liberalesso PB, D'Andrea KF, Cordeiro ML, Zeigelboim BS, Marques JM, Jurkiewicz AL. Effects of sleep deprivation on central auditory processing. BMC Neurosci. 2012;13:83.
40. Shtyrov Y, Smith ML, Horner AJ, et al. Attention to language: novel MEG paradigm for registering involuntary language processing in the brain. Neuropsychologia. 2012;50:2605–16.
41. Kundermann B, Spernal J, Huber MT, Krieg JC, Lautenbacher S. Sleep deprivation affects thermal pain thresholds but not somatosensory thresholds in healthy volunteers. Psychosom Med. 2004;66:932–7.
42. Haack M, Lee E, Cohen DA, Mullington JM. Activation of the prostaglandin system in response to sleep loss in healthy humans: potential mediator of increased spontaneous pain. Pain. 2009;145:136–41.
43. Furchtgott E, Willingham WW. The effect of sleep-deprivation upon the thresholds of taste. Am J Psychol. 1956;69:111–2.
44. Killgore WDS, McBride SA. Odor identification accuracy declines following 24 h of sleep deprivation. J Sleep Res. 2006;15:111–6.
45. McBride SA, Balkin TJ, Kamimori GH, Killgore WDS. Olfactory decrements as a function of two nights of sleep deprivation. J Sens Stud. 2006;21:456–63.
46. Penetar D, McCann U, Thorne D, et al. Caffeine reversal of sleep deprivation effects on alertness and mood. Psychopharmacology (Berl). 1993;112:359–65.
47. Tempesta D, Couyoumdjian A, Curcio G, et al. Lack of sleep affects the evaluation of emotional stimuli. Brain Res Bull. 2010;82:104–8.
48. Franzen PL, Gianaros PJ, Marsland AL, et al. Cardiovascular reactivity to acute psychological stress following sleep deprivation. Psychosom Med. 2011;73:679–82.
49. Minkel JD, Banks S, Htaik O, et al. Sleep deprivation and stressors: evidence for elevated negative affect in response to mild stressors when sleep deprived. Emotion. 2012;12(5):1015–20.
50. Kahn-Greene ET, Lipizzi EL, Conrad AK, Kamimori GH, Killgore WDS. Sleep deprivation adversely affects interpersonal responses to frustration. Pers Individ Dif. 2006;41:1433–43.
51. Killgore WDS, Kahn-Greene ET, Lipizzi EL, Newman RA, Kamimori GH, Balkin TJ. Sleep

deprivation reduces perceived emotional intelligence and constructive thinking skills. Sleep Med. 2007;9: 517–26.
52. Kamphuis J, Meerlo P, Koolhaas JM, Lancel M. Poor sleep as a potential causal factor in aggression and violence. Sleep Med. 2012;13:327–34.
53. Kahn-Greene ET, Killgore DB, Kamimori GH, Balkin TJ, Killgore WDS. The effects of sleep deprivation on symptoms of psychopathology in healthy adults. Sleep Med. 2007;8:215–21.
54. Gujar N, Yoo SS, Hu P, Walker MP. Sleep deprivation amplifies reactivity of brain reward networks, biasing the appraisal of positive emotional experiences. J Neurosci. 2011;31:4466–74.
55. Franzen PL, Buysse DJ, Dahl RE, Thompson W, Siegle GJ. Sleep deprivation alters pupillary reactivity to emotional stimuli in healthy young adults. Biol Psychol. 2009;80:300–5.
56. Rosales-Lagarde A, Armony JL, Del Rio-Portilla Y, Trejo-Martinez D, Conde R, Corsi-Cabrera M. Enhanced emotional reactivity after selective REM sleep deprivation in humans: an fMRI study. Front Behav Neurosci. 2012;6:25.
57. Baran B, Pace-Schott EF, Ericson C, Spencer RM. Processing of emotional reactivity and emotional memory over sleep. J Neurosci. 2012;32:1035–42.
58. Killgore WDS, McBride SA, Killgore DB, Balkin TJ. The effects of caffeine, dextroamphetamine, and modafinil on humor appreciation during sleep deprivation. Sleep. 2006;29:841–7.
59. McGlinchey EL, Talbot LS, Chang KH, Kaplan KA, Dahl RE, Harvey AG. The effect of sleep deprivation on vocal expression of emotion in adolescents and adults. Sleep. 2011;34:1233–41.
60. Benedict C, Brooks SJ, O'Daly OG, et al. Acute sleep deprivation enhances the brain's response to hedonic food stimuli: an fMRI study. J Clin Endocrinol Metabol. 2012;97:E443–7.
61. Brondel L, Romer MA, Nougues PM, Touyarou P, Davenne D. Acute partial sleep deprivation increases food intake in healthy men. Am J Clin Nutr. 2010;91:1550–9.
62. Morselli L, Leproult R, Balbo M, Spiegel K. Role of sleep duration in the regulation of glucose metabolism and appetite. Best Pract Res Clin Endocrinol Metab. 2010;24:687–702.
63. Benedict C, Hallschmid M, Lassen A, et al. Acute sleep deprivation reduces energy expenditure in healthy men. Am J Clin Nutr. 2011;93:1229–36.
64. St-Onge MP, McReynolds A, Trivedi ZB, Roberts AL, Sy M, Hirsch J. Sleep restriction leads to increased activation of brain regions sensitive to food stimuli. Am J Clin Nutr. 2012;95:818–24.
65. Diekelmann S, Born J. The memory function of sleep. Nat Rev Neurosci. 2010;11:114–26.
66. Walker MP, Stickgold R. Sleep, memory, and plasticity. Annu Rev Psychol. 2006;57:139–66.
67. Walker MP. The role of sleep in cognition and emotion. Ann N Y Acad Sci. 2009;1156:168–97.
68. Saletin JM, Walker MP. Nocturnal mnemonics: sleep and hippocampal memory processing. Front Neurol. 2012;3:59.
69. Walker MP. Sleep-dependent memory processing. Harv Rev Psychiatry. 2008;16:287–98.
70. Drummond SP, Brown GG, Gillin JC, Stricker JL, Wong EC, Buxton RB. Altered brain response to verbal learning following sleep deprivation. Nature. 2000;403:655–7.
71. Yoo SS, Hu PT, Gujar N, Jolesz FA, Walker MP. A deficit in the ability to form new human memories without sleep. Nat Neurosci. 2007;10:385–92.
72. Van Der Werf YD, Altena E, Schoonheim MM, et al. Sleep benefits subsequent hippocampal functioning. Nat Neurosci. 2009;12:122–3.
73. Harrison Y, Horne JA. Sleep loss and temporal memory. Q J Exp Psychol A. 2000;53:271–9.
74. Martella D, Plaza V, Estevez AF, Castillo A, Fuentes LJ. Minimizing sleep deprivation effects in healthy adults by differential outcomes. Acta Psychol (Amst). 2012;139:391–6.
75. Volkow ND, Fowler JS, Logan J, et al. Effects of modafinil on dopamine and dopamine transporters in the male human brain: clinical implications. JAMA. 2009;301:1148–54.
76. Mander BA, Santhanam S, Saletin JM, Walker MP. Wake deterioration and sleep restoration of human learning. Curr Biol. 2011;21:R183–4.
77. Ellenbogen JM, Hulbert JC, Stickgold R, Dinges DF, Thompson-Schill SL. Interfering with theories of sleep and memory: sleep, declarative memory, and associative interference. Curr Biol. 2006;16: 1290–4.
78. Fischer S, Diekelmann S, Born J. Sleep's role in the processing of unwanted memories. J Sleep Res. 2011;20:267–74.
79. Peigneux P, Laureys S, Fuchs S, et al. Are spatial memories strengthened in the human hippocampus during slow wave sleep? Neuron. 2004;44:535–45.
80. Harrison Y, Horne JA, Rothwell A. Prefrontal neuropsychological effects of sleep deprivation in young adults—a model for healthy aging? Sleep. 2000;23: 1067–73.
81. Harrison Y, Horne JA. The impact of sleep deprivation on decision making: a review. J Exp Psychol Appl. 2000;6:236–49.
82. Thomas M, Sing H, Belenky G, et al. Neural basis of alertness and cognitive performance impairments during sleepiness. I. Effects of 24 h of sleep deprivation on waking human regional brain activity. J Sleep Res. 2000;9:335–52.
83. Wu JC, Gillin JC, Buchsbaum MS, et al. Frontal lobe metabolic decreases with sleep deprivation not totally reversed by recovery sleep. Neuropsychopharmacology. 2006;31:2783–92.
84. Venkatraman V, Huettel SA, Chuah LY, Payne JW, Chee MW. Sleep deprivation biases the neural mechanisms underlying economic preferences. J Neurosci. 2011;31:3712–8.

85. Yoo SS, Gujar N, Hu P, Jolesz FA, Walker MP. The human emotional brain without sleep—a prefrontal amygdala disconnect. Curr Biol. 2007;17:R877–8.
86. Miyata S, Noda A, Ozaki N, et al. Insufficient sleep impairs driving performance and cognitive function. Neurosci Lett. 2012;469:229–33.
87. Jones K, Harrison Y. Frontal lobe function, sleep loss and fragmented sleep. Sleep Med Rev. 2001;5:463–75.
88. Pace-Schott EF, Hutcherson CA, Bemporad B, et al. Failure to find executive function deficits following one night's total sleep deprivation in university students under naturalistic conditions. Behav Sleep Med. 2009;7:136–63.
89. Tucker AM, Whitney P, Belenky G, Hinson JM, Van Dongen HP. Effects of sleep deprivation on dissociated components of executive functioning. Sleep. 2010;33:47–57.
90. Vandewalle G, Archer SN, Wuillaume C, et al. Functional magnetic resonance imaging-assessed brain responses during an executive task depend on interaction of sleep homeostasis, circadian phase, and PER3 genotype. J Neurosci. 2009;29:7948–56.
91. Horne JA. Sleep loss and "divergent" thinking ability. Sleep. 1988;11:528–36.
92. Killgore WDS, Kahn-Greene ET, Grugle NL, Killgore DB, Balkin TJ. Sustaining executive functions during sleep deprivation: a comparison of caffeine, dextroamphetamine, and modafinil. Sleep. 2009;32:205–16.
93. Gottselig JM, Adam M, Retey JV, Khatami R, Achermann P, Landolt HP. Random number generation during sleep deprivation: effects of caffeine on response maintenance and stereotypy. J Sleep Res. 2006;15:31–40.
94. Harrison Y, Horne JA. One night of sleep loss impairs innovative thinking and flexible decision making. Organ Behav Hum Decis Process. 1999;78:128–45.
95. Van Dongen HP, Caldwell Jr JA, Caldwell JL. Individual differences in cognitive vulnerability to fatigue in the laboratory and in the workplace. Prog Brain Res. 2011;190:145–53.
96. Ophir E, Nass C, Wagner AD. Cognitive control in media multitaskers. Proc Natl Acad Sci U S A. 2009; 106:15583–7.
97. Couyoumdjian A, Sdoia S, Tempesta D, et al. The effects of sleep and sleep deprivation on task-switching performance. J Sleep Res. 2010;19:64–70.
98. Haavisto ML, Porkka-Heiskanen T, Hublin C, et al. Sleep restriction for the duration of a work week impairs multitasking performance. J Sleep Res. 2010;19:444–54.
99. Sagaspe P, Sanchez-Ortuno M, Charles A, et al. Effects of sleep deprivation on color-word, emotional, and specific stroop interference and on self-reported anxiety. Brain Cogn. 2006;60:76–87.
100. Chuah YM, Venkatraman V, Dinges DF, Chee MW. The neural basis of interindividual variability in inhibitory efficiency after sleep deprivation. J Neurosci. 2006;26:7156–62.
101. Drummond SP, Paulus MP, Tapert SF. Effects of two nights sleep deprivation and two nights recovery sleep on response inhibition. J Sleep Res. 2006; 15:261–5.
102. Killgore WDS, Balkin TJ, Wesensten NJ. Impaired decision-making following 49 hours of sleep deprivation. J Sleep Res. 2006;15:7–13.
103. Killgore WDS, Lipizzi EL, Kamimori GH, Balkin TJ. Caffeine effects on risky decision-making after 75 hours of sleep deprivation. Aviat Space Environ Med. 2007;78:957–62.
104. Killgore WD, Grugle NL, Balkin TJ. Gambling when sleep deprived: don't bet on stimulants. Chronobiol Int. 2012;29:43–54.
105. Pace-Schott EF, Nave G, Morgan A, Spencer RM. Sleep-dependent modulation of affectively guided decision-making. J Sleep Res. 2012;21:30–9.
106. McKenna BS, Dickinson DL, Orff HJ, Drummond SP. The effects of one night of sleep deprivation on known-risk and ambiguous-risk decisions. J Sleep Res. 2007;16:245–52.
107. Venkatraman V, Chuah YM, Huettel SA, Chee MW. Sleep deprivation elevates expectation of gains and attenuates response to losses following risky decisions. Sleep. 2007;30:603–9.
108. Anderson C, Dickinson DL. Bargaining and trust: the effects of 36-h total sleep deprivation on socially interactive decisions. J Sleep Res. 2010;19:54–63.
109. Killgore WDS, Killgore DB, Day LM, Li C, Kamimori GH, Balkin TJ. The effects of 53 hours of sleep deprivation on moral judgment. Sleep. 2007; 30:345–52.
110. Tempesta D, Couyoumdjian A, Moroni F, Marzano C, De Gennaro L, Ferrara M. The impact of one night of sleep deprivation on moral judgments. Soc Neurosci. 2012;7:292–300.
111. Olsen OK, Pallesen S, Eid J. The impact of partial sleep deprivation on moral reasoning in military officers. Sleep. 2010;33:1086–90.
112. Killgore WDS. Effects of sleep deprivation on cognition. Prog Brain Res. 2010;185:105–29.
113. Walker MP, van der Helm E. Overnight therapy? The role of sleep in emotional brain processing. Psychol Bull. 2009;135:731–48.

Caffeine and Naps as Countermeasures for Sleep Loss

17

Yvonne Alameddine, Elizabeth B. Klerman, and Matt T. Bianchi

Introduction

Insufficient sleep impacts nearly every aspect of human physiology including cognition and performance. Health consequences, including increased risk of systemic and neuropsychiatric disorders as well as safety issues involving driving and occupational accidents, have been detailed in several reports, including a recent detailed cost analysis [1]. Polls conducted by the National Sleep Foundation reveal striking self-reported statistics of sleep-related problems and driving: 60 % of adult drivers reported feeling drowsy while at the wheel and 20 % fell asleep while driving. Impaired performance is a major concern for work productivity from absenteeism, but perhaps more commonly, presenteeism problems. Sleep deprivation can be compared to alcohol consumption in terms of the impairments in performance and reaction time [2–4]. In a now classic study, the performance decrement over 10–26 h of sustained wakefulness was similar to that obtained with alcohol ingestion, such that 17 h of wake was associated with performance impairment similar to that seen with a blood alcohol (BAC) level of 0.05 %, and after 24 h awake the impairment was similar to a 0.1 % BAC [4].

The goal of introducing countermeasures in those with sleep loss is to promote alertness and thus decrease the risk of sleep loss-related performance impairment. This can be accomplished in several ways, ranging from scheduling systems that facilitate adjustment of the circadian rhythm to atypical work schedules, to system-level safeguards designed to warn or prevent error occurrence associated with sleep loss and/or shift work. At the individual level, three countermeasures have dominated the experimental literature regarding effectiveness for increasing alertness and/or performance: naps, caffeine, and prescription-stimulant use.

Here we review the literature evaluating the utility of caffeine and napping to promote improved objective performance under conditions of sleep deprivation and sleep restriction; stimulant use in sleep medicine has been reviewed recently [5]. The use of prescription-stimulant therapy is beyond the scope of this chapter and should be considered only in the context of a formal sleep disorders evaluation [6]. Although countermeasures represent important consideration for those with sleepiness, it is important to recognize at the outset that symptoms often

Y. Alameddine, B.A.
Department of Neurology, Massachusetts General Hospital, Boston, MA, USA

E.B. Klerman, M.D., Ph.D.
Division of Sleep Medicine, Department of Medicine, Harvard Medical School, Brigham and Women's Hospital, Boston, MA, USA

M.T. Bianchi, M.D., Ph.D., M.M.Sc. (✉)
Division of Sleep Medicine, Department of Neurology, Massachusetts General Hospital, Boston, MA, USA
e-mail: mtbianchi@partners.org

M.T. Bianchi (ed.), *Sleep Deprivation and Disease: Effects on the Body, Brain and Behavior*,
DOI 10.1007/978-1-4614-9087-6_17, © Springer Science+Business Media New York 2014

associated with sleep loss (sleepiness, fatigue, poor concentration) may be due to a primary sleep disorder or primary medical disorder, as well as insufficient sleep opportunity. It is critical in particular to recognize the medical possibilities so as not to mask the underlying problem and delay diagnosis and/or treatment by initiating countermeasures targeting only the symptom, thus allowing the root cause to persist unaddressed.

Overview of Caffeine

Coffee Consumption and Regulation

Caffeine is the most widely consumed psychoactive substance in the world [7]. Among beverage formulations containing caffeine, the three most common types are coffee (71 %), soda (16 %), and tea (12 %) [8]. Common commercially available caffeine-containing products include soda, chocolate, ice cream, energy drinks, over-the-counter medications, and energy supplements. Natural sources of caffeine include over 60 plant species, the most common of which are coffee beans, tea leaves, kola nut, yerba mate, cacao, and guarana [8, 9]. The caffeine content of coffee and tea sources varies greatly, and the beverages derived from them may have different caffeine contents depending on the type of plant and growing conditions, as well as the brewing and processing methods [10, 11]. In the USA, regulations by the Food and Drug Administration (FDA) for indicating on the food label the amount of caffeine depend on whether the source is natural (as in coffee beans), or added (as in colas) [12, 13]. Interested readers are directed to one of many web sites cataloguing the caffeine content of food and beverages [14, 15]. In the USA, nearly 50 % adults drink coffee daily and 80 % of adults consume caffeine in some form [16]. Published FDA analysis indicates that the average amount of caffeine consumed per day among adults over the age of 22 in the US was 300 mg in 2008 [17]. The US Army Medical Research and Material Command (USAMRC) recommends caffeine in daily doses <600 mg to improve cognitive performance and alertness among military personnel [18]. The amount of coffee consumed per capita, however, greatly differs around the world. For example, annual consumption in the US totals 4.2 kg of coffee per person, while in Finland it is 12 kg [19].

Basic Caffeine Pharmacology

The impact of caffeine on sleep-wake patterns can be understood in the context of current theories of sleep-wake regulation. Many of these theories are based on the two-process model of Borbely and Achermann [20], which invokes the dual influence of circadian rhythms and sleep homeostasis. Recent work implicates adenosine as an important mediator of the sleep homeostatic process, whereby the drive for sleep increases with the duration of preceding time awake and decreases during sleep. Within this simplified construct, caffeine is postulated to counteract sleep drive associated with the homeostatic buildup of central nervous system adenosine through its actions as an adenosine receptor antagonist [21]. However, experimental evidence does not uniformly support this. For example, basal forebrain lesions in rodents that interrupted the homeostatic buildup of brain adenosine [22] did not alter homeostatic recovery sleep after deprivation, or the behavioral response to an adenosine antagonist. Pharmacological manipulation of adenosine A_1 receptors modulated sleep in rodents in a manner consistent with a role in sleep physiology [23]. However, mice engineered to lack adenosine A_1 receptors showed normal sleep and normal response to deprivation in one study [24], and a dissociation between impaired EEG-based slow wave activity (a marker of sleep drive) and intact recovery sleep duration after experimental sleep deprivation [25]. Thus, it may be that sleep homeostasis involves adenosine but also depends on other factors.

In vitro studies suggest that caffeine is an antagonist of the A_1 and A_{2A} adenosine receptors [26]. Adenosine receptors are present in the brain and nonneuronal tissues, which would explain the multisystem impact of caffeine consumption.

Adenosine receptor signaling is itself diverse and serves many central nervous system functions through a variety of second messenger pathways [27]. Caffeine has "off-target" activity, for example, directly modulating potassium channels [28], consistent with the increasing general evidence for molecular promiscuity [29]. Adenosine receptors also show promiscuity at the protein assembly level, as the A_1 and A_{2A} receptors form heteromeric complexes with dopamine D_1 and D_2 receptors [30, 31]. In addition, coffee contains other bioactive compounds and recent studies linking caffeine to lower mortality found similar effects with caffeinated and decaffeinated coffee consumption [32], although decaffeinated coffee still has some caffeine content. Together with the behavioral sleep experiments above, it is apparent that adenosine signaling, and by inference caffeine's actions in the adenosine system, are complex and require further elucidation.

Caffeine, Absorption, Distribution, Metabolism, Excretion

Caffeine pharmacokinetics is an important topic contributing to inter-individual differences in caffeine bioactivity [33]. Caffeine is readily absorbed after oral intake. In the serum, the protein-binding portion is 36 % in adults and lower in children. Cerebrospinal fluid (CSF) levels are similar to serum levels and tissue distribution is similar throughout the body. The main hepatic source of caffeine metabolism is CYP1A2 (which also is weakly inhibited by caffeine), with minor contributions by CYP2C9, CYP2D6, CYP2E1, and CYP3A4. Caffeine and its metabolites, theophylline, theobromine, and paraxanthine, are excreted in the urine. The average time for caffeine to reach peak plasma levels is 30–120 min and the elimination half-life is 4–5 h. The formulation (e.g., immediate versus sustained release) also impacts pharmacokinetics. Clearance rate is increased by >50 % in smokers [34, 35]. The half-life of caffeine nearly triples during pregnancy and doubles in those taking oral contraceptives possibly attributed to estradiol/progesterone effects on the CYP1A enzymes [36]. Fetal risks of caffeine are not likely to occur at routine consumption levels, but caffeine does cross the placenta and caffeine has a level C pregnancy risk classification. Although caffeine binds to the fat in breast milk, according to the American Academy of Pediatrics, caffeine is not associated with risk at levels of 1–2 cups of coffee per day while breastfeeding [37].

Adverse Effects Associated with Caffeine

Although caffeine is widely consumed in a fairly unregulated manner, caffeine ingestion can lead to side effects such as psychomotor disturbances, insomnia, headache, gastrointestinal upset, as well as cardiovascular changes such as palpitations, although the evidence for more severe considerations such as arrhythmia remains uncertain [38]. These adverse effects should be considered in a balance with the evidence reviewed below regarding potential benefits. Caffeine has also been found to exacerbate symptoms of underlying psychiatric problems such as schizophrenia, panic disorder, and anxiety [39]. Caffeinism, or caffeine intoxication, refers to chronic use of excessive caffeine. The Diagnostic and Statistical Manual of Mental Disorders IV criteria involve reporting five of the following 12 symptoms related to caffeine use: restlessness, excitement, nervousness, insomnia, facial flushing, gastrointestinal upset, diuresis, muscle twitching, psychomotor agitation, rambling thought or speech, cardiac arrhythmia or tachycardia, and periods of inexhaustibility. Three additional caffeine-related disorders are recognized: caffeine-induced anxiety disorder, caffeine-induced sleep disorder, and caffeine-related disorder not otherwise specified. Although the DSM-IV suggests that consumption of 250 mg may be associated with adverse effects, the literature is variable in this regard; some sources indicate significant side effects starting at 600–750 mg/day, with more significant impact occurring with >1,000 mg/day.

Caffeine has diuretic actions and thus concerns exist regarding the risks of dehydration. However, there is evidence that caffeine in moderate amounts does not negatively affect fluid balance especially for single doses under 250 mg [40]. In addition, habitual caffeine consumers may develop a tolerance to the diuresis effect [40].

Eliminating caffeine from the diet of someone who is a habitual caffeine user, especially if done abruptly, can produce withdrawal symptoms such as headache and rebound sleepiness [41, 42]. Changes in the number or affinity of adenosine receptors may occur with habitual caffeine consumption (with as little as 100 mg/day) which may contribute to tolerance and/or withdrawal effects [7].

Genetic Variation Relevant to Caffeine Effects

Genetic factors have also been implicated in caffeine countermeasure studies. Twin-based studies that link genetic polymorphisms of caffeine-metabolizing enzymes and target receptors to variations in caffeine response highlight the hereditary nature of caffeine response traits. A review of studies of twins found that overall heritability of traits associated with caffeine ranged from 0.30 to 0.60 in different populations [43]. Single-nucleotide polymorphisms (SNPs) in the CYP1A1-CYP1A2 gene region have been linked to habitual caffeine consumption and its consequent effects [44–47] in some but not all studies [48]. For example, the SNP rs762551 (CYP1A2*1F allele) has been linked to caffeine metabolism: individuals with the rs762551(A/A) genotype are considered to be "fast" metabolizers of caffeine, while those with the rs762551 (A/C) heterozygotes or rs762551 (C/C) homozygotes (CYP1A2*1C alleles) are "slow" metabolizers.

One study also reported, in addition to the CYP1A1/2 variant, caffeine consumption links to the NCAM-a gene, which has been implicated in addiction, and another site linked to hypertension near the gene ULK3 [49]. Polymorphism of the adenosine A_{2A} receptor has been linked to caffeine consumption, with homozygotes for the 1083C-to-T variant consuming less caffeine [48]. Another variant in the A_{2A} receptor, previously linked to panic disorder, was associated with the self-reported anxiogenic effects of caffeine in placebo-controlled studies [50], one of which also revealed links to a dopamine D_2 receptor variant [44]. Caffeine consumption patterns have also been linked to the aryl-hydrocarbon receptor (AHR) gene, an upstream inducer of CYP1A1-CYP1A2 transcription. The variants rs4410790 and rs6968865 were found to be associated with those who consume greater than 400 mg of caffeine per day [46]. Another study reported an association between the rs6968865(T) allele and increased coffee consumption, although the magnitude of this finding was marginal (0.2 cups) [51].

Countermeasure Studies Using Caffeine and/or Naps

Caffeine is commonly used to combat sleepiness [52]. While caffeine is not regulated in the same manner as prescription pharmaceuticals, it is useful to consider caffeine in a similar context as one would a prescription drug—that is, to balance the risks and benefits of use. Although most of the literature considers group-level effects of caffeine, substantial individual variability exists, as discussed above, and may contribute to variability in terms of the presence and magnitude of caffeine performance benefits. This variability may involve genetic polymorphisms and nongenetic factors such as age, recent caffeine history, or the degree of sleep loss. The presence of bright light may also augment the alerting impact of caffeine [53].

Napping is an alternative countermeasure for sleepiness and sleep loss. Despite its nonpharmacological nature, it is useful to consider the associated risks and benefits, as well as the potential for inter-individual variability and context-dependence of this balance. For example, risks associated with napping could include insomnia in the subsequent sleep period, or sleep inertia, wherein transient performance/cognitive impairment occurs in the time frame immediately after awakening. These risks may vary by

Table 17.1 Methodological considerations

General issues	*Caffeine studies*	*Nap studies*
Demographics (e.g., age, sex)	Habitual use amount and frequency	Baseline nap habits
Circadian time of intervention	Dose	Duration of opportunity
Sleep history	Delivery route	Capacity to nap
Genetic variation	Delivery rate	Sleep stages obtained
Sensitivity to sleep loss	Smoking	Sleep inertia
Nature of task/measurements	Pregnancy	
Effect size of intervention		
Impact on subsequent sleep		
Population (exclusions)		

individual and by context, and may be affected for example by sleep loss, baseline insomnia risk or presence, and/or the immediate functional demands upon awakening from the nap. Nap length and timing relative to planned sleep opportunities can affect the risks of sleep inertia and/or subsequent insomnia. Naps can be considered to be prophylactic if they occur before a shift of night or extended work, in a person who is at baseline well-rested, or to be recuperative if they occur in the setting of sleep deprivation. The biological capacity to achieve sleep during a nap opportunity is also an important consideration, as is the feasibility of interrupting a work shift for this purpose. What performance demands (if any) are required in the post-nap period should be considered, in light of the possible issue of sleep inertia. The magnitude of sleep loss also impacts the relative improvements that can be expected from naps of varied duration—the greater the loss, the longer the nap will need to be to serve a countermeasure function, as will be discussed below.

A variety of experimental paradigms have tested the potential benefits of caffeine and naps to improve performance and alertness under sleep loss conditions. Comparing results across the caffeine experiments can be challenging due to differences in caffeine dose, method and timing of administration, and acute or sustained release delivery. Similarly, comparing nap studies is challenging due to different duration and timing of naps. In any countermeasure study, the methods may differ according to the degree of sleep deprivation or restriction, the extent of the resulting impairment, and the outcome measurements used. Table 17.1 summarizes these kinds of considerations. The comparison groups may include placebo (such as a non-sleep work break), different doses of caffeine, or different nap durations.

Caffeine and Naps in Studies of Driving Performance

Operating a motor vehicle under conditions of sleep loss poses substantial accident risk, and sleep-related accidents have been shown to confer greater risk of injury. Caffeine is a commonly employed countermeasure to increase alertness while driving. Other countermeasures are commonly employed, but have not been effective when studied formally [54–56]. For example, in a Swedish national questionnaire study, subjects were asked to indicate their general countermeasure preferences used while driving to maintain alertness [57]. The top five countermeasures included: stop and take a short walk (54 %), turn up/on the radio (52 %), open the window (47 %), drink coffee (45 %), and engage the passenger in conversation (45 %). Driving performance is typically assessed using simulations in which lane drift or other metrics can be tracked as outcome measures that are assumed to reflect propensity for sleepiness-related accidents on the road.

The effects of caffeine on simulator and field driving performance have been evaluated alone and in studies also assessing nap effects. In a small study of sleep restriction, low dose caffeine (100 mg) improved simulated driving performance, but interestingly, self-rated performance did not correlate with these objective improvements [58].

Another pair of sleep restriction studies of simulated afternoon driving tested caffeine and nap against a placebo (decaffeinated coffee) "break" condition. In the first study [59], 150 mg of caffeine was compared against a nap, and both interventions showed benefit for driving performance, subjective alertness, and 4–11 Hz EEG power, but not eye blink rate (all accepted outcome metrics in the field). However, not all subjects slept during the 15 min opportunity in this report. In the second study [60], the combination of a 15 min nap opportunity and 150 mg caffeine was superior to a 200 mg caffeine condition, which showed improvement versus decaffeinated placebo. Finally, in an important follow-up study, a 200 mg dose of caffeine was less effective in the 5-h per night sleep restriction paradigm used in the above two studies compared to a 1-night total sleep deprivation protocol [61]. This may not be surprising, since the sleep debt is greater with total deprivation, although other studies have shown that cumulative restriction eventually reaches similar performance impairments as acute deprivation [62].

Whereas the above studies utilized standard caffeine dosing (e.g., single servings of coffee), other studies tested extended dosing of caffeine in simulated driving performance during sleep restriction. De Valck et al. conducted two studies of sustained release caffeine (300 mg) with or without a morning 30 min nap following caffeine administration [63, 64]. Sustained release caffeine improved objective driving performance and subjective sleepiness in the first sleep restriction study [63]. In the second study, sustained release caffeine (300 mg) was tested with or without a 30 min nap opportunity in a 2×2 placebo-controlled design [64]. The impact was difficult to interpret because the benefits were seen for only one driving metric, were evident at different times for the nap versus caffeine interventions, and there was no added benefit of their combination. Specifically, lane drift performance, but not speed deviation or accident liability, improved with caffeine but only in the afternoon testing period. In contrast, the same single driving metric improved in the nap intervention only in the morning testing period. Like the prior studies using a 15 min nap opportunity, there was little evidence of sleep inertia, since the driving performance improvements were assessed soon after the nap. The benefits of sustained release caffeine formulations have also been shown in other studies investigating vigilance and performance outcomes [65, 66].

Driving performance has also been examined in a pair of field studies. 200 mg of caffeine was tested against a 30 min nap opportunity in highway driving performance, by comparing early evening with nocturnal sessions (2:00–3:30 a.m.), with no intervening sleep [67]. Both interventions similarly improved subjective fatigue/sleepiness ratings as well as performance measures, without altering subsequent nocturnal sleep measured in the lab. Whereas this study involved young adult males, the follow-up study tested middle-aged versus young adults using the same nocturnal driving protocol [68]. The middle-age group responded better than the young group to coffee, but less well to the nap intervention. The young group responded similarly to the two interventions, and of note had 50 % more total sleep time and greater than twofold higher delta power during their naps (delta power is a biomarker of sleep homeostatic drive). In both groups, sleepiness improved after caffeine but not after the nap.

Caffeine and Naps in Studies of Sleepiness, Alertness, and Cognitive Performance

Standard and extended release caffeine and different duration naps have also been investigated in sleep restriction and sleep deprivation paradigms using outcomes of vigilance and cognitive performance. Napping generally shows benefits, but some studies have shown a negative sleep inertia effect in the post-nap period. Sleep inertia, characterized by subjective and/or objective impairments for 30-60 minutes after awakening, has been generally associated with longer duration naps. It is not consistently observed in napping countermeasure studies. In an evaluation of nap durations from 5 to 30 min after 1 night with 5-h sleep restriction, sleep inertia effects in the

20-min post-nap time reduced the performance benefits for the 30 min nap, and for certain cognitive tests after the 20 min nap [69]. Similar results were obtained in a related study comparing 10 and 30 min naps, in which the latter was associated with sleep inertia effects on performance [70]. In the setting of overnight total sleep deprivation, a 2-h nap improved objective sleep propensity as measured using the Multiple Sleep Latency Test (MSLT) [71] and showed greater benefit than a 15 min nap [72]. Caffeine has been tested, with or without a nap, over a range of sleep deprivation challenges. For example, 150 mg of caffeine improved simulated laparoscopy performance of medical students after overnight deprivation [73]. In two studies of 48–88 h sleep deprivation, hourly low dose caffeine (0.03 mg/kg/h) improved objective sleep propensity by MSLT during an 88-h extended wake paradigm and reduced sleep-inertia impairments in psychomotor vigilance task (PVT) performance immediately post-nap [74]. Multiple dose caffeine regimens improved performance, mood, subjective sleepiness, and sleep latency on MSLT during a 48 h sleep deprivation paradigm [75]. The improvements were dose-dependent across regimens, including a 400 mg single dose, a 150 mg dose every 6 h, or a 300 mg dose every 6 h, although in each case the benefit was short-lived compared to the results from the nap condition. Nap durations from 2 to 8 h also showed "dose" dependent improvements and the benefits were more durable. Interestingly, repeated small doses of caffeine, as well as short naps, were both better than single large caffeine doses in terms of performance, mood, and alertness. Also of note, performance was markedly impaired during conditions with more than 24 h of sleep deprivation, with marked reduction in observed benefits of either of these countermeasures.

Countering performance impairments during night or shift work is of particular interest given the increasing need for 24-h coverage in certain fields in modern society. The performance and objective sleepiness benefit of the combination of caffeine and nap was greater than either alone in a study that combined simulated and field shift work [76]. However, it is interesting to note that the benefit was greatest in the first 1–2 nights and decreased in the subsequent 2 nights, similar to the diminishing effect of (hourly low dose) caffeine under forced-desynchrony conditions with 28.57 h wake episodes [21]. Napping prior to a shift has been investigated before and during night shifts, although results have not always been positive [77], especially when there are sleep inertia impairments [78], which may be task-dependent [79]. A 30-min nap had no effect on performance or sleepiness in simulated shift-work paradigm, although the nap and no-nap groups both had a 2-h pre-shift prophylactic nap [80]. By comparison, a 3-h pre-shift nap improved objective performance and subjective sleepiness in a shift-work paradigm that incorporated a single night of sleep restriction [81].

The effect of naps in the field has been investigated in shift workers using self-reported sleep metrics as well as field testing. A 20-min nap opportunity improved performance metrics, after an initial lag attributed to sleep inertia in 12-h rotating-shift aircraft maintenance engineers. However, this benefit was only seen on the first night shift but not on subsequent nights. Self-reported naps among locomotive engineers revealed lower overnight sleep quality and increased insomnia complaints associated with napping [82]. It cannot be determined from this survey study whether the naps caused subsequent sleep problems, and whether napping was a reaction to shift-work-related sleep difficulties. In another survey study, there was a correlation of self-reported naps with decreased night-time motor vehicle accidents shift-working police officers [83]. In a combined laboratory and home-based study of elderly patients, a 90-min afternoon nap opportunity was associated with decreased nocturnal sleep time and efficiency, and a small improvement in evening MSLT scores from 11 to 15 min, both of which are in the normal range.

Caffeine Compared to Prescription-Stimulant Medications

Although a detailed review of this topic is beyond the scope of this chapter, and we do not intend to suggest that prescription medications be utilized as countermeasures for sleep loss, studies have compared the effect of these medications with that of caffeine in a variety of paradigms. Several studies have shown that 200–600 mg of caffeine was as effective as 200–400 mg modafinil in maintaining performance during long-duration sleep deprivation, with duration of benefit correlating with expected clearance pharmacokinetics. In other sleep deprivation experiments, the duration of benefit was shorter, and the reported side effects were more common, in caffeine compared to amphetamine stimulant [84]. The results of these studies differed in whether subsequent sleep architecture was impacted by these countermeasures. Decision making remains impaired despite improvements in vigilance with caffeine and prescription stimulants in a 24-44 h total sleep deprivation paradigm [85]. Interestingly, it has been reported that self-assessed performance under conditions of sleep deprivation may be overly optimistic compared to objective performance in the presence of modafinil or amphetamine [86].

Hypnotic-Assisted Napping

In a study of healthy young adult pilots undergoing 38 h total sleep deprivation three times with different countermeasures, the effects of a zolpidem-assisted nap intervention were compared to unassisted naps and forced rest periods on sleepiness, mood, and cognitive performance [86]. Zolpidem-assisted naps were equivalent to, and in some cases better than, non-assisted naps. It is unknown whether the improvements were due to increased total sleep during the naps, lower proportion of N1 sleep, or another effect of zolpidem not revealed in standard sleep metrics. However, not all studies support the role of hypnotic-assisted napping. Cohen et al. reported cognitive performance impairment during a simulated night shift work after a ramelteon-assisted evening nap [87].

Discussion

Both napping and caffeine reduce performance impairments associated with sleep deprivation, sleep restriction, or shift work. There are two main risks associated with napping in addition to the obvious work/schedule limitation that time must be allocated to the nap opportunity. First, naps may induce sleep inertia, which effectively extends the time required to institute this intervention. Therefore, there is a tradeoff: how much more recuperative would a nap be required to outweigh the additional time needed to resolve potential sleep inertia associated with the nap? The answer will depend on the operational setting, individual sensitivity to sleep deprivation, and potential for post-nap sleep inertia impairment. Second, napping may interfere with nocturnal sleep by causing insomnia at the time of the desired major sleep episode, presumably due to reduction of homeostatic sleep pressure. It is also noteworthy that the impact of napping on performance may vary according to the measurement task used. This creates a combinatorial challenge experimentally, since the task may interact with the nap timing and duration, each of which is also related to the baseline severity of sleep loss. Prophylactic naps may be best if used closer to the time of the extended or late shift of work. It may have advantages compared to on-the-job napping, because sleep inertia, if present, would not be happening at the job. However, sleep inertia following a pre-shift nap could potentially have important impact outside of the job, such as on driving to work after having a nap.

It is also interesting to note that several of the studies showed dissociations between subjective and objective outcome measures. It is frequently mentioned in the literature that self-reporting sleepiness under conditions of restriction or deprivation underestimates the objective impairments. One of the most dramatic examples of this dissociation is the study by Van Dongen et al. [62], in which objective performance impairments which continued to worsen daily exceeded subjective sleepiness reports which reached a plateau after a few days under conditions of sleep restriction. Although not all studies support this finding [88], the implications would be important considering that individuals routinely must judge their own sleepiness before participating in activities for which sleepiness might be dangerous, such as driving. Interestingly, dissociations between subjective sleepiness and objective performance occur in both directions. For example, in some cases when performance was improved by a countermeasure, there was no correlation with subjective report, including self-assessment of performance [58, 64], and in some cases the performance improvement was associated with increased subjective sleepiness [77]. Paradoxical effects of caffeine have been reported: increased subjective sleepiness despite improved objective alertness measures [21]. Different aspects of objective performance may be differentially responsive to countermeasures [63, 89]. These examples serve as a reminder of the complexities involved in these experiments, their interpretation, and extrapolation to other settings. In that regard, concerning any countermeasure for insufficient sleep, the extent to which results from controlled laboratory environments can generalize to the "real world" remains challenging to predict. For example, some environments may be associated with higher degrees of stimulation and/or higher stakes associated with performance, such as medical practice or police work. Individual differences in a person's interest in their job, or incentives related to performance, may also play important roles in the field setting that are difficult to reproduce in the experimental setting. The diverse experimental paradigms make comparisons across studies challenging. Experiments may differ in how sleepiness was measured (subjectively versus objectively, and, within each category, which metrics were used); whether these metrics and surrogates are equally valid or relevant for different populations; interventions, and outcomes. Table 17.1 lists some methodological considerations relevant not only to interpreting the literature, but also to considering potential interventions in operational settings.

As is true for any intervention in clinical research, the concept of efficacy should be distinguished from that of effectiveness. These concepts are similar to the terms external validity or ecological validity in other domains. Efficacy refers to the change in an outcome of interest by an intervention carried out under careful experimental conditions. Effectiveness, on the other hand, refers to the change in an outcome of interest when the intervention is applied in the "real world," where the constraints and controls of the experimental paradigms are often not maintained. Consider a drug that must be taken with food: it could show high efficacy in a trial where the staff administer the drug and meals to ensure absorption, whereas it could show lower effectiveness in a real-world trial in which the drug might not always be taken with food. Thus, in the experiments reviewed here, the details of the methods and inclusion/exclusion criteria directly impact the extent to which the efficacy results can translate into effectiveness.

Another important issue to consider is the magnitude of improvement seen with a countermeasure. When considering if a statistically significant countermeasure effect would be important operationally, the answer is likely to differ across different operational settings. For example, different settings might involve different degrees of risk tolerance, error impact, baseline frequency of errors, existence of safeguards, and so forth. An individual's baseline skill level may also be an important factor. Within the multidimensional framework of an operational setting, one would ideally want to estimate what portion of error/risk is attributable to sleep or circadian factors. For example, if 99 % of product assembly errors in a factory are due to moisture rusting the conveyor belts, an expensive sleep scheduling intervention for employees might not be the best place to allocate resources. On the other hand, if 30 % of motor vehicle accidents at night are due to sleepiness, and they often result in serious injury or death, then resource allocation focused on drowsy driving is more easily justified. Even if the risk is entirely attributed to sleep-related impairment, if the baseline error rate is very small, it may be difficult to demonstrate improvement with a sleep countermeasure. Investigating this balance may be quite complex in real-world settings, and the situation is of course further complicated by the reality of individual differences in vulnerability to the performance effects of sleep loss as well as in the beneficial impact of countermeasures.

Conclusion

The experiments outlined above indicate across a wide range of experimental paradigms that naps and caffeine are important countermeasures against the performance impairments associated with insufficient sleep. The relative impact of naps and caffeine depend on the many factors, some of which pertain to the operational setting and others relate to the individual suffering insufficient sleep. Because these countermeasures are of great interest in their application to modern operational settings in which insufficient sleep may be critical, it is important that the potential benefits should be weighed against potential risks for any countermeasure.

References

1. The price of fatigue. https://sleep.med.harvard.edu/file_download/100. Accessed March 2013.
2. Falleti MG, Maruff P, Collie A, Darby DG, McStephen M. Qualitative similarities in cognitive impairment associated with 24 h of sustained wakefulness and a blood alcohol concentration of 0.05%. J Sleep Res. 2003;12(4):265–74.
3. Williamson AM, Feyer AM. Moderate sleep deprivation produces impairments in cognitive and motor performance equivalent to legally prescribed levels of alcohol intoxication. Occup Environ Med. 2000; 57(10):649–55.
4. Dawson D, Reid K. Fatigue, alcohol and performance impairment. Nature. 1997;388(6639):235.
5. Bonnet MH, Balkin TJ, Dinges DF, et al. The use of stimulants to modify performance during sleep loss: a review by the sleep deprivation and Stimulant Task Force of the American Academy of Sleep Medicine. Sleep. 2005;28(9):1163–87.
6. Morgenthaler TI, Kapur VK, Brown T, et al. Practice parameters for the treatment of narcolepsy and other hypersomnias of central origin. Sleep. 2007;30(12): 1705–11.
7. James JE, Keane MA. Caffeine, sleep and wakefulness: implications of new understanding about withdrawal reversal. Hum Psychopharmacol. 2007; 22(8):549–58.
8. Frary CD, Johnson RK, Wang MQ. Food sources and intakes of caffeine in the diets of persons in the United States. J Am Diet Assoc. 2005;105(1):110–3.
9. Durrant KL. Known and hidden sources of caffeine in drug, food, and natural products. J Am Pharm Assoc (Wash). 2002;42(4):625–37.
10. Dorea JG, da Costa TH. Is coffee a functional food? Br J Nutr. 2005;93(6):773–82.
11. Heckman MA, Weil J, Gonzalez de Mejia E. Caffeine (1, 3, 7-trimethylxanthine) in foods: a comprehensive review on consumption, functionality, safety, and regulatory matters. J Food Sci. 2010;75(3):R77–87.
12. Why isn't the amount of caffeine a product contains required on a food label? http://www.fda.gov/AboutFDA/Transparency/Basics/ucm194317.htm. Accessed March 2013.
13. Select Committee on GRAS Substances (SCOGS) opinion: caffeine. http://www.fda.gov/Food/IngredientsPackagingLabeling/GRAS/SCOGS/ucm256650.htm. Accessed March 2013.
14. Caffeine content for coffee, tea, soda and more. www.mayoclinic.com/health/caffeine/AN01211. Accessed March 2013.
15. Caffeine content of food & drugs. www.cspinet.org/new/cafchart.htm#table_coffees; http://ndb.nal.usda.gov/ndb/foods/list. Accessed March 2013.
16. Caffeine and your body. http://www.fda.gov/downloads/Drugs/ResourcesForYou/Consumers/BuyingUsingMedicineSafely/UnderstandingOver-the-CounterMedicines/UCM205286.pdf. Accessed March 2013.
17. New caffeine report shows no measurable change in consumption trends of the U.S. population. http://www.fda.gov/downloads/AboutFDA/CentersOffices/OfficeofFoods/CFSAN/CFSANFOIAElectronicReadingRoom/UCM333191.pdf. Accessed March 2013.
18. Institute of Medicine. Caffeine for the sustainment of mental task performance: formulations for military operations. Washington, DC: National Academy Press; 2001.
19. Current Worldwide Annual Coffee Consumption per capita. www.ChartsBin.com/view/581. Accessed March 2013.
20. Achermann P, Borbely AA. Mathematical models of sleep regulation. Front Biosci. 2003;8:S683–93.
21. Wyatt JK, Cajochen C, Ritz-De Cecco A, Czeisler CA, Dijk DJ. Low-dose repeated caffeine administration for circadian-phase-dependent performance degradation during extended wakefulness. Sleep. 2004;27(3):374–81.
22. Blanco-Centurion C, Xu M, Murillo-Rodriguez E, et al. Adenosine and sleep homeostasis in the Basal forebrain. J Neurosci. 2006;26(31):8092–100.
23. Methippara MM, Kumar S, Alam MN, Szymusiak R, McGinty D. Effects on sleep of microdialysis of adenosine A1 and A2a receptor analogs into the lateral preoptic area of rats. Am J Physiol Regul Integr Comp Physiol. 2005;289(6):R1715–23.
24. Stenberg D, Litonius E, Halldner L, Johansson B, Fredholm BB, Porkka-Heiskanen T. Sleep and its homeostatic regulation in mice lacking the adenosine A1 receptor. J Sleep Res. 2003;12(4):283–90.
25. Bjorness TE, Kelly CL, Gao T, Poffenberger V, Greene RW. Control and function of the homeostatic sleep response by adenosine A1 receptors. J Neurosci. 2009;29(5):1267–76.

26. Lieberman HR, Tharion WJ, Shukitt-Hale B, Speckman KL, Tulley R. Effects of caffeine, sleep loss, and stress on cognitive performance and mood during U.S. Navy SEAL training. Sea-Air-Land. Psychopharmacology (Berl). 2002;164(3):250–61.
27. Benarroch EE. Adenosine and its receptors: multiple modulatory functions and potential therapeutic targets for neurologic disease. Neurology. 2008;70(3):231–6.
28. Reiser MA, D'Souza T, Dryer SE. Effects of caffeine and 3-isobutyl-1-methylxanthine on voltage-activated potassium currents in vertebrate neurones and secretory cells. Br J Pharmacol. 1996;118(8):2145–51.
29. Bianchi MT, Botzolakis EJ. Targeting ligand-gated ion channels in neurology and psychiatry: is pharmacological promiscuity an obstacle or an opportunity? BMC Pharmacol. 2010;10:3.
30. Fuxe K, Ferre S, Canals M, et al. Adenosine A2A and dopamine D2 heteromeric receptor complexes and their function. J Mol Neurosci. 2005;26(2–3):209–20.
31. Fuxe K, Agnati LF, Jacobsen K, et al. Receptor heteromerization in adenosine A2A receptor signaling: relevance for striatal function and Parkinson's disease. Neurology. 2003;61(11 Suppl 6):S19–23.
32. Freedman ND, Park Y, Abnet CC, Hollenbeck AR, Sinha R. Association of coffee drinking with total and cause-specific mortality. N Engl J Med. 2012;366(20):1891–904.
33. Caffeine drug information section. www.uptodate.com. Accessed Feb 2013.
34. Kroon LA. Drug interactions with smoking. Am J Health Syst Pharm. 2007;64(18):1917–21.
35. de Leon J, Diaz FJ, Rogers T, et al. A pilot study of plasma caffeine concentrations in a US sample of smoker and nonsmoker volunteers. Prog Neuropsychopharmacol Biol Psychiatry. 2003;27(1):165–71.
36. McKim EM. Caffeine and its effects on pregnancy and the neonate. J Nurse Midwifery. 1991;36(4):226–31.
37. American Academy of Pediatrics Committee on Drugs. Transfer of drugs and other chemicals into human milk. Pediatrics. 2001;108(3):776–89.
38. Pelchovitz DJ, Goldberger JJ. Caffeine and cardiac arrhythmias: a review of the evidence. Am J Med. 2011;124(4):284–9.
39. Fredholm BB, Battig K, Holmen J, Nehlig A, Zvartau EE. Actions of caffeine in the brain with special reference to factors that contribute to its widespread use. Pharmacol Rev. 1999;51(1):83–133.
40. Maughan RJ, Griffin J. Caffeine ingestion and fluid balance: a review. J Hum Nutr Diet. 2003;16(6):411–20.
41. Hewlett P, Smith A. Effects of repeated doses of caffeine on performance and alertness: new data and secondary analyses. Hum Psychopharmacol. 2007;22(6):339–50.
42. Ozsungur S, Brenner D, El-Sohemy A. Fourteen well-described caffeine withdrawal symptoms factor into three clusters. Psychopharmacology (Berl). 2009;201(4):541–8.
43. Yang A, Palmer AA, de Wit H. Genetics of caffeine consumption and responses to caffeine. Psychopharmacology (Berl). 2010;211(3):245–57.
44. Childs E, Hohoff C, Deckert J, Xu K, Badner J, de Wit H. Association between ADORA2A and DRD2 polymorphisms and caffeine-induced anxiety. Neuropsychopharmacology. 2008;33(12):2791–800.
45. Womack CJ, Saunders MJ, Bechtel MK, et al. The influence of a CYP1A2 polymorphism on the ergogenic effects of caffeine. J Int Soc Sports Nutr. 2012;9(1):7.
46. Josse AR, Da Costa LA, Campos H, El-Sohemy A. Associations between polymorphisms in the AHR and CYP1A1-CYP1A2 gene regions and habitual caffeine consumption. Am J Clin Nutr. 2012;96(3):665–71.
47. Rodenburg EM, Eijgelsheim M, Geleijnse JM, et al. CYP1A2 and coffee intake and the modifying effect of sex, age, and smoking. Am J Clin Nutr. 2012;96(1):182–7.
48. Cornelis MC, El-Sohemy A, Campos H. Genetic polymorphism of the adenosine A2A receptor is associated with habitual caffeine consumption. Am J Clin Nutr. 2007;86(1):240–4.
49. Amin N, Byrne E, Johnson J, et al. Genome-wide association analysis of coffee drinking suggests association with CYP1A1/CYP1A2 and NRCAM. Mol Psychiatry. 2012;17(11):1116–29.
50. Alsene K, Deckert J, Sand P, de Wit H. Association between A2a receptor gene polymorphisms and caffeine-induced anxiety. Neuropsychopharmacology. 2003;28(9):1694–702.
51. Sulem P, Gudbjartsson DF, Geller F, et al. Sequence variants at CYP1A1-CYP1A2 and AHR associate with coffee consumption. Hum Mol Genet. 2011;20(10):2071–7.
52. Roehrs T, Roth T. Caffeine: sleep and daytime sleepiness. Sleep Med Rev. 2008;12(2):153–62.
53. Wright Jr KP, Badia P, Myers BL, Plenzler SC. Combination of bright light and caffeine as a countermeasure for impaired alertness and performance during extended sleep deprivation. J Sleep Res. 1997;6(1):26–35.
54. Reyner LA, Horne JA. Evaluation "in-car" countermeasures to sleepiness: cold air and radio. Sleep. 1998;21(1):46–50.
55. Phipps-Nelson J, Redman JR, Rajaratnam SM. Temporal profile of prolonged, night-time driving performance: breaks from driving temporarily reduce time-on-task fatigue but not sleepiness. J Sleep Res. 2011;20(3):404–15.
56. Schwarz JF, Ingre M, Fors C, et al. In-car countermeasures open window and music revisited on the real road: popular but hardly effective against driver sleepiness. J Sleep Res. 2012;21(5):595–9.
57. Anund A, Kecklund G, Peters B, Akerstedt T. Driver sleepiness and individual differences in preferences for countermeasures. J Sleep Res. 2008;17(1):16–22.

58. Biggs SN, Smith A, Dorrian J, et al. Perception of simulated driving performance after sleep restriction and caffeine. J Psychosom Res. 2007;63(6):573–7.
59. Horne JA, Reyner LA. Counteracting driver sleepiness: effects of napping, caffeine, and placebo. Psychophysiology. 1996;33(3):306–9.
60. Reyner LA, Horne JA. Suppression of sleepiness in drivers: combination of caffeine with a short nap. Psychophysiology. 1997;34(6):721–5.
61. Reyner LA, Horne JA. Early morning driver sleepiness: effectiveness of 200 mg caffeine. Psychophysiology. 2000;37(2):251–6.
62. Van Dongen HP, Maislin G, Mullington JM, Dinges DF. The cumulative cost of additional wakefulness: dose-response effects on neurobehavioral functions and sleep physiology from chronic sleep restriction and total sleep deprivation. Sleep. 2003;26(2):117–26.
63. De Valck E, Cluydts R. Slow-release caffeine as a countermeasure to driver sleepiness induced by partial sleep deprivation. J Sleep Res. 2001;10(3):203–9.
64. De Valck E, De Groot E, Cluydts R. Effects of slow-release caffeine and a nap on driving simulator performance after partial sleep deprivation. Percept Mot Skills. 2003;96(1):67–78.
65. Beaumont M, Batejat D, Pierard C, et al. Slow release caffeine and prolonged (64-h) continuous wakefulness: effects on vigilance and cognitive performance. J Sleep Res. 2001;10(4):265–76.
66. Patat A, Rosenzweig P, Enslen M, et al. Effects of a new slow release formulation of caffeine on EEG, psychomotor and cognitive functions in sleep-deprived subjects. Hum Psychopharmacol. 2000;15(3):153–70.
67. Philip P, Taillard J, Moore N, et al. The effects of coffee and napping on nighttime highway driving: a randomized trial. Ann Intern Med. 2006;144(11):785–91.
68. Sagaspe P, Taillard J, Chaumet G, Moore N, Bioulac B, Philip P. Aging and nocturnal driving: better with coffee or a nap? A randomized study. Sleep. 2007;30(12):1808–13.
69. Brooks A, Lack L. A brief afternoon nap following nocturnal sleep restriction: which nap duration is most recuperative? Sleep. 2006;29(6):831–40.
70. Tietzel AJ, Lack LC. The short-term benefits of brief and long naps following nocturnal sleep restriction. Sleep. 2001;24(3):293–300.
71. Vgontzas AN, Pejovic S, Zoumakis E, et al. Daytime napping after a night of sleep loss decreases sleepiness, improves performance, and causes beneficial changes in cortisol and interleukin-6 secretion. Am J Physiol Endocrinol Metab. 2007;292(1):E253–61.
72. Helmus T, Rosenthal L, Bishop C, Roehrs T, Syron ML, Roth T. The alerting effects of short and long naps in narcoleptic, sleep deprived, and alert individuals. Sleep. 1997;20(4):251–7.
73. Aggarwal R, Mishra A, Crochet P, Sirimanna P, Darzi A. Effect of caffeine and taurine on simulated laparoscopy performed following sleep deprivation. Br J Surg. 2011;98(11):1666–72.
74. Van Dongen HP, Price NJ, Mullington JM, Szuba MP, Kapoor SC, Dinges DF. Caffeine eliminates psychomotor vigilance deficits from sleep inertia. Sleep. 2001;24(7):813–9.
75. Bonnet MH, Gomez S, Wirth O, Arand DL. The use of caffeine versus prophylactic naps in sustained performance. Sleep. 1995;18(2):97–104.
76. Schweitzer PK, Randazzo AC, Stone K, Erman M, Walsh JK. Laboratory and field studies of naps and caffeine as practical countermeasures for sleep-wake problems associated with night work. Sleep. 2006;29(1):39–50.
77. Rosa RR. Napping at home and alertness on the job in rotating shift workers. Sleep. 1993;16(8):727–35.
78. Sallinen M, Harma M, Akerstedt T, Rosa R, Lillqvist O. Promoting alertness with a short nap during a night shift. J Sleep Res. 1998;7(4):240–7.
79. Hofer-Tinguely G, Achermann P, Landolt HP, et al. Sleep inertia: performance changes after sleep, rest and active waking. Brain Res Cogn Brain Res. 2005;22(3):323–31.
80. Tremaine R, Dorrian J, Lack L, et al. The relationship between subjective and objective sleepiness and performance during a simulated night-shift with a nap countermeasure. Appl Ergon. 2010;42(1):52–61.
81. Macchi MM, Boulos Z, Ranney T, Simmons L, Campbell SS. Effects of an afternoon nap on nighttime alertness and performance in long-haul drivers. Accid Anal Prev. 2002;34(6):825–34.
82. Pilcher JJ, Popkin SM, Adkins K, Roether L. Self-report naps in irregular work schedules. Ind Health. 2005;43(1):123–8.
83. Garbarino S, Mascialino B, Penco MA, et al. Professional shift-work drivers who adopt prophylactic naps can reduce the risk of car accidents during night work. Sleep. 2004;27(7):1295–302.
84. Killgore WD, Rupp TL, Grugle NL, Reichardt RM, Lipizzi EL, Balkin TJ. Effects of dextroamphetamine, caffeine and modafinil on psychomotor vigilance test performance after 44 h of continuous wakefulness. J Sleep Res. 2008;17(3):309–21.
85. Killgore WD, Grugle NL, Balkin TJ. Gambling when sleep deprived: don't bet on stimulants. Chronobiol Int. 2012;29(1):43–54.
86. Baranski JV, Pigeau RA. Self-monitoring cognitive performance during sleep deprivation: effects of modafinil, d-amphetamine and placebo. J Sleep Res. 1997;6(2):84–91.
87. Cohen DA, Wang W, Klerman EB, Rajaratnam SM. Ramelteon prior to a short evening nap impairs neurobehavioral performance for up to 12 hours after awakening. J Clin Sleep Med. 2010;6(6):565–71.
88. Horne J. The end of sleep: 'sleep debt' versus biological adaptation of human sleep to waking needs. Biol Psychol. 2011;87(1):1–14.
89. Asaoka S, Fukuda K, Murphy TI, Abe T, Inoue Y. The effects of a nighttime nap on the error-monitoring functions during extended wakefulness. Sleep. 2012;35(6):871–8.

Fatigue in the Workplace 18

Gregory Belenky, Amanda Lamp, Anna Hemp, and Jennifer L. Zaslona

The Fog of Fatigue and Its Remedy: Sleep

Charles Lindberg describes nearly falling asleep while on his solo flight across the Atlantic [1]: "My mind clicks on and off, as though attached to an electric switch with which some outside force is tampering. I try letting one eyelid close at a time while I prop the other open with my will. But, the effort is too much. Sleep is winning. My whole body argues dully that nothing life can attain is quite so desirable as sleep. My mind is losing resolution and control." Winston Churchill commented on the value of napping [2]: "Nature has not intended mankind to work from eight in the morning until midnight without that refreshment of blessed oblivion which, even if it only lasts 20 min, is sufficient to renew all the vital forces." The American soldier and historian of small unit operations, S.L.A. Marshall speaking of the interaction of fear and mental and physical fatigue commented [3]: "Reduced to this condition, the soldier fails to dig a foxhole; even though he knows that he is in danger. The officer fails to properly inspect his position. Troops fail to reconnoiter the immediate area of their bivouac. Commanders hesitate to give orders and defer important decisions."

G. Belenky, M.D. (✉) • A. Lamp, B.S. • A. Hemp
Sleep and Performance Research Center, Washington State University, Spokane, WA, USA

J.L. Zaslona, B.Sc.
Sleep/Wake Research Centre, Massey University, Wellington, New Zealand

The Operational Environment

The operational environment, broadly construed, is a system in which the performance of the human embedded in the system is critical to a successful outcome. Further, there are time boundaries (a temporal envelope) during which the correct decision must be reached or the system will fail. This dependence on a correct and timely human response is captured in the "observe, orient, decide, act" loop conceptualized by the American Air Force fighter pilot and military theoretician John Boyd [4]. First applied to explain the superiority of American fighter pilots over their adversaries during the Korean War, Boyd's conceptualization applies to any operation in which the performance of the human–in–the–loop is critical to a successful outcome. In the parlance of operations research, most operational settings are complex and tightly coupled—a small error can set off a cascading sequence of failures [5]. Examples of operational settings include all modes of transportation, resource extraction (mining, drilling, pumping), energy generation, manufacturing, financial markets, military operations, and medicine. Most involve, at least at times, extended hours, shift work, and nighttime operations. High reliability operational settings are ones in which the operating

M.T. Bianchi (ed.), *Sleep Deprivation and Disease: Effects on the Body, Brain and Behavior*, DOI 10.1007/978-1-4614-9087-6_18, © Springer Science+Business Media New York 2014

personnel remain mindful in day-to-day operations and maintain presence of mind in an emergency [6]. For example, operations on the deck of an aircraft carrier are considered high reliability. For most of us, the work setting is a workstation in a climate-controlled space with little or no operational risk. In a high-risk operational settings (e.g., in-flight, in nuclear power plants, in mining, in health care, etc.), the consequences of an error, incident, or accident can be catastrophic.

The Problem of 24/7 Operations: The Earth at Night

Figure 18.1 is a composite image of the earth at night showing the pattern and extent of 24/7 human activity and enterprise [7]. It presents, in a compelling way, the activity driving extended work hours and backside of the clock (nighttime) operations supporting economic and other forms of human activity. When the United States Army developed and fielded third-generation night vision devices in the 1980s, it adopted the slogan—"We own the night." In a wry commentary, an Army Colonel observed—"And now we have to staff it."

Sleep and the Short-, Mid-, and Long-Term Effects of Sleep Loss

Humans and all other mammals, as well as birds, reptiles, fish, insects, and possibly even jellyfish, sleep. Thus, it appears that any animal that has one or more assemblies of nerve cells (neuronal assemblies) is capable of, and has the need for, sleep. In the fruit fly, sleep deprivation leads to rebound sleep during recovery, degraded performance during the sleep deprivation, and shortened life span when the sleep loss continues over days just as it does in humans [8]. After over a hundred years of experimental sleep loss studies in humans, we know that extended wakefulness degrades performance, that recovery sleep restores it, and that approximately 8 h of actual sleep time (with a range of 7–9 h) in every 24 h is optimal for sustaining complex mental operations and performance. We understand much of the brain regulation of sleep stages. Nevertheless, what it is that goes wrong in the brain during sleep loss and how that is restored by recovery sleep remain as unanswered questions.

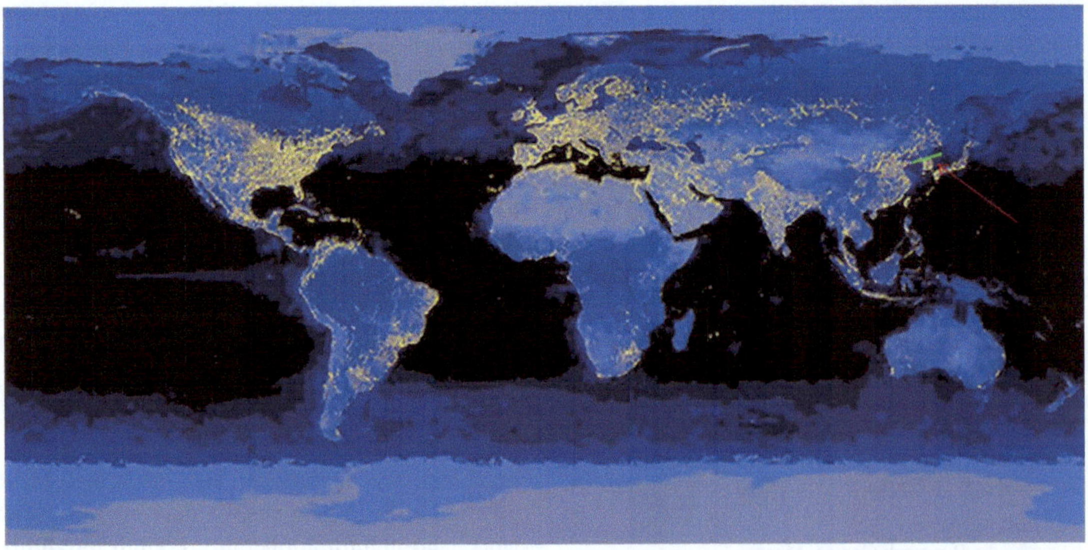

Fig. 18.1 The earth at night—visual depiction of human 24/7 activity (http://apod.nasa.gov/apod/ap001127.html)

The risks from sleep loss (acute total sleep deprivation and chronic, partial sleep restriction) manifest over the short, mid, and long term. In the short-term (minutes, hours, days), sleep loss degrades performance and leads to error, incident, and accident. In the mid-term (weeks, months), sleep loss degrades planning, strategizing, and making good life decisions. In the long-term (over years) sleep loss leads to weight gain, metabolic syndrome, type II diabetes, and inflammation and hypertension leading to cardiovascular disease. Further, sleep loss may lead to mild cognitive impairment, a precursor of Alzheimer's disease. We all accept that diet and exercise are important for performance, health, and well-being. It is time to add sleep to the list.

Fatigue: Operationally Defined

An operational definition of fatigue is crucial to good research because it defines how to measure fatigue. We measure fatigue both subjectively and objectively. Subjectively, we operationally define fatigue as a person reporting "I am tired" or endorsing the high end of a fatigue scale, e.g., the Samn-Perelli Fatigue Scale. Objectively, we operationally define fatigue as degraded performance. Performance can be measured by added metrics or embedded metrics. Added metrics are metrics extraneous to the task, e.g., the psychomotor vigilance task (PVT). The PVT is a reaction time test that is sensitive to attentional lapses and has other desirable psychometric properties [9–11]. The high rate of stimulus presentation makes the PVT unforgiving of even momentary lapses in attention and thus sensitive to total sleep deprivation and sleep restriction, circadian periodicity, and time on task (a component of workload), all of which affect vigilance performance. On the PVT, time on task effects can emerge in just a few minutes even in well-rested individuals.

Embedded metrics are metrics integrated into the work task itself, e.g., lane deviation in driving or flight operational quality assurance (FOQA) in commercial aviation. Embedded metrics have the advantage of face validity and of not interrupting the normal flow of work.

The Components of Fatigue

Laboratory and field studies indicate that fatigue is the final common pathway integrating the interacting effects of sleep/wake history (time awake, sleep loss), circadian rhythm (time of day), and workload (time on task, task intensity, and task complexity). There appear to be trait-like (enduring over time) individual differences in response to all three factors.

The Science of Circadian Rhythms

Figure 18.2 shows the circadian rhythm in core body temperature (Core Tb (deg)) over 24 h [12]. The circadian clock drives the circadian rhythm in humans and other animals. Anatomically, the circadian clock is in the suprachiasmatic nucleus in the hypothalamus deep in the brain. Genes control the period of this clock. Most humans have an intrinsic circadian rhythm of slightly more than 24 h. The circadian clock in the suprachiasmatic nucleus anticipates earth's rotational dynamics. The circadian clock is entrained (synchronized) by the light/dark cycle, specifically by light exposure. The retina of the eye contains specialized (nonvisual) receptors that are sensitive to blue light (they are literally "blue sky" detectors) [13]. There are circadian rhythms in core body temperature, performance, and sleep propensity. Normally, these rhythms are roughly in synchrony. Performance is better when body temperature is rising or high and worse when body temperature is falling or low. Conversely, it is easier to fall asleep and stay asleep when body temperature is falling or low and harder to fall asleep and stay asleep when body temperature is rising or high. The so-called window of circadian low (WOCL), roughly between the hours of 04:00 and 06:00, contains the low point in body temperature, the low point in performance, and the high point in sleep propensity.

The circadian clock in the suprachiasmatic nucleus in the hypothalamus, when synchronized to the light/dark cycle, serves to consolidate sleep during the light or dark period (depending on

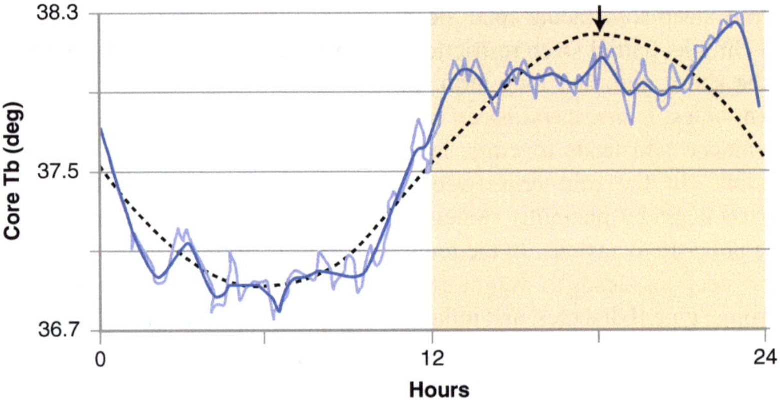

Fig. 18.2 The core body temperature as a marker of circadian rhythm (From Mistlberger and Rusak [12], Reprinted with permission from Elsevier)

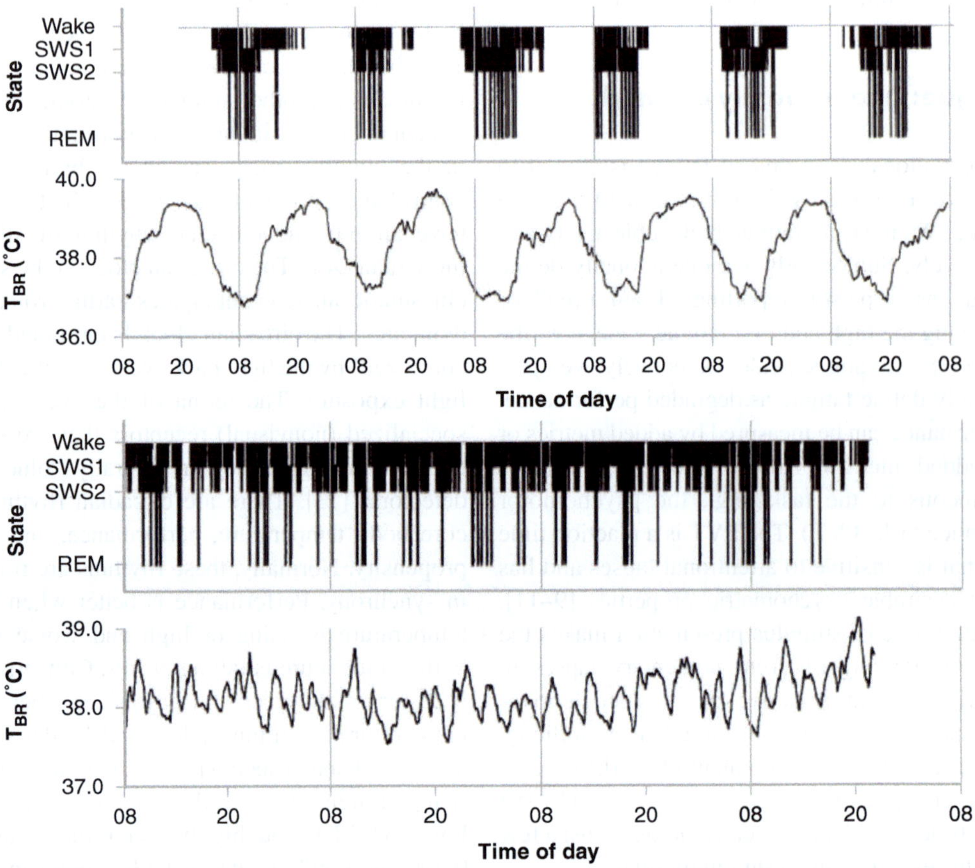

Fig. 18.3 The circadian rhythm consolidates sleep (Reprinted with permission from Edgar et al. [14])

whether the animal in question is nocturnal or diurnal). In the top half of Fig. 18.3, the graph shows the circadian rhythm in sleep (upper panel of top half) and core body temperature (lower panel of top half) in a monkey with an intact suprachiasmatic nucleus [14]. In this monkey, sleep consolidates in and around the low point in body temperature. In the bottom half of Fig. 18.3, the graph shows the loss of the circadian rhythm in sleep (upper panel of bottom half) and core body temperature (lower panel of bottom half) in a monkey whose suprachiasmatic nucleus has been selectively destroyed. In this monkey, there is no longer a circadian rhythm in body temperature and therefore sleep distributes itself evenly across the 24 h of the day/night cycle.

Individual Differences in Sensitivity to Sleep Loss

There are clear trait-like, enduring individual differences in sensitivity to sleep loss [15] (see Fig. 18.4). The left panel shows the average performance over 40 h of wakefulness of eight less-vulnerable individuals (triangles) and seven more-vulnerable individuals (circles). Demonstrating the persistence (and hence trait-like characteristics) of sensitivity and vulnerability, the right panel shows the consistency in sensitivity/vulnerability (compare the diamonds to the squares) from one sleep deprivation bout to another sleep deprivation bout 1 month later. Despite the differences in individual vulnerability of performance to sleep loss (see Fig. 18.5; left panel), this is not reflected in self-perceived subjective sleepiness (Fig. 18.5, right panel) [16]. Thus, one's own subjective sense of sleepiness is not a good predictor of how one is actually performing.

Furthermore, systematic, trait-like individual differences in phase angle and amplitude of circadian rhythm (e.g., morningness, eveningness, and age) may contribute to fatigue and are evident when measured by both self-report and by objective performance [17, 18].

Figure 18.6 further reinforces the concept of individual variations in response to sleep loss. One can see the average PVT response time (in black) for the 3-h sleep opportunity group in the sleep dose-response study [19]. Contrast this with the performance of individual subjects in this study. One subject, whose data are represented by the triangles, was unaffected by having the sleep opportunity restricted to 3 h/night. In further contrast to the average performance in the 3-h sleep opportunity group, the filled and unfilled diamonds represent data from two individuals who were more sensitive to sleep loss than the average. Further evidence of individual differences is found when comparing older and younger adults. When well-rested, younger individuals respond more quickly in a reaction time test than older individuals, but under conditions of sleep loss older individuals respond more quickly than younger ones [20].

Figure 18.7 shows performance measured as speed on the PVT. PVT speed is shown here as

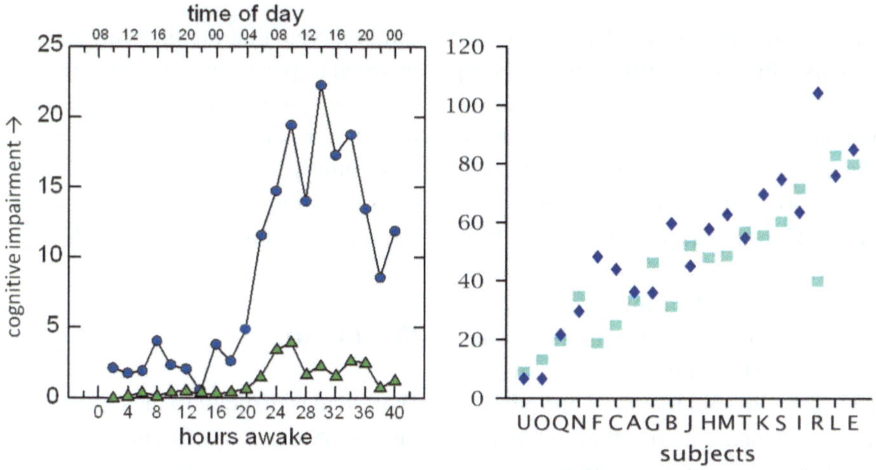

Fig. 18.4 Trait individual differences in vulnerability to performance impairment from sleep loss (Reprinted with permission from Van Dongen et al. [15])

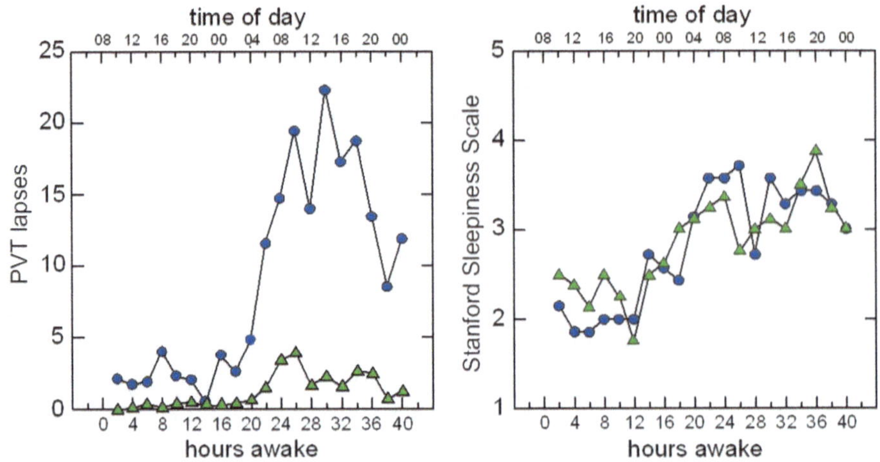

Fig. 18.5 Mismatch between subjective sleepiness and objective performance deficits during sleep deprivation (Reprinted with permission from Van Dongen et al. [16])

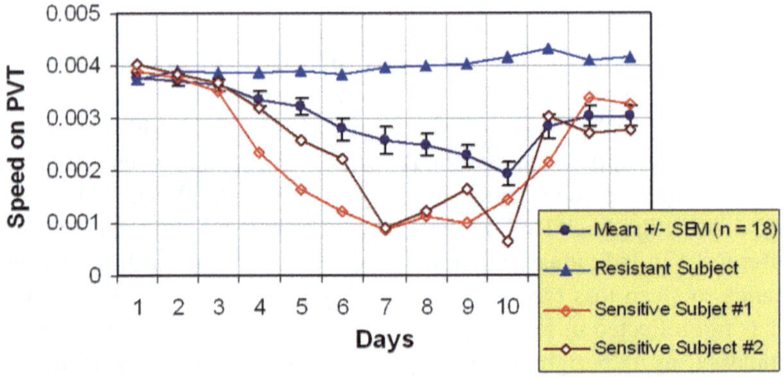

Fig. 18.6 Individual variability in resistance to sleep restriction based on PVT response time (From Balkin et al. [19])

the reciprocal of reaction time (1/reaction time (1/RT)) as it is affected by time awake (sleep loss), time of day (circadian rhythm), and time on task (a component of workload). In this study, 49 young healthy nonsmoking volunteers (mean age 22.4, range 18–30; 13 women) were deprived of sleep for over 42 h and tested on the PVT for 10 min at 2 h intervals [21]. We added some marks to Fig. 18.7 to aid in interpretation. The straight line approximates the overall linear effect of time awake (sleep loss) on performance (speed on the PVT). The sinusoidal curve approximates the effect of the circadian rhythm on performance. The minute-by-minute average speed on the 10 min PVT are pulled out and expanded (to equivalent scale) for the second PVT (after 1.5 h awake) and the thirteenth PVT (after 25.5 h awake). Note that the time on task effect (decline in speed of performance across the duration of the PVT) is evident even when the person is well-rested and is amplified after 24 h without sleep. In summary, the study depicted in the graph captures the time awake, time of day, and time on task interacting to create the fatigued state.

Workload

Workload is difficult to measure in the field or the laboratory due to an absence of an adequate operational definition. Time on task is an element of workload and some studies have defined workload in this way. Taking breaks during the shift can alleviate fatigue resulting from time on task

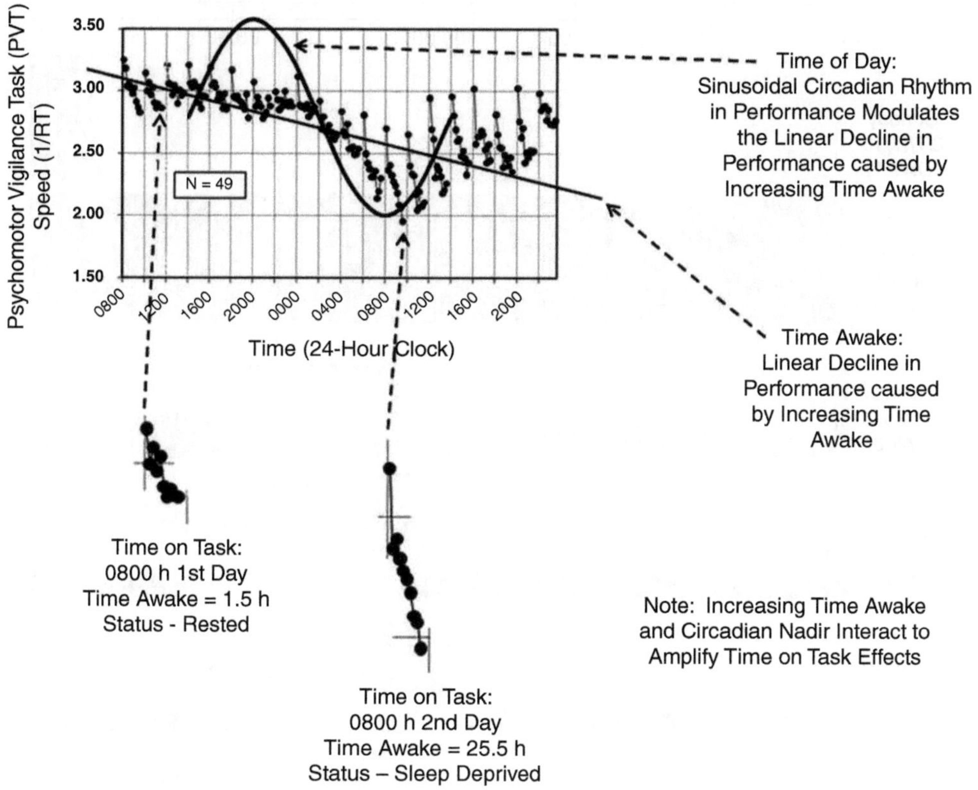

Fig. 18.7 Fatigue as the integration of sleep loss, circadian rhythm, and workload modified to highlight the interaction of time awake, time of day, and time on task (Modified with permission from Wesensten et al. [21])

and so recovery from time on task effects does not necessarily require sleep [22]. On the other hand, sleep is essential to remedy the decline in performance and fatigue associated with time awake [23]. The probability of an accident caused by fatigue is increased by working long hours or overtime shifts [24]. Task performance is influenced by the interaction of circadian phase, workload, and loss of sleep.

Executive Function

A study that looked at the effects of sleep deprivation on executive function found that sleep deprivation reduced accuracy and swiftness of task switching and saw an increase in errors compared to normal sleep. One night of recovery sleep was enough to reverse the effects of sleep deprivation on these tasks [25]. Sleep deprivation can reduce the ability to deal with unforeseen or difficult situations involving ambiguity, distractions, and evaluating risk. This appears to be a consequence of decline in "supervisory executive functions" of the prefrontal cortex [26]. For example, in aviation it would be expected that fatigue would be greater during a series of flights which have multiple take-offs and landings compared to a flight of the same length with only one take-off and landing. The multiple take-offs and landings in between the initial take-off and final landing would be expected to engage the prefrontal cortex more than flying the plane continuously at cruise for the same duration.

Field Measurement of Sleep and Performance

The scientific study of sleep and performance requires the objective measurement of sleep and performance. In the laboratory, we use polysomnography, the combination of electroencephalographic, electrooculographic, and

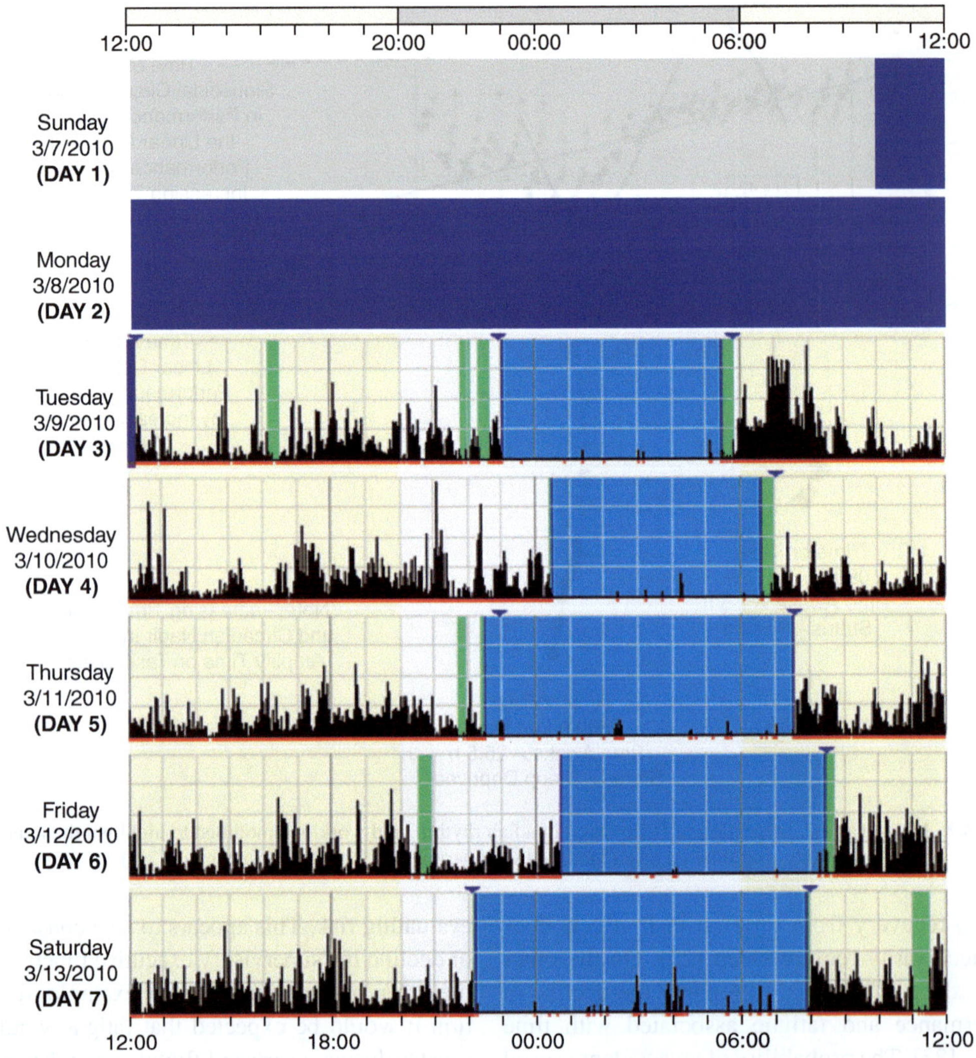

Fig. 18.8 Actigraphy data—*left* to *right* is noon to noon, *top* to *bottom* is days in sequence. Wake periods are determined by increased activity (*vertical black lines*); resting waking by *lime green* shading; sleep by *sky blue* shading

electromyographic recording, to determine the placement and duration of sleep periods as well as the stages of each sleep. In the field, we use actigraphy, the measurement of nondominant wrist movements summed in 1-min bins, to determine the placement and duration of main sleep and nap periods and to determine total sleep (the sum of main sleep plus naps) in 24 h.

The actigraph is an unobtrusive wristwatch-size device worn on the nondominant (usually left) wrist. Actigraphy uses limb movement to infer whether the person being studied is awake or asleep. It cannot, however, determine the stage of sleep. This measurement of total sleep time is considered adequate for fieldwork based on data suggesting that total sleep time in successive 24 h periods, not sleep stage distribution, determines recuperation from sleep loss [27]. The actigraph also has the virtue of being able to determine continuous sleep/wake history for up to 6 months in current models, enabling the examination of sleep in the context of work, community, family, and recreational activity and vice versa. Actigraphy can be used in combination with sleep diaries to accurately measure the sleep/wake history in an individual.

Figure 18.8 is a sleep/wake history as measured by a wrist actigraph. From left to right is a

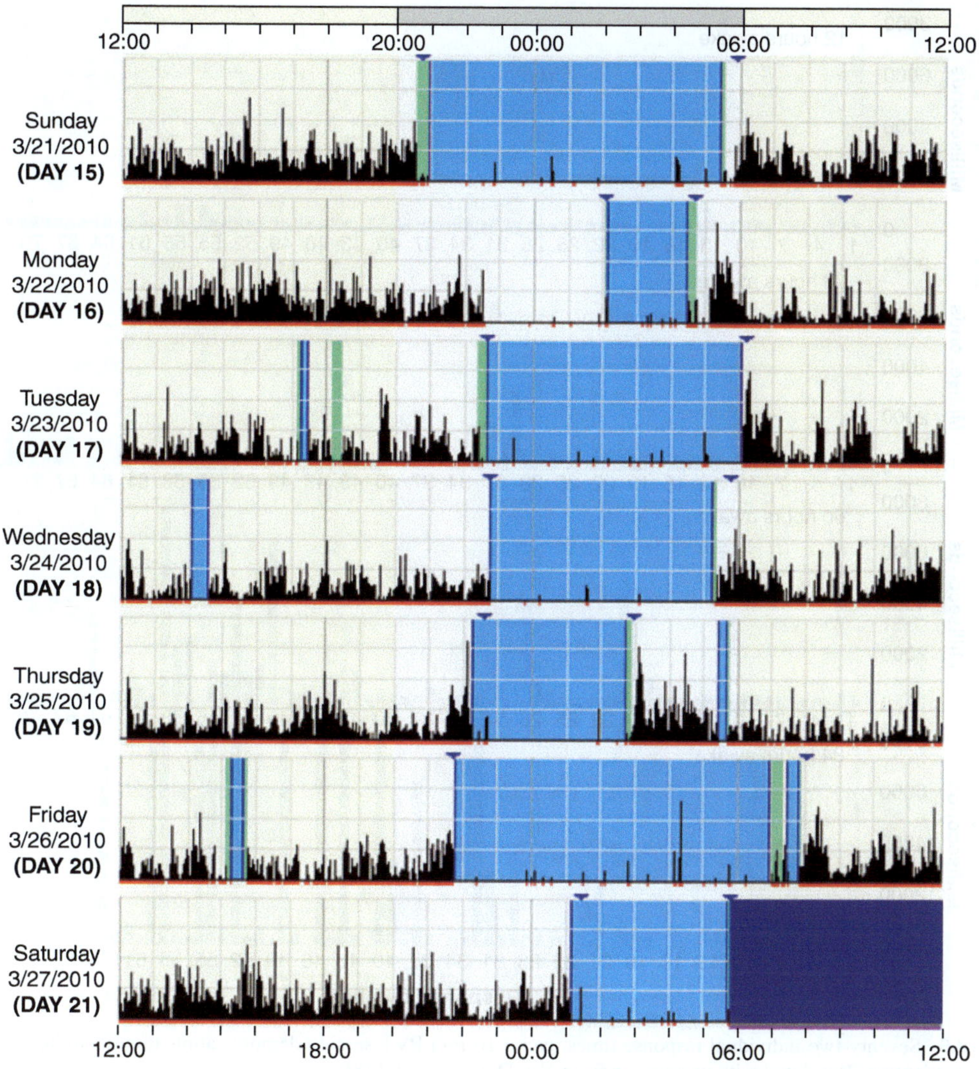

Fig. 18.8 (continued)

24-h period, measured from noon on one day to noon on the next day. Successive days run from top to bottom. The sky blue boxes indicate scored sleep by actigraphy. The lime green boxes indicate inactivity (rest) but not sleep. We excluded from analysis the dark blue areas at the beginning and end of the record as the actigraph software determined that the actigraph was off the volunteer's wrist during those intervals.

To measure performance in the laboratory, we use a battery of cognitive performance tests including tests of attention and vigilance, e.g., the PVT. For the field measurement of performance, we have programmed the PVT on a smartphone. In a typical smartphone implementation, the study participant holds the smartphone in his/her hands and focuses attention on the screen. When the required stimulus (e.g., a bull's eye) appears, the participant responds by pressing the designated button. The time it takes for the participant to press the button after seeing the stimulus, the latency to the button press, is the participant's score on that presentation. Typically, a well-rested, undistracted person will respond in 250 ms.

The PVT has other useful psychometric properties. For example, performance on the PVT is

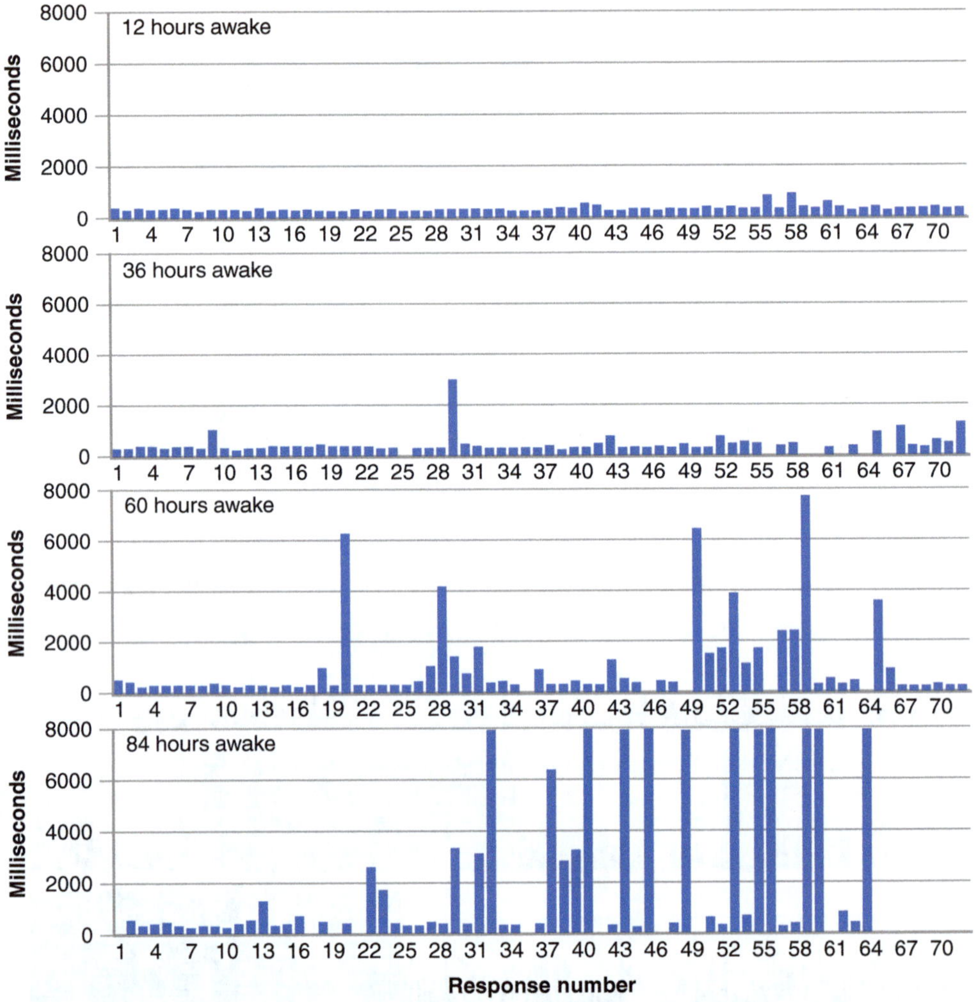

Fig. 18.9 Seventy-two individual response times over a 10-min PVT session demonstrating attentional lapses during sleep deprivation (Reprinted with permission from Van Dongen et al. [28])

independent of IQ and there is virtually no improvement through learning beyond a few practice sessions.

Figure 18.9 depicts attentional lapses in a single person across the 10 min of a PVT after 12 h awake, 36 h awake, and 60 h awake. Note that this is the response-by-response time in milliseconds for each stimulus presented across the 10 min of the PVT [28]. A slight increase in response latency is evident even during the PVT at 12 h awake indicating a time on task effect degradation of performance even when well-rested. Longer response latency becomes increasingly evident at 36 h awake and 60 h awake. Conversely, performance for the first ten or so randomly presented stimuli does not change across increasing sleep deprivation. Time-on-task unmasks the underlying sleepiness and degraded performance.

Our team has used the PC-based PVT in a laboratory study of the relative effectiveness of sleep that is either split or consolidated in sustaining performance. We have used the smartphone-based PVT in field studies of sleep during ultra-long-range flights in commercial aviation and in field studies of sleep during types of motorcoach operations. Currently, we are using the smartphone-based PVT in field studies of sleep and performance during flights with multiple take-offs and landings

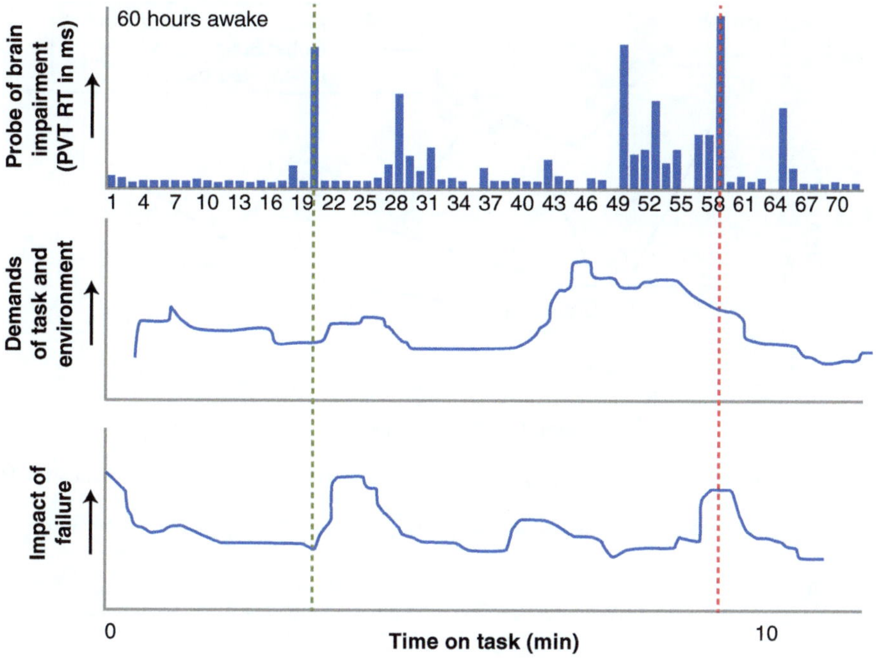

Fig. 18.10 Framework for relating PVT to predict workplace risk: the risk is greatest at the intersection of PVT lapses, increased demand, and increased impact of failure (*red line*). In the absence of this combination, the risk might be less (*green line*) (Reprinted with permission from Van Dongen et al. [28])

in commercial aviation. Given this extensive use of the PVT in laboratory and field studies, the question that arises is how lapses on the PVT translate into errors, incidents, and accidents in actual operations. This is a particularly important area of research since PVT lapses are common in experimental sleep deprivation settings while errors, incidents, and accidents are rare in field settings. Figure 18.10 depicts what we think is happening in the field environment to turn lapses in attention into accidents [28]—when system demands for timely, accurate performance coincide with lapses in attention that is when errors, incidents, and accidents occur.

A sleep/wake history in itself, whether determined by polysomnography or actigraphy, is not enough to predict performance, as circadian rhythm phase, workload, and individual differences are all contributing factors, at times synergistic and at other times antagonistic. When the first actigraph was developed for field studies of sleep and performance at the Walter Reed Army Institute of Research, the novel technological wonder was presented to U.S. Army General Max Thurman. He harrumphed and said, "I do not care how much they sleep; I want to know how well they perform." This started the search for a way to encapsulate the known scientific factors underlying fatigue into a mathematical model predicting performance. This mathematical model would need to integrate at a minimum the effects of sleep/wake history and circadian rhythm phase in order to predict performance. The model inspired by General "Max" became the basis of a current, commercially available, and widely used sleep/performance prediction model—the Sleep, Activity, Fatigue, and Effectiveness/Fatigue Avoidance Scheduling Tool (SAFTE/FAST) [29].

Total Sleep Deprivation and Performance

Total sleep deprivation degrades performance and the circadian rhythm modulates this decline. Figure 18.11 shows the effects of 85 h

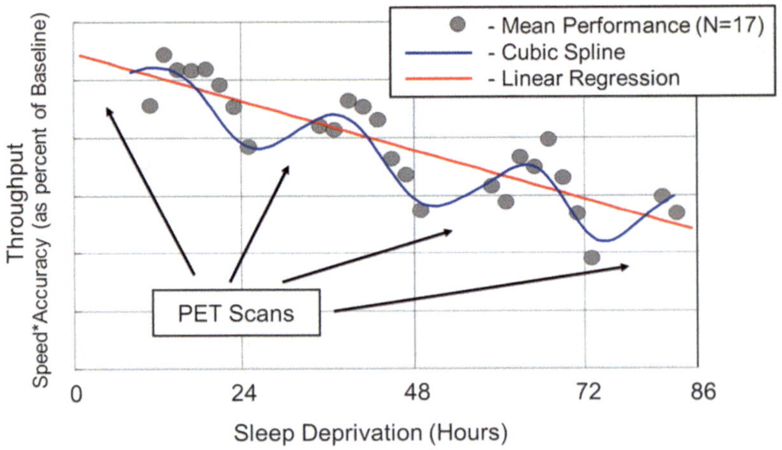

Fig. 18.11 Eighty-five hours of total sleep deprivation: effect on performance (Adapted with permission from Thomas et al. [29])

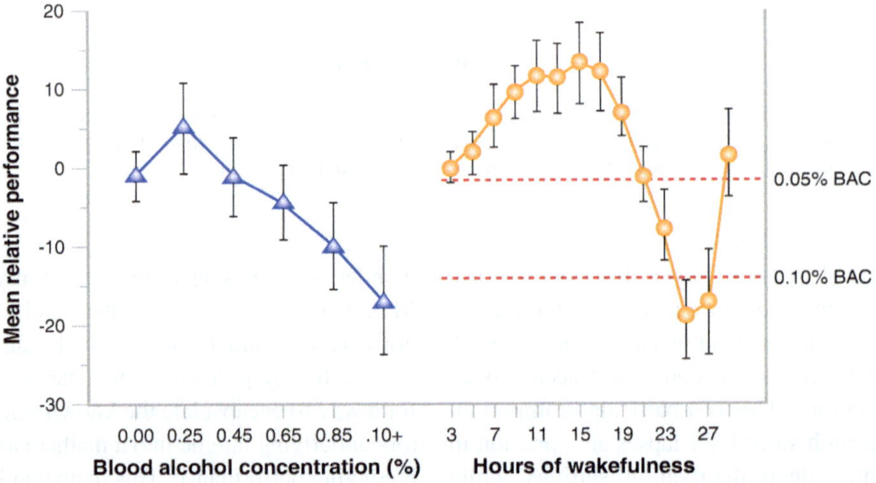

Fig. 18.12 Comparing the performance impact of sleep deprivation and alcohol intoxication (Reprinted with permission from Dawson and Redi [31])

of total sleep deprivation on performance in 17 volunteers, with performance measured as throughput—the product of speed and accuracy—on a serial addition/subtraction task [30]. The grey circles are the actual average performance data on the serial addition/subtraction task. The solid straight line shows the linear decline in performance across the 85 h of total sleep deprivation, with the decline in performance being approximately 17 % for each successive 24 h awake. The solid sinusoidal line shows that circadian rhythmicity modulates the linear decline in performance in a sinusoidal fashion.

Being 24 h sleep-deprived is, on some tasks, the equivalent of being legally drunk [31]. Figure 18.12 shows, in a study comparing the effects of varying levels of sleep deprivation with alcohol intoxication, that performance on a tracking task after having been awake for 24–27 h is similar to that seen when more than legally drunk (blood alcohol concentration greater than 0.10 %). In the United States, the standard for being legally drunk is blood alcohol concentration of 0.08 %.

Brain Imaging Studies of Sleep

One study examined regional brain activation using positron emission tomography (PET) and radiolabeled water as the tracer, during waking, NREM sleep, REM sleep, and subsequent waking [32] (see Fig. 18.13). Brain metabolism decreased by ~30 % from waking to NREM (slow wave) sleep and returned to waking levels in most brain regions (except the prefrontal cortex) with the transition from NREM to REM sleep. The prefrontal cortex (the most frontal of cortical areas) remains deactivated until 20–30 min after awakening, probably representing the neurophysiological basis underlying sleep inertia, the feeling of grogginess when first awakening in the morning or from a long nap.

Brain Imaging Studies of Total Sleep Deprivation

In order to characterize the changes in brain activation accompanying sleep deprivation, 17 subjects were deprived of all sleep for 85 h [30]. PET was used with fluorodeoxyglucose (FDG) as a tracer to measure regional brain glucose uptake, a correlate of regional brain activation. Volunteers were scanned when rested, and after 24, 48, and 72 h of sleep deprivation. From well-rested to 24 h sleep deprivation there was a whole brain decrease in glucose uptake, and hence brain activation, of 6 %. Larger decreases of 12–14 % were found in regional brain activation in the prefrontal cortex, parietal association cortex, and thalamus. These brain areas are involved in anticipation, planning, and focused attention [30] (see Fig. 18.14).

Sleep Restriction and Performance

While fatigue is most obvious in the laboratory in the context of total sleep deprivation combined with adverse circadian phase and high workload, in real world operations, total sleep deprivation is rare. A more common problem is chronic sleep restriction. Sleep restriction refers to sleeping less than the optimal 8 h of sleep/24 h, but still getting some sleep, over days and weeks. Many adults in North America are chronically sleep-restricted, sleeping on average around 6 h/night, with slightly more or less sleep depending on gender and ethnicity [33]. To provide data for the

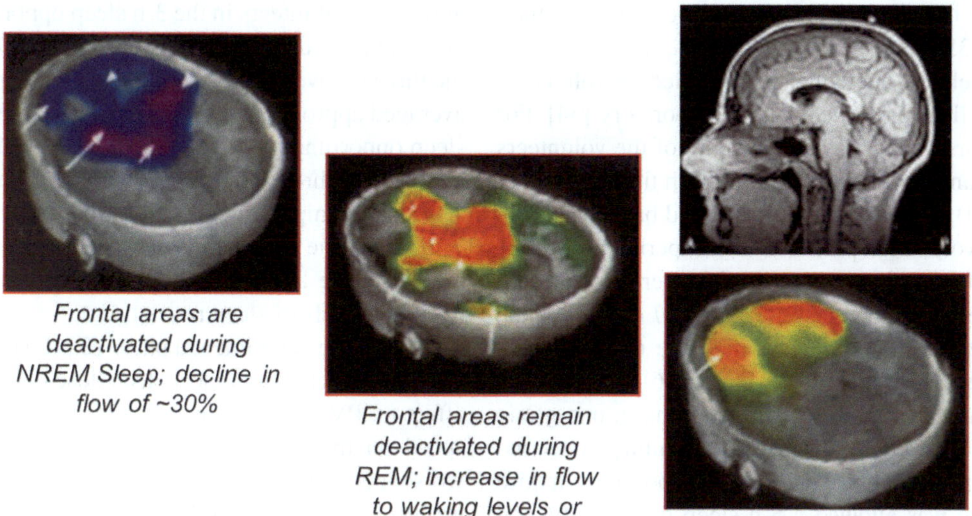

Fig. 18.13 Brain metabolism during NREM (slow wave) and REM sleep (Reprinted with permission from Braun et al. [32])

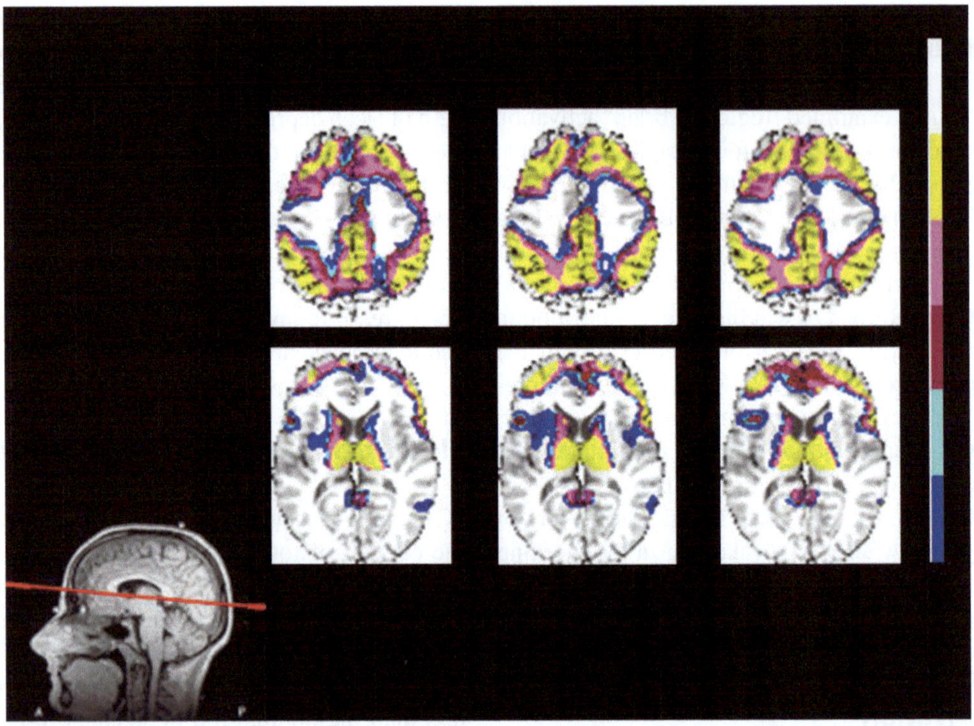

Fig. 18.14 Brain metabolism at 24, 48, and 72 h of sleep deprivation showing changes from well-rested baseline, color-coded to reflect *z*-score increases (Reprinted with permission from Thomas et al. [30])

development of mathematical models predicting performance from sleep/wake history, the effects of different degrees of sleep restriction over days were investigated in a sleep dose-response study [34, 35].

Belenky and colleagues studied 68 volunteers who lived for 2 weeks in the laboratory [34]. For the first 3 days (adaptation), all of the volunteers had an 8-h sleep opportunity (8 h time in bed per night). During the adaptation and baseline phase, the volunteers practiced the experimental tasks. On the fourth day, baseline data were collected on the experimental tasks. The next 7 days were the experimental phase in which the 68 volunteers were divided into four groups of 16–18 volunteers each. During the experimental phase, one group was allowed a 9-h sleep opportunity, a second group was allowed a 7-h sleep opportunity, a third group was allowed a 5-h sleep opportunity, and the fourth group was allowed a 3-h sleep opportunity on each of the nights of the experimental phase. Volunteers in the 9-h sleep opportunity group averaged 7.9 h of sleep each night, volunteers in the 7-h sleep opportunity group averaged 6.3 h of sleep each night, volunteers in the 5-h sleep opportunity group averaged 4.7 h of sleep each night, and volunteers in the 3-h sleep opportunity group averaged 2.9 h of sleep each night. During the three recovery nights, volunteers in all groups averaged approximately 7 h sleep during their 8-h sleep opportunity. All volunteers were awakened at 07:00 h throughout all phases of the study. Thus, the manipulation of sleep opportunity (3, 5, 7, or 9 h time in bed) during the 7-day experimental phase had the desired effect of creating different levels of sleep restriction.

During the experimental phase (E1–E7), it was found that there was a clear sleep dose-dependent effect on PVT performance. Figure 18.15 depicts speed on the PVT with lower speed indicating worse performance. The 9-h sleep opportunity group maintained stable performance across the days of the study. Performance in the 7-h sleep opportunity group declined over time while performance in the 5-h sleep opportunity group declined even more. Performance in the 3-h sleep

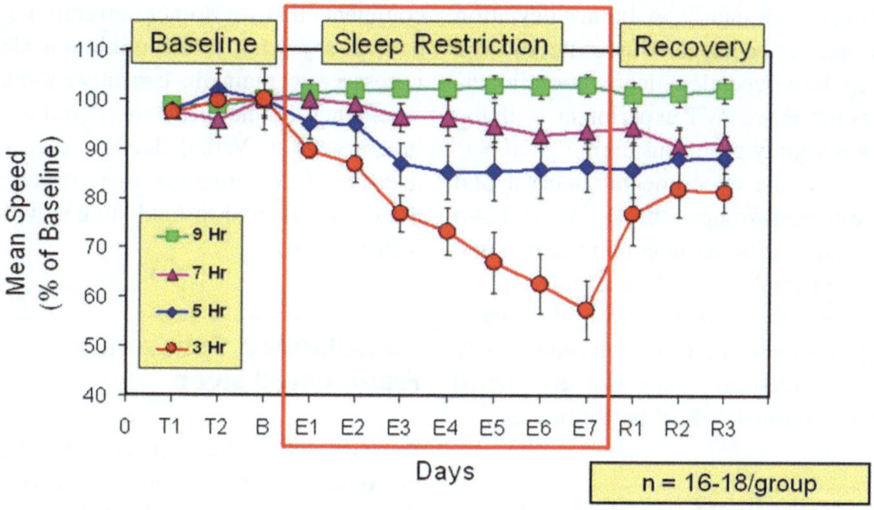

Fig. 18.15 Psychomotor vigilance task (PVT) performance speed during sleep restriction (From Belenky et al. [34])

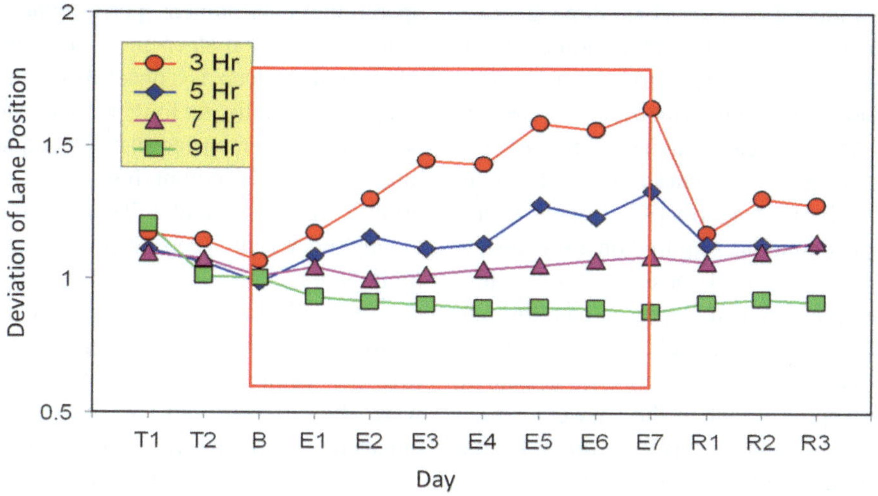

Fig. 18.16 Lane deviation while driving in the driving simulator during sleep restriction and recovery (From Balkin et al. [19])

opportunity group declined the most. Both the 5- and 7-h sleep opportunity groups appeared to decline over the first few days and then show stable, although degraded, performance on the PVT. In contrast, the 3-h sleep opportunity group continued to decline across the 7 days of the experimental interval. None of the three conditions of sleep restriction recovered to baseline performance levels during the recovery period (R1–R3). These findings suggest that if a person gets more than 4 h time in bed/night the brain can adjust and will, after a few days, stabilize at a lower level of performance, and that full performance recovery with return to normal 8 h time in bed per night may take more than 3 days [34].

Balkin and colleagues [19] reported on the same study the findings for driving simulator performance. The volunteers were all professional drivers holding commercial driver's licenses (CDLs). The performance findings were similar for the driving simulator as for the PVT (see Fig. 18.16). Lane deviation was measured as the driving performance metric. A higher deviation indicates worse performance. The results showed similar sleep dose-dependent degradation in performance as the above PVT experiment, with the 9-h sleep opportunity group sustaining good performance across the experimental interval and the sleep-restricted groups (the 7-, 5-, and 3-h sleep opportunity groups) degrading across the experimental interval (E1–E7). In addition, similar to the PVT experiment above, the sleep-restricted groups, when allowed 8 h time in bed/night during the recovery period (R1–R3), failed to recover to baseline levels of performance.

Executive Thinking Versus Logical Thinking and Performance

The highest mental operations are dependent on the prefrontal cortex of the brain and consist of logical thinking (deductive, critical reasoning) and executive thinking (innovative, creative thinking) [35]. Logical thinking is remarkably resistant to sleep loss, whereas executive thinking is more sensitive to sleep loss [35]. Logical thinking, the typical thinking required on an IQ test, is applicable when all of the possible answers to a problem are presented and a person can, through a systematic, logical approach, deduce which of the presented alternatives is correct. Executive thinking is applicable when the answers cannot be deduced easily and there is irrelevant information intertwined with the necessary information, requiring the person to distinguish signal from noise. Executive thinking enables the individual to update and change plans or solutions if new information is presented during the process of planning or answering the question(s) at hand. Success in operational settings is dependent on effective executive thinking that in turn depends on obtaining adequate sleep. Whether caffeine or other stimulant drugs can mitigate the effects of sleep loss on executive function is an open question. Horne [36], however, found that the executive thinking during sleep loss was degraded and did not substantially improve after the administration of caffeine. This was the case even though subjective sleepiness was reduced. Horne [36] comments that we do not currently have enough data to say what is the minimum sleep length necessary to maintain executive thinking in an emergency, but he speculates that it is at least 4 h in every 24 h. Verbal fluency tests are a good measure of executive function; however, they are not easily adapted to field studies with repeated measures [9].

Consolidated, Split, and Fragmented Sleep

As indicated earlier, operational fatigue is the outcome of the interaction of sleep loss, circadian rhythm phase, and workload. In addition, sleep loss is not simply acute total sleep deprivation but also chronic sleep restriction. Similarly, in the operational environment, performance is largely a function of total sleep in 24 h, irrespective of whether that sleep is consolidated in one long sleep bout or split. As long as total sleep in 24 h is adequate, a person can sustain adequate performance. A study comparing a no nap group, 10-min nap group, and a 30-min nap group following nocturnal sleep restriction showed the group that had no nap following sleep restriction showed a plateau or decline of performance in the objective and subjective alertness measures over the testing period [38]. The subjects who were allowed a 10-min nap showed subsequent enhancement in cognitive performance and subjective alertness throughout the hour following the napping. Conversely, after taking a 30-min nap alertness and performance seemed to deteriorate; however, some improvement was shown towards the end of testing. This decline in performance for the 30-min nap group could have been due to sleep inertia [38].

Figure 18.17 is a view from the flight deck of a commercial jetliner flying over the North Pole from the U.S. to China. Flight crew performance in such long-range flights depends on sleep obtained before the flight, during the flight, during the layover, and during the return flight making this the ideal venue for the study of fatigue and fatigue risk management. In-flight sleep and layover sleep are often not taken in a

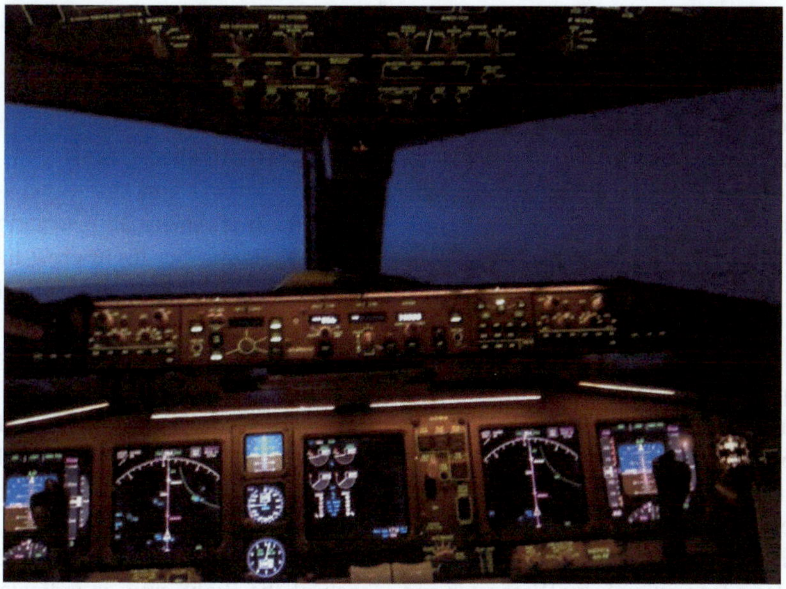

Fig. 18.17 View from the flight deck of a Boeing 777 while flying over the North Pole from Newark, New Jersey to Hong Kong, China

consolidated block but split into main sleep and one or two naps.

Studies have shown that under conditions of overall sleep restriction, split sleep is as restorative as consolidated sleep [39, 40]. These findings [39, 40] on the value of short duration sleep are supported by studies of controlled napping in-flight on the flight deck in commercial aviation pilots [41]. On trips back and forth over the Pacific Ocean, a single 40-min nap opportunity on the flight deck improved performance during the subsequent landing. The 40-min nap opportunity on average yielded approximately 26 min of actual sleep.

Sleep can range from consolidated (one sleep bout/24 h), through split (two or three sleep bouts/24 h), to fragmented (punctuated by awakenings every 2–3 min) [42]. Whereas split sleep can retain its recuperative value, fragmented sleep loses its recuperative value. The cross over point at which a bout of sleep appears to sustain the same recuperative value minute by minute as fully consolidated sleep appears to be about 20 min. Thus, if sleep is fragmented, broken by a brief awakening, every 20 min (three times an hour) its minute-by-minute recuperative value will be the same as it is for fully consolidated sleep, e.g., 8 h of continuous sleep. However, as fragmentation increases in frequency recuperative value erodes (see Fig. 18.18).

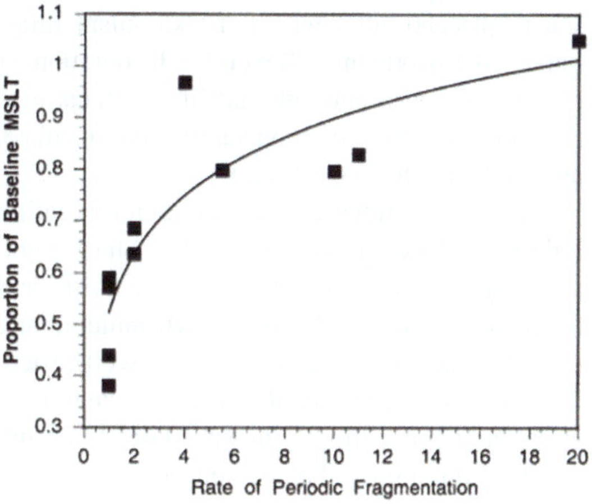

Fig. 18.18 Actigraphy data—*left* to *right* is noon to noon, *top* to *bottom* is days in sequence; active waking is shown by absence of *lime green* or *sky blue* shading, resting waking by *lime green* shading, and sleep by *sky blue* shading. *Dark blue* at the beginning and end indicates that the actigraph was off wrist. (**a**) Actigraph L, (**b**) Actigraph R (From Bonnet and Arand [42], Reprinted with permission from Elsevier)

Mitigating Strategies

Ample sleep opportunity and effective use of the opportunity at periods of higher circadian sleep propensity is the most effective way to overcome fatigue. When this is not possible, taking advantage of sleep opportunities at periods of lower circadian sleep propensity can be helpful. If sleep is elusive for whatever reason, a temporary solution can be found in the use of sleep-inducing drugs. If sleep is not possible, stimulants may be used to maintain performance temporarily in spite of sleep loss and/or when working during the circadian trough.

One of the few studies comparing the relative effects of different stimulant drugs under conditions of total sleep deprivation is by Wesensten and colleagues [44]. In this study, a drug (d-amphetamine, caffeine, modafinil, or placebo) was given to a volunteer a little before midnight after 65 h of total sleep deprivation. For the first 2 h, in comparison to placebo, all three of the stimulant drugs improved performance. Beyond 2 h, duration of effects was consistent with half-life, with caffeine the shortest acting, d-amphetamine intermediate, and modafinil the longest acting.

Other countermeasures effective in mitigating fatigue include bright (especially blue) light, strict environmental control of light, noise, and temperature in the sleeping environment, and ensuring that workers arrive at work well-rested. The most effective countermeasures center on sleep and involve modifying schedules to ensure adequate duration and placement of sleep opportunity with respect to circadian rhythm and sleep propensity.

Another useful mitigating strategy is preloading sleep. Preloading sleep before periods of sleep restriction results in a swifter recovery after chronic sleep restriction [45]. Early starts that truncate sleep can affect alertness even days later. If pilots, for example, are anticipating a challenging flight, they need to ensure that they have preloaded (pre-augmented in terms of total duration) sleep in the days leading up to the flight. In the case of a night flight it may be wise to nap in the afternoon prior to the flight to ensure maximum sleep.

Sleep and Performance in Operations

The Guantanamo Crash

In the crash of American International Flight 808 at Guantanamo, the flight crew had been awake for at least 18 h prior to the crash. The flight crew chose the more difficult approach (hooked arrow) as opposed to the easier one (straight arrow) (see Fig. 18.19). The hard right banking turn is the more difficult approach because of the danger of stalling the right wing during the turn while avoiding Cuban airspace during the approach to the turn. Figure 18.20 shows the reconstructed sleep wake histories of the flight crew; sleep for each of the flight crew is indicated by the solid horizontal bars at the base of each of the three plots. The flight crew had been awake all night and was awake throughout the day up until the time of the crash a little after 16:00 h. The time of the crash is indicated on the figure by the large arrow. The sleep wake histories in Fig. 18.20 reconstructed during the accident investigation were used as inputs to the SAFTE/FAST sleep/performance prediction model to predict the effectiveness of the flight crew at the time of the crash [46] (see Fig. 18.20). For the Captain, who was the flying pilot, the predicted effectiveness at the time of the crash was 71 %. Figure 18.21 is a transcript of the conversation between the crew members as they approached the runway. The Captain's dialogue is bolded. The "strobe light" that the Captain is referring to is a marker on the ground that shows the boundary between American and Cuban airspace. In fact, although the Captain was not aware of it, the strobe was not working on this day. This transcript provides excellent insight into one of the cognitive deficits that characterizes sleep loss—perseveration, repeating the same failed or failing solution. Note that even though the Captain was clearly warned that his airspeed was dangerously slow, the Captain kept looking for the strobe rather than focusing on the primary task of flying the airplane. The Captain ignored the basics of aviation to—in order of priority—aviate, navigate, and

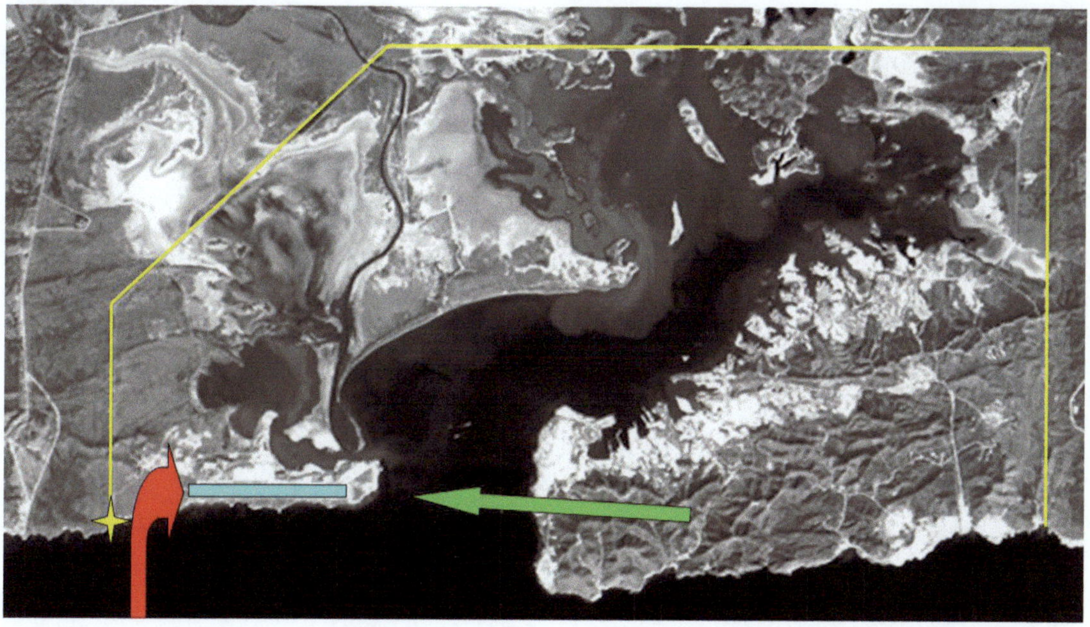

Fig. 18.19 Landing approaches at Guantanamo Bay, Cuba: the straight (*green*) approach versus curved (*red*) approach to the landing strip (*blue*)

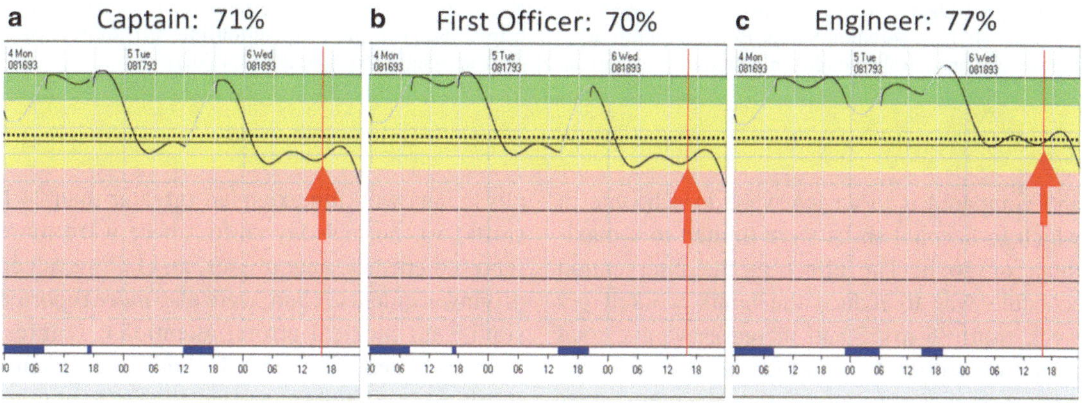

Fig. 18.20 Accident investigation—American International Flight 808 (SAFTE/FAST model) showing performance prediction at the time of the crash for the captain, copilot, and engineer; by the model predictions, all three members of the flight crew were moderately impaired. The colors represent relative impairment with *pink* indicating severe impairment, *yellow* indicating moderate impairment, and *green* indicating no impairment. The *horizontal dotted* represents the estimated threshold of serious accident risk

communicate. He was navigating rather than aviating. In trying to find the strobe light, the Captain was stuck perseverating instead of trying new possible solutions. Perseverating is a characteristic of the prefrontal cortical dysfunction associated with sleep loss.

Harvard Work Hours Health and Safety Group Studies

A Harvard group studied physicians in postgraduate training (interns and residents) in the traditional schedule that allows for 36-h shifts in the hospital

Engineer:	Slow, Airspeed
Co-Pilot:	Check the turn.
Captain:	**Where's the strobe?**
Co-Pilot:	Right over here.
Captain:	**Where?**
Co-Pilot:	Right inside there, right inside there.
Engineer:	You know, we're not gettin' our airspeed back there.
Captain:	**Where is the strobe?**
Co-Pilot:	Right down there.
Captain:	**I still don't see it.**
Engineer:	#, we're never goin' to make this.
Captain:	**Where do you see a strobe light?**
Co-Pilot:	Right over here.
Captain:	Gear, gear down, spoilers armed.
Engineer:	Gear down, three green spoilers, flaps, checklist
???:	*There you go, right there, lookin' good.*
Captain:	***Where's the strobe?***
Co-Pilot:	*Do you think you're gonna make this?*
Captain:	***Yeah... if I can catch the strobe light.***
Co-Pilot:	*500, you're in good shape.*
Engineer:	*Watch the, keep your airspeed up.*
Co-Pilot:	*140. [sound of stall warning]*
???:	*Don't – stall warning.*
Captain:	***I got it.***
Co-Pilot:	*Stall warning.*
Engineer:	*Stall Warning*
Captain:	***I got it, back off.***
???:	*Max power!*
???:	*There it goes, there it goes!*
???:	*Oh no!*

Fig. 18.21 Transcript of the conversation from the crew as they approached the runway at Guantanamo Bay (From US National Transportation Safety Board. Aircraft accident report: uncontrolled collision with terrain American International Airways Flight 808. Washington, DC: US National Transportation Safety Board; 1994. Available at http://libraryonline.erau.edu/online-full-text/ntsb/aircraft-accident-reports/AAR94-04.pdf)

and compared it to an intervention schedule in which in-hospital shifts were limited to a maximum of 16 h. The effect of the intervention schedule was to reduce the hours worked per week from 85 to 65 and increase average total sleep time from 6.6 to 7.4 h/24 h. Also, when on duty on the intervention schedule the participants had a lighter workload (fewer admissions, less patient days, and increased distribution of work to non-intern providers) [47, 48]. The intervention schedule had dramatic effects by reducing serious medical errors from 136/1,000 patient days to 100/1,000 patient days. There was an even more dramatic selective decrease in diagnostic errors. Diagnostic errors were reduced from 18.6/1,000 patient days to 3.3/1,000 patient days, a more than fivefold reduction. Other studies by the same group complemented these findings of the differences between the traditional and intervention schedule with survey data. In postdoctoral physicians working extended (greater than 24 h shifts) vs. normal day shifts, there were more reported crashes, near misses, and falling asleep driving accidents. There were also more reported significant medical errors, attentional failures, fatigue-related preventable adverse events resulting in a fatality, and needle stick injuries with the physicians working the extended shifts [49–51].

The Crash of Comair 5191

In the Comair 5191 crash in Lexington, KY, the flight crew became misoriented to the topography of the airport and the Air Traffic Controller did not correct their error. They attempted to take off from the wrong runway, a general aviation runway that was much too short for their aircraft. The plane crashed at the end of the runway killing

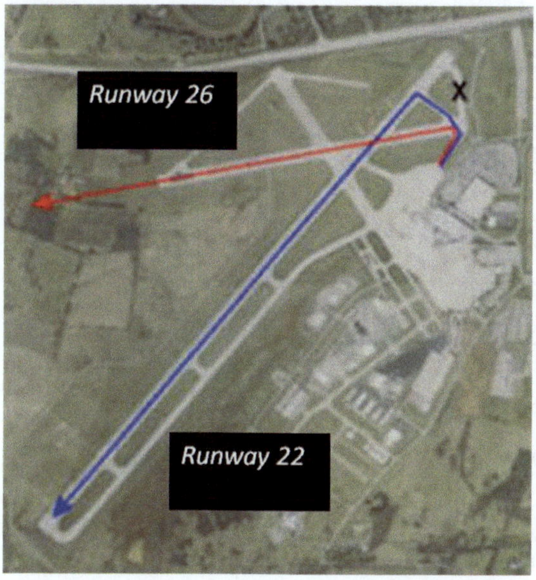

Fig. 18.22 Aerial view of the airport with both the correct taxi and runway (Runway 22) and the incorrect taxi and runway marked (Runway 26) (http://en.wikipedia.org/wiki/Comair_Flight_191)

all but one on board. Figure 18.22 is an aerial photograph of the airport with both the correct taxi and runway (Runway 22) and the incorrect taxi and runway (Runway 26) marked. The flight crew lined up the aircraft on Runway 26. Comair 5191 crashed at approximately 06:00 h. The Air Traffic Controller had worked an early morning shift the day before (06:30–14:30 h). He had the mandated by regulation 8 h off and went back on duty at 23:30 h. He was scheduled to work through to 07:00 h the morning of the crash. Thus, he was sleep-deprived and working at an adverse circadian phase at the time of the crash. The Captain and First Officer had an early start restricting their total sleep opportunity and were working at an adverse circadian phase. Thus, the Air Traffic Controller and the Captain and First Officer were sleep-deprived and working at an adverse circadian phase at the time of the crash. While we cannot say definitively that fatigue played a role in the choice of the wrong runway, it seems likely that if the personnel involved had been less fatigued (a function of sleep loss and adverse circadian phase) they might have realized the error in time to correct it [52].

Models Predicting Performance

At its most basic, performance is dependent on sleep/wake history and circadian phase. Mathematical models that predict performance and sleep/wake history are thus generally two-process models. An example of a two-process model is the SAFTE/FAST model, which is currently used in commercial applications.

Customizability is an important aspect in fatigue modeling. Sleep tactics, habitual sleep length, equipment malfunctions and failures, transfer times, unexpected delays, longer flight duration (e.g., from prevailing winds), and variations in the instrument landing systems are all factors that should be taken into account when customizing a fatigue model (in this instance for the aviation industry).

In modeling performance, the diurnal type (morning type—prefer to get up early and go to bed early vs. evening type—prefer to get up late and stay up late) of the individual should be taken into consideration and used as a basis for scheduling, as evening types tolerate night-shift work better than morning types [53]. Also, current models do not take into account the possibility of the presence of sleep disorders in the population being modeled but hopefully this information will be integrated into future models.

Another limitation of the current models is the use of "bright lines" such as the 77.5 used in the SAFTE/FAST model. In theory, a bright line is the point above which the individual is "safe" and below which the risk of an error, incident, or accident in an operational setting is greatly increased. In reality, risk increases gradually with both increasing blood alcohol concentration and increasing sleep loss. Whether considering blood alcohol levels or sleep loss, these bright lines are convenient fictions simplifying reality and enforcement. Relative numbers that take into account a linear progression with incremental changes or comparing schedules (for example, comparing a schedule where the safety is unknown to a schedule that is known to be safe) are alternatives to bright lines.

Model verification, validation, and certification should be conducted by a neutral third party

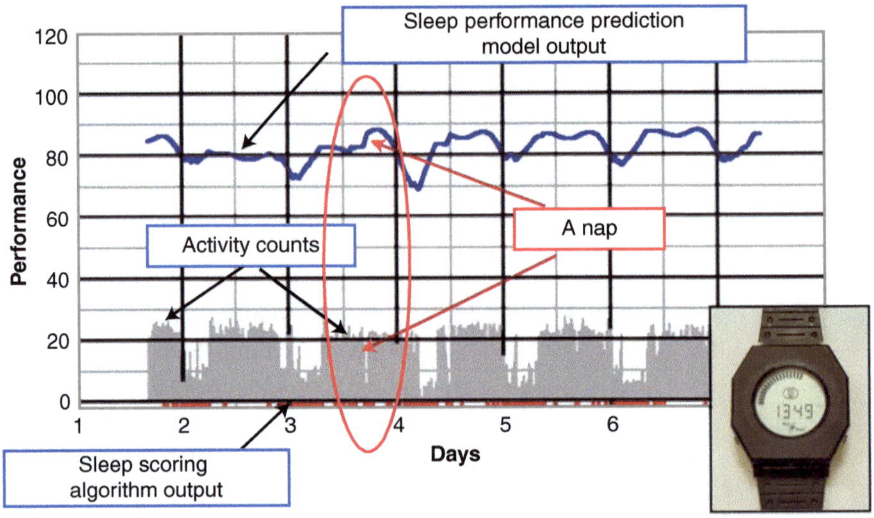

Fig. 18.23 Predicting performance from actigraphically derived sleep/wake history

rather than left to the modelers themselves. Models can predict performance based on objectively measured sleep/wake history or (as is the case with some models) the model can first estimate placement and quantity of sleep and use this to provide the sleep/wake history input to the main performance prediction module of the model. In general, two-process models using objectively measured sleep/wake history are reliable in predicting relative performance, e.g., the safety/performance of one schedule vs. another. In contrast, models that use as inputs model-generated sleep estimates are not as reliable.

In Fig. 18.23, we see a prediction of human performance based on actigraphically measured sleep/wake history and estimated circadian phase. Plotted as vertical lines is the raw actigraph record (activity counts; arm movements summed in 1-min bins). Plotted as horizontal bars just below the actigraph record is the sleep/wake history scored from the actigraph record (sleep scoring algorithm output). Plotted in the upper portion of the graph is the sleep/performance prediction model output. Note the actigraphically recorded nap (break in vertical lines) and the increase in the predicted performance subsequent to it (curve in upper graph).

In the future, we will have objective measures of sleep/wake history, accurate measures of circadian phase, and validated sleep/performance prediction models integrated into rostering and scheduling software, providing fatigue-mitigating schedules and enabling turn-key fatigue risk management.

Observations on Working the Night Shift

The typical night-shift worker will get off work in the morning, commute home, and then sleep well for 4–5 h. However, around 13:00 h the typical night-shift worker will wake up because his/her circadian rhythm is increasingly stimulating wakefulness as his/her homeostatic drive for sleep is diminishing. Thus, the interaction of the two processes (homeostatic drive for sleep; circadian drive for wakefulness) will, in night-shift workers, effectively truncate daytime off-duty sleep to around 5 h. In complementary fashion, when going on shift in the evening the night-shift worker initially performs well as body temperature is high and he/she has not yet had extended hours awake. However, performance rapidly decreases across the night shift as the circadian drive for alertness diminishes in the early morning hours and the drive for sleep increases with increasing time awake. Again, performance improves when body temperature is rising or high and sleep propensity is greater when body temperature is falling or low.

The New Science of Fatigue Risk Management

We are entering an age in which we will increasingly embed ourselves in robotic systems that monitor us, assist us, and sustain us [54]. The flight deck of a modern commercial jet aircraft is suggestive of such an environment, with radio traffic to air traffic control, text messages to and from airline headquarters, and streaming telemetry to ground stations, all in the service of a safe and timely flight. A component of these evolving robotic systems will be personal biomedical status monitoring, including actigraphic assessment of sleep/wake history and assessment by some technology yet to be determined of circadian rhythm phase angle and amplitude. These quantitative assessments will serve as input to mathematical models encapsulating sleep science and predicting performance. Such models will be validated against metrics of operational performance including both embedded (e.g., FOQA) and added (e.g., PVT) metrics. Validated model predictions for individuals in an operational environment can be integrated into the rostering and scheduling software while being optimized against other constraints (e.g., flight duty time limitations, labor management agreements, etc.) to provide turn-key fatigue risk management [55].

Full integration of fatigue risk management into rostering and scheduling software will likely depend upon the development of ubiquitous, personal biomedical status monitoring. Such personal biomedical status monitoring would involve: (1) the measurement of sleep and waking (sleep/wake history) to detect sleep loss and to sum up sleep obtained in every 24 h, probably by means of actigraphy; (2) the measurement of circadian rhythm phase and amplitude by some technology yet to be developed; and (3) the use of these metrics as inputs to a mathematical model predicting performance. The predictions could be validated against measures of real world performance such as FOQA in commercial aviation or lane deviation in commercial trucking. These metrics and models would be integrated into the optimization function of commercially available rostering and scheduling software (e.g., Carmen) so schedules would minimize fatigue [55].

Fatigue risk management should be embedded within the corporate structure of safety management, as it is a safety management system. In one conceptualization, a fatigue risk management system (FRMS) is a multi-tiered, defense in depth against fatigue risk [23]. Tier 1 uses computer-based rostering and scheduling with integrated predictive modeling ensuring that there is adequate opportunity for sleep propensity both in terms of duration and in terms of placement with respect to the circadian rhythm. Tier 2 uses self-report and the wrist-worn actigraph to ensure that personnel make adequate use of the sleep opportunity available. Tier 3 uses self-report, coworker report, and added (e.g., PVT) and embedded (e.g., FOQA) objective performance metrics to ensure that, given the opportunity for sleep and the use made of it, the person has the ability to perform well.

Summary and Conclusions

The operational environment is one in which human performance is critical and failure consequential. Extended work hours and shift work are common in operational environments and those who "own the night" are forced to confront the problems of staffing it and dealing with fatigue.

Fatigue, defined subjectively by self-report and objectively by degraded performance, is a function of the interaction of sleep loss (sleep deprivation; sleep restriction), the circadian rhythm in performance and sleep propensity, and workload. How sleep loss, adverse circadian phase, and high workload degrade performance remains a fundamental mystery in human and general mammalian neurobiology. There are tantalizing hints that sleep loss decreases neuronal firing in the brain as measured by brain energy consumption and that recuperation during sleep is associated with a general reduction in neuronal firing and brain metabolism in particular in the prefrontal cortex—the seat of anticipation, planning, and the integration of reason and emotion.

From a behavioral standpoint, sleep restriction degrades performance in a sleep dose-dependent manner with even mild sleep restriction degrading performance over days. Obtaining sufficient sleep in a 24 h period is crucial to sustaining performance both short and long term. For equivalent total sleep time, sleep split into two or three sleep bouts appears to be as recuperative as more consolidated sleep. In contrast, fragmented sleep (sleep interrupted more frequently than every 20 min) loses recuperative value with increasing in fragmentation. Studies in the 24/7 workplace (e.g., the Harvard studies of physicians in post-graduate training) indicate that increased sleep opportunity improves performance, particularly performance depending on complex mental processes, e.g., medical diagnosis.

Fatigue results in error, incident, or accident when a fatigue-induced lapse in attention coincides with a workplace demand for good performance. This is where a FRMS comes into play. Fatigue risk management has both short and long-term objectives. The short-term objective is to reduce the immediate fatigue risk [43]. The long-term objective is to improve health and well-being across a person's working life, particularly in terms of reducing obesity, insulin resistance, metabolic syndrome, type II diabetes, hypertension, cardiovascular disease, and cognitive decline [56, 57]. The science of fatigue and sleep can be instantiated into mathematical models predicting performance from sleep/wake history, circadian phase, and workload. Models incorporating the first two factors (two-process models) are already in commercial use. Such models are being integrated into existing industrial strength rostering and scheduling software enabling turn-key fatigue risk management. In such a turn-key system, the model would replace prescriptive hours of service regulations and labor management agreements. In fatigue risk management, the mathematical model becomes the regulatory rule.

References

1. Lindbergh CA. The spirit of Saint Louis. New York, NY: Scribner; 1953. p. 233.
2. Churchill WS. The gathering storm. New York, NY: Houghton Mifflin Company; 1948. p. 375.
3. Marshall SLA. The soldier's load and the mobility of a nation. Quantico, VA: The Marine Corps Association; 1980. p. 48.
4. Wikipedia [Internet]. 2012. http://en.wikipedia.org/wiki/John_Boyd_(military_strategist)
5. Perrow C. Normal accidents: living with high risk technologies. Princeton, NJ: Princeton University Press; 1999. p. 334.
6. Weick KE, Sutcliffe KM. Managing the unexpected: resilient performance in an age of uncertainty. 2nd ed. San Francisco, CA: Willey; 2007. p. 2.
7. Mayhew C, Simmon R. (NASA/GSFC), NOAA/GSFC, DMSP Digital Archive [Internet]. 2000. http://apod.nasa.gov/apod/ap001127.html
8. Greenspan RJ, Tononi G, Cirelli C, Shaw PJ. Sleep and the fruit fly. Trends Neurosci. 2001;24(3):142–6.
9. Balkin TJ, Bliese PD, Belenky G, Sing H, Thorne DR, Thomas M, et al. Comparative utility of instruments for monitoring sleepiness-related performance decrements in the operational environment. J Sleep Res. 2004;13(3):219–27. PubMed PMID: WOS:000223642500003. English.
10. Dorrian J, Rogers NL, Dinges DF. Psychomotor vigilance performance: neurocognitive assay sensitive to sleep loss. In: Kushida CA, editor. Sleep deprivation: clinical issues, pharmacology, and sleep loss effects. New York, NY: Marcel Dekker; 2005. p. 39–70.
11. Dinges DF, Powell JW. Microcomputer analyses of performance on a portable, simple visual RT task during sustained operations. Behav Res Meth Instr. 1985;17(6):652–5.
12. Mistlberger RE, Rusak B. Circadian rhythms in mammals: formal properties and environmental influences. In: Kryger M, Roth T, Dement WC, editors. Principles and practice of sleep medicine. 5th ed. St. Louis, MO: Elsevier Saunders; 2011. p. 363–75.
13. Dacey DM, Lee BB. The 'blue-on' opponent pathway in primate retina originates from a distinct bistratified ganglion cell type. Nature. 1994;367:731–5.
14. Edgar DM, Dement WC, Fuller CA. Effect of SCN lesions on sleep in squirrel-monkeys—evidence for opponent processes in sleep wake regulation. J Neurosci. 1993;13(3):1065–79.
15. Van Dongen HPA, Baynard MD, Maislin G, Dinges DF. Systematic interindividual differences in neurobehavioral impairment from sleep loss: evidence of trait-like differential vulnerability. Sleep. 2004;27(3):423–33.
16. Van Dongen HPA, Maislin G, Dinges DF. Dealing with inter-individual differences in the temporal dynamics of fatigue and performance: importance and techniques. Aviat Space Environ Med. 2004;75(3 Suppl):A147–54.
17. Brock MA. Chronobiology and aging. J Am Geriatr Soc. 1991;39(1):74–91.
18. Kerkhof GA, Van Dongen HPA. Morning-type and evening-type individuals differ in the phase position of their endogenous circadian oscillator. Neurosci Lett. 1996;218(3):153–6.
19. Balkin T, Thorne D, Sing H, Thomas M, Redmond D, Williams J, Hall S, Belenky G. Effects of sleep schedules

on commercial vehicle driver performance. Washington, DC: U.S. Department of Transportation; 2000. Report No.: DOT-MC-00-133. Contract No.: DTFH61-94-Y-00090.
20. Bliese PD, Wesensten NJ, Balkin TJ. Age and individual variability in performance during sleep restriction. J Sleep Res. 2006;15(4):376–85.
21. Wesensten NJ, Belenky G, Thorne DR, Kautz MA, Balkin TJ. Modafinil vs. caffeine: effects on fatigue during sleep deprivation. Aviat Space Environ Med. 2004;75(6):520–5.
22. Knutson KL, Spiegel K, Penev P, Van Cauter E. The metabolic consequences of sleep deprivation. Sleep Med Rev. 2007;11(3):163–78.
23. Dawson D, McCulloch K. Managing fatigue: it's about sleep. Sleep Med Rev. 2005;9(5):365–80.
24. Dembe AE, Erickson JB, Delbos RG, Banks SM. The impact of overtime and long work hours on occupational injuries and illnesses: new evidence from the United States. Occup Environ Med. 2005;62(9): 588–97.
25. Couyoumdjian A, Sdoia S, Tempesta D, Curcio G, Rastellini E, De Gennaro L, et al. The effects of sleep and sleep deprivation on task-switching performance. J Sleep Res. 2010;19(1):64–70. PubMed PMID: WOS:000274712400010. English.
26. Horne J. Working throughout the night: beyond 'sleepiness'—impairments to critical decision making. Neurosci Biobehav Rev. 2012;36(10):2226–31.
27. Ancoli-Israel S, Cole R, Alessi C, Chambers M, Moorcroft W, Pollak CP. The role of actigraphy in the study of sleep and circadian rhythms. Sleep. 2003;26(3):342–92.
28. Van Dongen HPA, Hursh SR. Fatigue, performance errors, and accidents. In: Kryger M, Roth T, Dement WC, editors. Principles and practice of sleep medicine. 5th ed. St. Louis, MO: Elsevier Saunders; 2011. p. 734–7.
29. Hursh SR, Redmond DP, Johnson ML, Thorne DR, Belenky G, Balkin TJ, et al. Fatigue models for applied research in warfighting. Aviat Space Environ Med. 2004;75(3 Suppl):A44–53; discussion A4-60. PubMed PMID: 15018265.
30. Thomas M, Sing H, Belenky G, Holcomb H, Mayberg H, Dannals R, et al. Neural basis of alertness and cognitive performance impairments during sleepiness. I. Effects of 24 h of sleep deprivation on waking human regional brain activity. J Sleep Res. 2000;9(4):335–52.
31. Dawson D, Reid K. Fatigue, alcohol and performance impairment. Nature. 1997;388(6639):235.
32. Braun AR, Balkin TJ, Wesensten NJ, Carson RE, Varga M, Baldwin P, et al. Regional cerebral blood flow throughout the sleep-wake cycle—an (H_2O)-O-15 PET study. Brain. 1997;120:1173–97. PubMed PMID: WOS:A1997XM39500008. English.
33. Lauderdale DS, Knutson KL, Rathouz PJ, Yan LJL, Hulley SB, Sidney S, et al. Re: "Objectively measured sleep characteristics among early-middle-aged adults: the CARDIA study"—the authors reply. Am J Epidemiol. 2007;165(2):232-U8. PubMed PMID: WOS:000243495400017. English.
34. Belenky G, Wesensten NJ, Thorne DR, Thomas ML, Sing HC, Redmond DP, et al. Patterns of performance degradation and restoration during sleep restriction and subsequent recovery: a sleep dose-response study. J Sleep Res. 2003;12(1):1–12. PubMed PMID: 12603781.
35. Van Dongen HPA, Maislin G, Mullington JM, Dinges DF. The cumulative cost of additional wakefulness: dose-response effects on neurobehavioral functions and sleep physiology from chronic sleep restriction and total sleep deprivation. Sleep. 2003;26(2): 117–26.
36. Horne J. Sleepfaring. Oxford: Oxford University Press; 2006. p. 70–86.
37. Harrison Y, Horne JA. The impact of sleep deprivation on decision making: a review. J Exp Psychol Appl. 2000;6(3):236–49.
38. Tietzel AJ, Lack LC. The short-term benefits of brief and long naps following nocturnal sleep restriction. Sleep. 2001;24(3):293–300.
39. Mollicone DJ, Van Dongen HPA, Dinges DF. Optimizing sleep/wake schedules in space: sleep during chronic nocturnal sleep restriction with and without diurnal naps. Acta Astronaut. 2007;60(4–7):354–61.
40. Mollicone DJ, Van Dongen HPA, Rogers NL, Dinges DF. Response surface mapping of neurobehavioral performance: testing the feasibility of split sleep schedules for space operations. Acta Astronaut. 2008;63(7–10):833–40.
41. Rosekind MR, Graeber RC, Dinges DF, et al. Crew factors in flight operations IX: effects of planned cockpit napping on crew performance and alertness in long-haul operations. NASA Technical Report 108839 [Internet]. 1994. http://humanfactors.arc.nasa.gov/zteam/PDF_pubs/Flight_Ops/Cockpit_Rest_IX/c-rest_opsumm.pdf
42. Bonnet MH, Arand DL. Clinical effects of sleep fragmentation versus sleep deprivation. Sleep Med Rev. 2003;7(4):297–310.
43. Gander P, Hartley L, Powell D, Cabon P, Hitchcock E, Mills A, et al. Fatigue risk management: organizational factors at the regulatory and industry/company level. Accid Anal Prev. 2011;43(2):573–90. PubMed PMID: WOS:000287617200007. English.
44. Wesensten NJ, Killgore WD, Balkin TJ. Performance and alertness effects of caffeine, dextroamphetamine, and modafinil during sleep deprivation. J Sleep Res. 2005;14(3):255–66.
45. Rupp TL, Wesensten NJ, Bliese PD, Balkin TJ. Banking sleep: realization of benefits during subsequent sleep restriction. Sleep. 2009;32(3):311–21.
46. Hursh SR, Balkin TJ. Response to commentary on fatigue models for applied research in warfighting. Aviat Space Environ Med. 2004;75(3):A57–60.
47. Landrigan CP, Rothschild JM, Cronin JW, Kaushal R, Burdick E, Katz JT, et al. Effect of reducing interns' work hours on serious medical errors in intensive care units. N Engl J Med. 2004;351(18):1838–48. PubMed PMID: 15509817.
48. Lockley SW, Cronin JW, Evans EE, Cade BE, Lee CJ, Landrigan CP, et al. Effect of reducing interns' weekly

work hours on sleep and attentional failures. N Engl J Med. 2004;351(18):1829–37. PubMed PMID: 15509816.
49. Barger LK, Cade BE, Ayas NT, Cronin JW, Rosner B, Speizer FE, et al. Extended work shifts and the risk of motor vehicle crashes among interns. N Engl J Med. 2005;352(2):125–34. PubMed PMID: WOS:000226251700005. English.
50. Barger LK, Ayas NT, Cade BE, Cronin JW, Rosner B, Speizer FE, et al. Impact of extended-duration shifts on medical errors, adverse events, and attentional failures. PLoS Med. 2006;3(12):2440–8. PubMed PMID: WOS:000243482500035. English.
51. Ayas NT, Barger LK, Cade BE, Hashimoto DM, Rosner B, Cronin JW, et al. Extended work duration and the risk of self-reported percutaneous injuries in interns. JAMA. 2006;296(9):1055–62. PubMed PMID: 16954484.
52. Pruchnicki SA, Wu LJ, Belenky G. An exploration of the utility of mathematical modeling predicting fatigue from sleep/wake history and circadian phase applied in accident analysis and prevention: the crash of Comair Flight 5191. Accid Anal Prev. 2011;43(3):1056–61.
53. Drake CL, Wright KP. Shift work, shift work disorder, and jet lag. In: Kryger M, Roth T, Dement WC, editors. Principles and practice of sleep medicine. 5th ed. St. Louis, MO: Elsevier Saunders; 2011. p. 784–98.
54. Belenky G, Akerstedt T. Introduction to occupational sleep medicine. In: Kryger M, Roth T, Dement WC, editors. Principles and practice of sleep medicine. 5th ed. St. Louis, MO: Elsevier Saunders; 2011. p. 734–7.
55. Romig E, Klemets T. Fatigue risk management in flight crew scheduling. Aviat Space Environ Med. 2009;80(12):1073–4.
56. Van Cauter E, Spiegel K, Tasali E, Leproult R. Metabolic consequences of sleep and sleep loss. Sleep Med. 2008;9 Suppl 10:S23–8.
57. Mullington JM, Haack M, Toth M, Serrador JM, Meier-Ewert HK. Cardiovascular, inflammatory, and metabolic consequences of sleep deprivation. Prog Cardiovasc Dis. 2009;51(4):294–302.

Sleep Deprivation and Economic Burden

19

Tracy L. Skaer

Introduction

Sleep disorders can have an intensely negative effect on an individual's health-related quality-of-life (HRQOL), workplace productivity, and overall daily functioning [1]. Approximately 35–40 % of the US adult population annually report having difficulty falling asleep or daytime sleepiness resulting in significant morbidity and mortality [1, 2]. An estimated 50–70 million people in the United States complain of night-time sleep loss associated with daytime impairment [3]. The resulting annual workplace costs due to illness-related absenteeism, presenteeism, reduced productivity, and workplace accidents amounts to a significant society burden [4–7]. Presenteeism refers to reduced performance or productivity while at work and is usually measured by worker self-report. As an example, annual insomnia-related workplace costs in the US civilian workforce are estimated to be between $15–92 billion [7, 8]. Kessler, et al. found annual loses in work performance associated with insomnia to be 357 million days and $91.7 billion without controlling for comorbid illness [9]. Comorbidity accounts for about one third of these losses, such that the net annual costs for insomnia equate to 252.7 million days and $63.2 billion annual in the United States [9].

T.L. Skaer (✉)
Department of Pharmacotherapy,
College of Pharmacy, Washington State University,
Spokane, WA, USA

Insomnia

Epidemiology

Insomnia is the most prevalent sleep disorder, especially among the elderly [10, 11]. Epidemiological studies indicate that occasional sleep disturbances occur in approximately one third of the population, with about 6–10 % of these cases meeting diagnostic criteria for insomnia [12, 13]. Insomnia is more often diagnosed in women (55–60 %) than in men (40–45 %) [12–16]. It can occur acutely (transient insomnia) or become a chronic disorder (occurring at least ≥3 times per week; usually 1–6 months in duration, and with some degree of daytime dysfunction) [14]. In addition to International Classification of Sleep Disorders (ICSD) guidelines, insomnia is also classified based on etiology and includes primary insomnia that is not caused by any known physical or mental conditions (i.e., idiopathic, environmental, travel, shift work, grief), and secondary insomnia resulting from other medical and psychiatric illnesses, medications, or other sleep disorders [15].

Etiology and Comorbidity

Common causes and/or comorbid precursors of insomnia include situational events (e.g., work or financial stress, major life events, interpersonal conflicts, jet lag, shift work), medical conditions (e.g., chronic pain, cardiovascular disease,

M.T. Bianchi (ed.), *Sleep Deprivation and Disease: Effects on the Body, Brain and Behavior*,
DOI 10.1007/978-1-4614-9087-6_19, © Springer Science+Business Media New York 2014

respiratory disorders, endocrine disorders, gastroesophageal reflux, peptic ulcer disease, epilepsy, Parkinson's disease, Alzheimer's disease, pregnancy), psychiatric disorders (e.g., mood and/or anxiety disorders, substance abuse), and medications (e.g., anticonvulsants, selective serotonin reuptake inhibitors, steroids, stimulants) [17]. Table 19.1 lists some common medications with insomnia as a potential adverse effect [17].

Chronic insomnia is frequently associated with medical and/or psychiatric conditions [18–20]. More than 40 % of individuals with persistent or chronic insomnia are reported to have a mental illness, with depression as the most commonly reported psychiatric-related comorbid illness [19–21]. For some patients, symptoms of insomnia may be a predictor for the onset of depression [22]. Thus, given the potential for insomnia or its symptoms to reflect and/or trigger the onset of psychiatric disease, a complete diagnostic evaluation is warranted [18–20].

A study conducted in Quebec, Canada ($n=953$, mean age 43.7 years, 60 % females, 58 % married, 76.4 % worked day shifts, 55.9 % full-time employees), showed that individuals with a diagnosis of insomnia were 2.8 times more likely to have at least one chronic health problem, were more likely to have recently consulted their healthcare provider, and more likely to have been prescribed prescription medication for the treatment of insomnia, mood, and/or anxiety disorders than those experiencing a normal sleep pattern [23]. Significant differences ($p<0.05$) in self-reported chronic health problems, including COPD, diabetes, arthritis, headaches, chronic pain, and hypertension, were discerned in those with insomnia compared to subjects with a normal sleep pattern (see Table 19.2). Interactions with healthcare providers were substantially higher ($p<0.05$) for those with insomnia than those experiencing a normal sleep pattern, specifically for psychiatrists, social-workers, acupuncturists, psychologists pharmacists, general practitioners, and other specialists (see Table 19.3). Additionally, individuals with insomnia were nearly 1.8 times more likely to self-administer over-the-counter (OTC) medications, and 4.8 times more likely to consume alcohol to induce sleep than those without insomnia ($p<0.05$).

Table 19.1 Medication-induced insomnia[a]

Antidepressants
Fluoxetine
Bupropion
Imipramine
Phenelzine
Protriptylene
Antipsychotics
Aripiprazole
Risperidone
Stimulants
Methylphenidate
Methamphetamine
Theophylline
Nicotine
Caffeine
Antihypertensives
Beta-Blockers (e.g., propranolol, pindolol)
Beta-Agonists
Albuterol
Salbutamol
Antiretroviral
Efavirenz
Emtricitabine
Miscellaneous
Anabolic steroids
Corticosteroids
Donepezil
Fluoroquinolones (e.g., Ciprofloxacin, levofloxacin, gemifloxacin, moxifloxacin)
Galantamine
Thyroid hormone
Over-the-counter medications
Dextromethorphan
Caffeine-containing products
Cough and cold preparations with decongestants (e.g., pseudoephedrine)
Loratidine in combination with pseudoepedrine
As a result of withdrawal reactions
Benzodiazepines
Opiates
Illicit drugs (e.g., cocaine, heroin, and marijuana)

[a]List of medications is not all-inclusive
OTC over the counter

Table 19.2 Incidence (% affected) and likelihood or odds of significant insomnia-related chronic health problems in Quebec Canada Provence in 2002

Chronic illness	Normal sleep (%)	Insomnia sleep (%)	Odds ratio[a]
COPD	0.4	3.1	11.26
Diabetes	2.5	4.8	4.57
Arthritis	5.6	26	3.88
Headaches/migraines	11	21.2	3.44
Chronic pain	13.3	26	3.28
Hypertension	7.3	15.4	2.46

[a]Likelihood or odds of insomniacs having other concomitant chronic health problems versus those with normal sleep

Table 19.3 Incidence (% affected) and likelihood or odds of significant healthcare provider interactions in Quebec Canada Province in 2002

Healthcare provider	Normal sleep (%)	Insomnia(%)	Odds ratio[a]
Psychiatrists	14.1	20	13.92
Social workers	0.8	5.9	11.09
Acupuncturists	0.2	3.7	9
Psychologists	2.5	14.1	5.3
Pharmacists	20	36.3	2.27
General practitioner	31.7	48.2	1.88
Other specialists	18.2	30.9	1.85

[a]Likelihood or odds of insomniacs having significant healthcare provider interaction versus those with normal sleep

Impact on the Workplace

The majority of studies investigating the burden of insomnia have utilized self-report and involved small sample sizes [24–26]. Nevertheless, findings stemming from these investigations have been highly consistent. Patients with insomnia utilize emergency department services, outpatient physician services, and OTC medications to a greater degree than those without insomnia [24–26]. HRQOL is diminished for individuals with insomnia; and those with chronic insomnia report increased expenses for healthcare, as well as greater physical and social disability [26–28].

Higher rates of absenteeism, reduced productivity, and a higher potential for nonmotor vehicle on-the-job accidents and falls are observed among individuals with insomnia [23]. Absenteeism and nonmotor vehicle accidents were 1.7 and 4.8 times higher among patients with insomnia ($p<0.05$) [23]. Psychiatric comorbidity was present for 8.4 % of those experiencing a normal sleep pattern compared with 36.1 % of those with insomnia ($p<0.05$). Interestingly, when comparisons were repeated for the subgroup of individuals without psychiatric comorbidity, all comparisons (individuals with insomnia versus those experiencing a normal sleep pattern) remained significant for those with insomnia (consultation with a healthcare provider (OR = 1.82), presence of chronic health conditions (OR = 2.09), use of prescribed medications (OR = 2.91), use of OTC medications (OR = 2.41), and reduced productivity (OR = 3.82)), with the exception of absences from work [23].

Additionally, research in Norway involving 6,599 workers (aged 40–45 years) with a 4-year follow-up period found insomnia to be a strong predictor (OR = 4.56) of permanent work disability, which remained significant (OR = 1.88) after controlling for sleep duration, as well as other possible confounders, including mental health (anxiety and depression), somatic health (myocardial infarction, stroke, diabetes, asthma, multiple sclerosis, chronic bronchitis, osteoporosis, or fibromyalgia), and somatic symptoms [27].

Economic Consequences

A US study [8] conducted from 1999 to 2003 utilized claims data for healthcare services, information regarding absenteeism, and short-term disability records to assess the cost of untreated insomnia among adults. The probability of being diagnosed with insomnia was greater for females and increased by about 0.08 % per year of age. Direct and indirect costs combined (controlling for other disease-state processes) over a 6-month period were estimated to be significantly $1,253 higher ($p<0.05$) among individuals aged 18–64 years with insomnia than in those without insomnia [8]. Among the elderly (aged ≥65 years) costs were $1,143 greater in those with insomnia ($p<0.05$) [8]. The average cost for absenteeism was $3,041 for patients eventually diagnosed with or treated for insomnia, versus $2,637 for those not experiencing insomnia; a significant difference of $405 ($p<0.05$) [8].

The total annual cost of insomnia within the province of Quebec, Canada, was estimated to be $6.6 billion Canadian dollars (CAD). Total expenditures (2002 values) included direct costs associated with insomnia-motivated healthcare consultations, transportation for these consultations, prescription medication, OTC medications, and alcohol consumption as a sleep aid, as well as substantial indirect costs of insomnia-related productivity losses of $5 billion CAD and $970.6 million CAD in absenteeism (see Table 19.4). The average annual expenditure for a patient diagnosed with insomnia was $5,010 as compared to $1,431 CAD for those presenting with insomnia symptoms and $421 CAD for those obtaining recommended amounts of sleep [23]. The authors concluded that the economic burden of insomnia was very high, with 76 % of all insomnia-related expenses attributed to absenteeism and reduced productivity. Moreover, it was hypothesized that the total societal cost of untreated insomnia was greater than the direct cost of treatment.

Table 19.4 Annualized insomnia-motivated healthcare expenditures in Quebec Canada Providence (2002 values)

Expenditure	Amount in $CAD
Total Provence (direct and indirect)	$6.6 billion
Productivity Loses	$5 billion
Absenteeism	$970.6 million
Alcohol consumption as a sleep aid	$339.8 million
Healthcare consultations	$191.2 million
Transportation for consultations	$36.6 million
Prescription medications	$16.5 million
OTC medications	$1.8 million
Average annual expenditure per patient[a]	$5,010
Insomnia diagnosis	$1,531
Presenting with insomnia symptoms	$421
Normal sleepers	

[a]Includes direct and indirect expenditures

Recently published results from the American Insomnia Survey ($N=4,990$, administered October 29, 2008 through July 31, 2009) found that patients with insomnia were significantly more likely to be involved in workplace accidents and/or errors controlling for other chronic conditions (OR = 1.4, $p<0.05$) [29]. The average costs of these insomnia-related accidents ($32,062) and errors ($21,914) were significantly greater than those associated with other accidents and errors ($p<0.05$). Insomnia was estimated to be associated with 7.2 % of all costly workplace accidents and errors and 23.7 % of all the costs of these incidents [29]. The researchers concluded that these proportions are higher than for any other chronic illness, with annualized US population projections of 274,000 costly insomnia-related workplace accidents and errors translating to a combined value of US $31.1 billion [29].

Given the above results, insomnia is among the most costly of all health problems in respect to workplace human capital. Unfortunately employers have yet to invest widely in workplace insomnia screening and treatment programs [29]. Employees, not employers, are currently enduring the majority of the burden because of capped limits on worker benefits (e.g., absence days due to sickness and employer-paid short-term disability benefits) or by insurance (e.g., health care costs and long-term disability benefits) [29]. Employers should recognize that insomnia may significantly influence costs of other important uncapped workplace outcomes, most importantly workplace accidents and errors that can involve equipment damage, operational disruptions, and litigation [29].

Sleep-Disordered Breathing

Description and Comorbidities

Sleep-disordered breathing (SDB) including snoring, obstructive sleep apnea (OSA), and obesity hypoventilation syndrome (OHS) are common disorders that impact a significant proportion of the population [30]. SDB is characterized by periodic complete or partial upper airway obstruction during sleep, causing intermittent cessation of breathing, or reductions in airflow [31–33]. The resulting sleep fragmentation and repetitive hypoxemia leads to excessive daytime sleepiness, the potential for neurocognitive impairment, and increased risk for motor vehicle and occupational accidents [31–33]. SDB is associated with significant cardiovascular morbidity and mortality including increased risk of hypertension and heart failure [34–36]. SDB can have a deleterious effect on social functioning and quality-of-life (QOL) [30].

OSA with comorbid diabetes, hypertension, and ischemic heart disease often results in increased healthcare utilization—especially among those classified as obese—prior to a formal diagnosis of OSA itself [37–41]. Interestingly, healthcare expenditures for OSA decline significantly once the illness is properly treated with weight reduction and/or continuous positive airway pressure (CPAP) [42, 43]. Unfortunately, poor adherence rates to CPAP are high—ranging from 46 to 83 %—especially among patients of low socioeconomic status [32]. Thus, early recognition and prompt diagnosis of OSA, along with intensified patient education, are essential if we are to meet the objectives of a reduction in morbidity, mortality, and fiscal burden [32, 44–46].

Gender Influences

While OSA has typically been described as a problem for middle-aged men, more diagnostic information regarding OSA in women is now available [47–50]. Results stemming from a case–control study [47] indicate that woman with OSA utilize more health services than men and have concomitant low Functional Outcomes of Sleep Questionnaire (FOSQ) score, poor perceived health status, and use of psychoactive medication further increased health service expenditures.

Research conducted in the Manitoba Canada examined healthcare utilization in three matched groups of females (obese with OSA, obese controls, and healthy-weight controls) for the 10 years leading up to a diagnosis of OSA [50]. Physician fees and office visits progressively increased significantly in the 10 years prior to diagnosis of OSA. Physician expenditures 1 year prior to a diagnosis of OSA among obese individuals were significantly higher than among obese controls ($547.49 ± 34.79 CAD vs. $248.85 ± 10.88 CAD, respectively; 2003 values). Moreover, the use of medical testing and psychotherapy were significantly higher among obese woman diagnosed with OSA than among obese controls. The authors concluded that obese women with OSA utilized more health services than healthy-weight controls and significantly more healthcare services than obese controls [50].

Similar results were reported in a study of Canadian males conducted over a 5-year period [49]. Preexisting ischemic heart disease at the time of a diagnosis of OSA predicted a fivefold increase ($p < 0.05$) in healthcare expenditures as compared to those without preexisting ischemic heart disease [49]. The authors concluded that treatment of OSA was responsible for an observed reversal in the upward trend of increasing healthcare expenditures seen with untreated OSA.

Economic Consequences

Considering the evidence provided, SDB may create a significant socioeconomic burden. Unfortunately, most of the existing research estimating socioeconomic impact of SDB has been conducted solely using questionnaires in select patient populations or by a model-based approach [25, 51–57]. Moreover, indirect cost accounting was not obtained or evaluated. Therefore, economic information and assumptions in these studies have focused solely on direct costs.

Jennum and Kjelberg [58] recently published data from the National Patient Registry (NPR) in Denmark (1996–2006) finding that snoring ($N = 12,045$), and especially OSA ($N = 19,438$) and obstructive hypoventilation syndrome (OHS, $N = 755$), had significantly ($p < 0.05$) higher rates of health-related contact, medication use, and unemployment than controls ($N = 77,752$). The increased socioeconomic costs were calculated from evaluations of direct and indirect expenditures. The presence of higher severity of OSA was associated with higher expenditures and patients with OHS had the highest unemployment rate ($p < 0.001$). The annual increased expenditures (direct and indirect costs) for patients with snoring, OSA, and OHS were €705, €3,890, and €3,263, respectively. Interestingly, the socioeconomic changes appeared up to 8 years prior to initial diagnosis of OSA and OHS and increased further with disease progression. During the 2-year observation period, CPAP treatment reduced mortality in those with OSA but not in OHS patients. Thus, early disease detection for SDB patients is required to potentially reduce morbidity and mortality.

Impact on Quality-of-life

HRQOL and the impact of OSA treatment on three negative health consequences of untreated OSA (strokes, myocardial infarctions, and motor vehicle accidents) was the subject of recently published research [59]. A "hypothetical" Markov model was constructed to compare expenditures and cost-effectiveness of different diagnostic and therapeutic strategies over a 10-year period and the expected lifetime of the patient. Baseline calculations were completed for hypothetical average cohort of 50-year-old males with a 50 % pretest probability of having moderate-to-severe OSA defined as an apnea/hypopnea index (AHI) ≥ 15 events per hour. The researchers found that CPAP therapy had an incremental cost-effectiveness ratio (ICER) of $15,915 per HRQOL years gained for the lifetime horizon. Full-night polysomnography (PSG) in conjunction with CPAP therapy was found to be the most economically efficient strategy at any willingness-to-pay level greater than $17,151 per-HRQOL years gained as it was utilized more frequently than all other strategies via comparison. Split-night PSG and unattended home monitoring can be cost-effective alternatives when full-night PSG is not available.

CPAP Adherence

In light of the fact that poor adherence is a common problem among CPAP users, especially those of low socioeconomic status, Tarasik and colleagues investigated the use of financial incentives to enhance CPAP acceptance in the poor population [60]. The study was conducted over 2 years beginning in February, 2009 ($N = 137$ receiving incentives, age 50.8 ± 10.6 years, AHI 38.7 ± 19.9 events; $N = 121$ controls, age $50.9 + 10.3$ years, AHI 39.9 ± 22). The control group had a co-payment of $330–660 and the financial incentive group paid a subsidized price of $55. CPAP acceptance, measured after the 2-week adaptation period, was 45 % higher ($p = 0.02$) in the financial incentive population including a low socioeconomic stratum ($N = 113$, adjusting for age, gender, BMI, tobacco smoking). Family and friends who had positive experience with CPAP also greatly influenced (average Odds Ratio at 95 % Confidence Interval = 3.43) CPAP adherence in the low socioeconomic subpopulation. In the average/high income patients ($N = 145$), CPAP acceptance was affected by living with a partner/spouse (average Odds Ratio at 95 % Confidence Interval = 8.82), AHI (>30 vs. <30) (average OR = 3.16), but not by the financial incentive. There was no significant difference in CPAP adherence at 1-year follow-up for financial incentive and control groups at 35 and 39 %, respectively. Finally, CPAP adherence rate was found to be sensitive to level of education (average OR = 1.28) and AHI (>30 vs. <30, average OR = 5.25).

Shift-Work Disorder

Social Impact

Excessive daytime sleepiness and fatigue are common symptoms and have contributed to a large number of industrial and motor vehicle accidents. Fatigued employees are less efficient, work more slowly, and are less effective, thereby increasing the probability of making a significant error [2, 61]. Some of the world's worst environmental disasters (e.g., Union Carbide Corp plant in Bhopal, India, Chernobyl nuclear plant in Ukraine, Exxon Valzez oil tanker in Alaska) occurred when workers were fatigued [2].

In the United States, the cost of shift-worker disorder (SWD) is estimated in the billions of dollars [2]. Individuals working extended shifts are 2–6 times more likely to be involved in a motor vehicle accident or near-miss incident when returning home from the work site than those with an average shift duration [62]. Shift and night workers are at higher risk of cardiovascular and gastrointestinal disease, mental illness (primarily depression and anxiety), and cancer (breast, prostate, and colorectal), and they have a reduced HRQOL [63–75].

Economic Consequences

Research on the economic impact of SWD is very limited. A study conducted in Australia in 2006 examined the cost of fatigue among train drivers and discerned that drivers reporting a moderate or high state of fatigue utilized more fuel (4 % and 9 %, respectively) than did drivers reporting a low level of fatigue [76]. Increased levels of fatigue translated into weekly increases in fuel costs of $3,512 Australian dollars (AUS). Highly fatigued train drivers also engaged in heavier braking and maximum speed violations. Thus, the more fatigued the driver, the lower the level of safety, and the higher the fiscal burden.

Impact on Quality-of-life and Social Interactions

Research completed in US Air Force radar controllers demonstrated that shift workers in general experienced higher levels of anxiety ($p<0.001$) and irritability ($p<0.05$), than did day workers [68]. Moreover, the researchers found that SWD imparted a significantly greater detriment to quality-of-life than did shift work alone. QOL for shift workers was significantly poorer than that of shift workers without this disorder for the Sickness Impact Profile (SIP) domains of sleep and rest ($p<0.001$), emotional behavior ($p<0.01$), social interaction ($p<0.01$), alertness behavior ($p<0.001$), home management ($p<0.05$), work ($p<0.05$), and recreational pastimes ($p>0.01$).

Drake and colleagues completed a large epidemiologic study of the general US population and found that those with SWD were more likely to be unable to attend social and family interactions due to sleep problems than those without SWD [67]. Permanent night workers with SWD missed 8.6 days of family or social activity each month compared with 1.5 days in those without SWD; rotating-shift workers with SWD missed 10.1 days of family and social activity each month versus 1 day in their coworkers without SWD.

SWD-related costs due to lost productivity and accidents are likely to be substantial. Studies evaluating the economic impact of SWD are not available at this time. However, costs have been documented on the two key symptoms of SWD, excessive sleepiness and insomnia; these findings suggest by extrapolation the amount of economic burden SWD represents.

Restless Legs Syndrome

Description and Epidemiology

Restless legs syndrome (RLS) is characterized by an irresistible urge to move the legs while resting [77]. This urge is usually accompanied or prompted by uncomfortable sensations (i.e., creeping, burning, throbbing) in the legs [77]. Symptoms begin or worsen during periods of rest or inactivity, are partially or totally relieved by movement, and are worse in the evening or at night [77]. RLS is one of the most common neurological disorders with an adult prevalence ranging from 2.5 to 10 % in the general population of Western industrialized nations (e.g., Europe 9.6 %, US 11.1 %) [78, 79]. Women are affected twice as often as men and are more likely to experience severe symptoms [80, 81]. The incidence of RLS advances with age, and thus it is more common and severe in the elderly [77, 80–82]. RLS has a higher incidence in pregnant women, patients undergoing dialysis, and those with Parkinson's disease, type 2 diabetes, or multiple sclerosis [83–87].

Economic Consequences

A German study conducted in 2006 provides some insight into the potential magnitude of RLS [88]. A total of 519 RLS patients (mean age 65.2±11.1 years, 63 % female) were administered a questionnaire that assessed healthcare resource consumption, as well as socioeconomic, demographic, clinical, and health status. Patients also completed the International RLS severity scale (IRLS), Epworth Sleepiness scale (ESS), EQ-5D, and Beck Depression Inventory (BDI). The average total costs (direct and indirect) were €2,090 over the 3-month observation period. The average direct medical and nonmedical expenditures were €780 with €300 attributed to medications and €354 to hospitalizations. The average indirect expenditures as a result of loss of productivity were €1,308. Based on the average prevalence of RLS in the German population and the average total costs per patient, the authors estimate the annual cost of RLS in Germany to be €1.7 billion. In comparison, the annual costs for diabetes and Parkinson's disease in Germany are approximately €31.4 billion and €3 billion, respectively [89, 90]. Additionally, the study found that disease severities measured via IRLS and ESS were significant cost-driving factors ($p<0.01$, $p<0.04$, respectively).

Allen and colleagues [89] found that primary RLS sufferers had a significant productivity loss ($p<0.0001$) ranging from 20 to 50 % with direct correlation to RLS severity. RLS significantly disrupted ability to work and, when severe, becomes disabling. The RLS-related productivity loss in this study was reported by the authors as similar to research completed on bipolar disorder. The authors also reported that all RLS-related expenditures increased with RLS severity, resulting in significantly higher decrements in health status. Mean direct annualized costs were $350.54 per primary RLS subject ($N=251$) and $490.70 per primarily RLS sufferer ($N=131$; defined as the number of primary RLS subjects who completed their RLS questionnaire and were symptomatic for ≥2 times per week with moderate-to-severe distress). Medical visits accounted for $186.95 per primary RLS subject and $273.62 per RLS sufferer. Medication expenditures, assuming a 50 % compliance rate, per primary RLS subject and RLS sufferer were $128.86 and $170.70, respectively. Given this data, using the RLS prevalence rate reported at 6.5 % [89] out of 302.2 million US citizens [90] and $400 annually per patient, the annualize estimate of direct expenditures (indirect costs were not studied) for RLS in the United States in 2007 dollars would be about $7.8 billion. It is important to note that the 6.5 % incidence was conservative. This research did not include all types of RLS and therefore the overall burden of RLS in the United States could be as much as $12.1 billion in direct costs using a 10 % prevalence rate.

Impact on Quality-of-life

The burden of RLS on HRQOL is considerable and comparable to other chronic illnesses (e.g., diabetes, arthritis, hypertension, acute myocardial infarction) [91, 92]. A US study examining HRQOL among patients with RLS ($n=158$; mean age 53 years; 65 % female) found that patients with RLS scored significantly below adjusted population norms on the SF-36 [90]. Five of the eight scales, including physical function, role physical, bodily pain, general health, and vitality, were significantly lower than the adjusted population norms by ≥0.8 standard deviations [91].

Conclusion

Sleep deprivation impacts both physical and mental health and has been associated with significant economic consequences. That said, to date there exists a paucity of data as to the direct and indirect cost structure associated with sleep disorders. In order to care for patients presenting with sleep-related illness, and to reduce the consequential economic burden, accurate screening efforts in the community and at the work site should be developed and employed. Affected individuals should be immediately referred for appropriate treatment.

References

1. National Institutes of Health. NIH state-of-the-science conference statement on manifestations and management of chronic insomnia in adults. NIH Consens State Sci Statements. 2005;22(2):1–30.
2. Hossain JL, Shapiro CM. The prevalence, cost implications, and management of sleep disorders: an overview. Sleep Breath. 2002;6:85–102.
3. Roth T. Prevalence, associated risks, and treatment patterns of insomnia. J Clin Psychiatry. 2005;66 Suppl 9:10–3. quiz 42-3.
4. Daley M, Morin CM, LeBlanc M, Gregoire JP, Savard J. The economic burden of insomnia: direct and indirect costs for individuals with insomnia syndrome, insomnia symptoms, and good sleepers. Sleep. 2009;32(1):55–64.
5. Metlaine A, Legar D, Choudat D. Scocioeconomic impact of insomnia in working populations. Ind Health. 2005;43(1):11–9.
6. Chilcott LA, Shapiro CM. The socioeconomic impact of insomnia. An overview. Pharmacoeconomics. 1995;10 Suppl 1:1–14.
7. Kleinman NL, Brook RA, Doan JF, Melkonian AK, Baran RW. Health benefit costs and absenteeism due to insomnia from the employer's perspective: a retrospective, case control, database study. J Clin Psychiatry. 2009;70(8):1098–104.
8. Ozminkowsk R, Wang S, Walsh J. The direct and indirect costs of untreated insomnia in adults in the United States. Sleep. 2007;30(3):263–73.
9. Kessler RC, Berglund PA, Coulouvrat C, et al. Insomnia and the performance of US workers: results from the American Insomnia Survey. Sleep. 2011;34(9):1161–71.
10. National Sleep Foundation. Sleep in America poll: sleep and aging. 2003. http//:www.sleepfoundation.org/sites/default/files/2003SleepPollExecSumm.pdf Accessed 08 Nov 2012.
11. Foley DJ, Monjan A, Simonsick EM, et al. Incidence and remission of insomnia among elderly adults: an epidemiologic study of 6,800 persons over three years. Sleep. 1999;22 Suppl 2:S366–72.
12. Morin CM, LeBlanc M, Daley M, et al. Epidemiology of insomnia: prevalence, self-help treatments and consultation initiated, and determinants of health-seeking behaviors. Sleep Med. 2006;7(2):123–30.
13. Ohayon MM. Epidemiology of insomnia; what we know and what we still need to learn. Sleep Med Rev. 2002;5(2):97–111.
14. Doghramaji K. The epidemiology and diagnosis of insomnia. Am J Manag Care. 2006;12(8 Suppl): S214–20.
15. Goldberg LD. Managing insomnia in an evolving marketplace. Am J Manag Care. 2006;12(8 Suppl): S212–3.
16. National Sleep Foundation. Sleep in America poll: women and sleep. 2007. http://www.sleepfoundation.org/sites/default/files/Summary_Of_Findings%20-%20FINAL.pdf Accessed 09 Nov 2012.
17. Malangu N. Drugs inducing insomnia as an adverse effect. In: Sahoo S, editor. Can't sleep? Issues of being an insomniac. Rijeka: Inteck; 23–36; 2012. http://www.intechopen.com/books/can-t-sleep-issues-of-being-an-insomniac/drugs-inducing-insomnia-as-an-adverse-effect. doi:10.5772/30921
18. Sateia MJ, Doghramji K, Hauri PJ, et al. Evaluation of chronic insomnia. Sleep. 2000;23(1):1–39.
19. Skaer TL, Robison LM, Sclar DA, et al. Psychiatric comorbidity and pharmacological treatment patterns among patients presenting with insomnia: an assessment of office-based encounters in the USA in 1995 and 1996. Clin Drug Investig. 1999;18(2):161–7.
20. Skaer TL, Sclar DA, Robison LM. Complaint of insomnia in the United States 1995-1998: prevalence, psychiatric comorbidity, and pharmacologic treatment patterns. Int J Psychiatry Clin Pract. 2001;7(4): 145–51.
21. McCall WV. A psychiatric perspective on insomnia. J Clin Psychiatry. 2001;62 Suppl 10:27–32.
22. Ancoli-Isreal S. The impact and prevalence of chronic insomnia and other sleep disturbances associated with chronic illness. Am J Manag Care. 2006;12 Suppl 8:S221–9.
23. Daley M, Morin CM, LeBlanc M, et al. Insomnia and its relationship to health-care utilization, work absenteeism, productivity, and accidents. Sleep Med. 2009;10(4):427–38.

24. Hatoum HT, Kong SX, Kania CM, et al. Insomnia, health-related quality of life and healthcare resource consumption: a study of managed-care organization enrollees. Pharmacoeconomics. 1998;14(6):629–37.
25. Hillman DR, Murphy AS, Antic R, et al. The economic cost of sleep disorders. Sleep. 2006;29(3):299–305.
26. Simon GE, VonKorff M. Prevalence, burden, and treatment of insomnia in primary care. Am J Psychiatry. 1997;154(10):1417–23.
27. Silvertsen B, Overland S, Pallesen S, et al. Insomnia and long sleep duration are risk factors for later work disability. The Hordaland Health Study. J Sleep Res. 2009;18(1):122–8.
28. Leger D, Guilleminault C, Bader G, et al. Medical and socio-professional impact of insomnia. Sleep. 2002;25(6):625–9.
29. Shahly V, Berglund PA, Coulouvrat C, Fitzgerald T, Hajak G, et al. The associations of insomnia with costly workplace accidents and errors. Arch Gen Psychiatry. 2012;69(10):1054–63.
30. Jennum P, Riha RL. Epidemiology of sleep apnoea/hypopnea syndrome and sleep-disordered breathing. Eur Respir J. 2009;33(4):907–14.
31. Gottlieb DJ, Whitnes CW, Bonekar WH, et al. Relation of sleepiness to respiratory disturbance index: the Sleep Heart Health Study. Am J Respir Crit Care Med. 1999;159(2):502–7.
32. Weaver TE, Chasens ER. Continuous positive airway pressure treatment for sleep apnea in older adults. Sleep Med Rev. 2007;11(2):99–111.
33. Norman D, Loredo JS. Obstructive sleep apnea in older adults. Clin Geriatr Med. 2008;24(1):151–65.
34. Nieto FJ, Young TB, Lind BK, et al. Association of sleep-disordered breathing, sleep apnea, and hypertension in a large community-based study. Sleep Heart Health Study. JAMA. 2000;283(14):1829–36.
35. Peppard PE, Young T, Palta M, et al. Prospective study of the association between sleep-disordered breathing and hypertension. N Engl J Med. 2000;342(19):1378–84.
36. Pk L, Here P, Hoffstein V. Obstructive sleep apnea syndrome as a risk factor for hypertension: population study. BMJ. 2000;320(7233):479–82.
37. Young T, Peppard PE, Gottlieb DJ. Epidemiology of obstructive sleep apnea: a population health perspective. Am J Respir Crit Care Med. 2002;165(9): 1217–39.
38. Katzmarzyk PT, Janssen I. The economic costs associated with physical inactivity and obesity in Canada: an update. Can J Appl Physiol. 2004;29(1):90–115.
39. Wolf AM, Colditz GA. Current estimates of the economic cost of obesity in the United States. Obes Res. 1998;6(2):97–106.
40. Detournay B, Fagnani F, Phillippo M, et al. Obesity morbidity and health care costs in France: an analysis of the 1991–1992 Medical Care Household Survey. Int J Obes Relat Metab Disord. 2000;24(2):151–5.
41. Smith R, Ronald J, Delaive K, et al. What are obstructive sleep apnea patients being treated for prior to this diagnosis? Chest. 2002;121(1):164–72.
42. Santamaria J, Iranzo A, Ma Mantserrat J, et al. Persistent sleepiness in CPAP treated obstructive sleep apnea patients: evaluation and treatment. Sleep Med Rev. 2007;11(3):195–207.
43. Tarasiuk A, Greenberg-Dotan S, Brin YS, Simon T, Tail A, Reuveni H. Determinants affecting health-care utilization in obstructive sleep apnea syndrome patients. Chest. 2005;128(3):1310–4.
44. Simon-Tuval T, Reuveni H, Greenberg-Dontan S, et al. Low socioeconomic status is a risk factor for CPAP acceptance among adult OSAS patients requiring treatment. Sleep. 2009;32(4):545–52.
45. Olsen S, Smith S, Oei T, et al. Health belief model predicts adherence to CPAP before experience with CPAP. Eur Respir J. 2008;32(3):710–7.
46. Reuveni H, Tarasiuk A, Wainstock T, et al. Awareness level of obstructive sleep apnea syndrome during routine unstructured interviews of a standardized patient by primary care physicians. Sleep. 2004;27(8):1518–25.
47. Greenberg-Dotan S, Reuveni H, Simon-Tuval T, et al. Gender differences in morbidity and health care utilization among adult obstructive sleep apnea patients. Sleep. 2007;30(9):1173–80.
48. Banno K, Manfreda J, Walld R, et al. Healthcare utilization in women with obstructive sleep apnea syndrome 2 years after diagnosis and treatment. Sleep. 2006;29(10):1307–11.
49. Albarrak M, Banno K, Sabbagh AA, et al. Utilization of heathcare resources in obstructive sleep apnea syndrome: a 5-year follow-up study in men using CPAP. Sleep. 2005;28(10):1306–11.
50. Banno K, Ramsey C, Walld R, et al. Expenditure on health care in obese women with and without sleep apnea. Sleep. 2009;32(2):247–52.
51. Weatherly HL, Griffin SC, McDaid C, et al. An economic analysis of continuous positive airway pressure for the treatment of obstructive sleep apnea-hypopnea syndrome. Int J Technol Assess Health Care. 2009;25(1):26–34.
52. McDaid C, Griffin SC, Weatherly H, et al. Continuous positive airway pressure devices for the treatment of obstructive sleep-aponea syndrome: a systematic review and economic analysis. Health Technol Assess. 2009;13(4):iii-iv,xi-xiv,1-119,143-274.
53. Tan MC, Ayas NT, Mulgrew A, et al. Cost-effectiveness of continuous positive airway pressure therapy in patients with obstructive sleep apnea-hypopnea in British Columbia. Can Respir J. 2008;15(2):159–65.
54. Guest JF, Healter MT, Morga A, et al. Cost-effectiveness of using continuous positive airway pressure in the treatment of severe obstructive sleep apnoea/hypopnea syndrome in the UK. Thorax. 2008;63(1):860–5.
55. Al Ghanim N, Comondore VR, Fleetham J, et al. The economic impact of obstructive sleep apnea. Lung. 2008;186(1):7–12.
56. Wittmann V, Rodenstein DO. Health care costs and the sleep apnea syndrome. Sleep Med Rev. 2004;8(4): 269–79.

57. Dougles NJ, George CF. Treating sleep apnoea is cost effective. Thorax. 2002;57(1):93.
58. Jennum P, Kjellberg J. Health, social and economical consequences of sleep-disordered breathing: a controlled national study. Thorax. 2011;66(7):560–6.
59. Pietzsch JB, Garner A, Cipriano LE, Linehan LJ. An integrated health-economic analysis of diagnostic and therapeutic strategies in the treatment of moderate-to-severe obstructive sleep apnea. Sleep. 2011;34(6):695–705.
60. Tarasiuk A, Reznor G, Greenberg-Dotan S, Reuveni H. Financial incentive increases CPAP acceptance in patients from low socioeconomic background. PLoS One. 2012;7(3):e33178.
61. Pilcher JJ, Huffcutt AI. Effects of sleep deprivation on performance: a meta-analysis. Sleep. 1996;19(4):318–26.
62. Berger LK, Cade BE, Ayas NT, et al. Extended work shifts and the risk of motor vehicle crashes among interns. N Engl J Med. 2005;352(2):125–34.
63. Boggild H, Knutsson A. Shift work, risk factors and cardiovascular disease. Scand J Work Environ Health. 1999;25(2):85–99.
64. Knutsson A. Health disorders of shift workers. Occup Med(Lond). 2003;3(2):103–8.
65. Schwartz JRL, Roth T. Shift work sleep disorder: burden of illness and approaches to management. Drugs. 2006;66(18):2357–70.
66. Folkard S, Tucker P. Shift work, safety and productivity. Occup Med. 2003;53(2):95–101.
67. Drake CL, Roehrs T, Richardson G, et al. Shift work sleep disorder: prevalence and consequences beyond that of symptomatic day workers. Sleep. 2004;27(8):1453–62.
68. Puca FM, Perrucci S, Prudenzano MP, et al. Quality of life in shift work syndrome. Funct Neurol. 1996;5(8):261–8.
69. Megdal SP, Kroenke CH, Laden F, et al. Night work and breast cancer risk: a systematic review and meta-analysis. Eur J Cancer. 2005;41(13):2023–32.
70. Schernhammer BS, Laden P, Spelzer FE, et al. Night-shift work and risk of colorectal cancer in the Nurses' Health Study. J Natl Cancer Inst. 2003;95(11):825–8.
71. Schernhammer BS, Kroenke CH, Laden F, Hankinson SE. Night work and breast cancer risk. Epidemiology. 2006;17(1):108–11.
72. Davis S, Mirick DK. Circadian distruption, shift work and the risk of cancer: a summary of the evidence and studies in Seattle. Cancer Causes Control. 2006;17(4):539–45.
73. Stevens RG, Black DE, Brainard GC, et al. Meeting report: the role of environmental lighting and circadian disruption in cancer and other diseases. Environ Health Perspect. 2007;115(9):1357–62.
74. Anistmov VN. The light-dark cycle regimen and cancer development. Neuro Endocrinol Lett. 2002;23(1):28–36.
75. Anistmov VN, Da B, Popovich IG, et al. Effect of exposure to light-at-night on life span and spontaneous carcinogenesis in female GBA mice. Int J Cancer. 2004;111(4):475–9.
76. Dorrian J, Hussey F, Dawson D. Train driving efficiency and safety: examining the cost of fatigue. J Sleep Res. 2007;15(1):1–1.
77. Smith JE, Tolson JM. Recognition, diagnosis, and treatment of restless legs syndrome. J Am Acad Nurse Pract. 2008;20(8):396–401.
78. Garcia-Borreguero D, Egatz R, WInkelmann J, et al. Epidemiology of restless legs syndrome: the current status. Sleep Med Rev. 2006;10(3):153–67.
79. Allen RP, Wahers A, Montplaisir J, et al. Restless legs syndrome prevalence and impact: REST general population study. Arch Intern Med. 2005;165(11):1286–95.
80. Berger K, Luedemann J, Trenkwalder C, et al. Sex and the risk of restless legs syndrome in the general population. Arch Intern Med. 2004;164(2):196–202.
81. Phillips B, Young T, Finn L, et al. Epidemiology of restless legs symptoms in adults. Arch Intern Med. 2000;160(14):2137–41.
82. Spiegelhalder K, Hornyak M. Restless legs syndrome in older adults. Clin Geriatr Med. 2008;24(1):167–80.
83. Gomez-Esteban JC, Zarrantz JJ, Tijero R, et al. Restless legs syndrome in Parkinson's disease. Mov Disord. 2007;22(13):1912–6.
84. Suzuki K, Ohida T, Sone T, et al. The prevalence of restless legs syndrome among pregnant women in Japan and the relationship between restless legs syndrome and sleep problems. Sleep. 2003;26(6):672–7.
85. Kavanagh D, Siddiqui S, Geddes CC. Restless legs syndrome in patients on dialysis. Am J Kidney Dis. 2005;43(5):763–71.
86. Chasens ER. Understanding sleep in persons with diabetes. Diabetes Educ. 2007;33(3):435–41.
87. Merlino G, Fraticci L, Valente M, et al. Association of restless legs syndrome in type 2 diabetes: a case-control study. Sleep. 2007;30(7):866–71.
88. Dodel R, Happo S, Peglau I, et al. Health economic burden of patients with restless legs syndrome in a German ambulatory setting. Pharmacoeconomics. 2010;29(5):381–93.
89. Allen RP, Bharmal M, Calloway M. Prevalence and disease burden of primary restless legs syndrome: results of a general population survey in the United States. Mov Disord. 2011;26(1):114–20.
90. Population Reference Bureau. World Population Data Sheet. 2007. http://www.prb.org/Publications/Datasheets/2007/2007WorldPopulationDataSheet.aspx. Accessed 12 Nov 2012.
91. Abetz L, Allen R, Follet A, et al. Evaluating the quality of life of patients with restless legs syndrome. Clin Ther. 2004;26(6):925–35.
92. Kushiba C, Blaisdell B, Ferini-Strambi L. Burden of restless legs syndrome on health related quality of life. Qual Life Res. 2007;16(4):617–24.

Index

M.T. Bianchi (ed.), *Sleep Deprivation and Disease: Effects on the Body, Brain and Behavior*, DOI 10.1007/978-1-4614-9087-6, © Springer Science+Business Media New York 2014

MIX
Papier aus verantwortungsvollen Quellen
Paper from responsible sources
FSC® C105338

If you have any concerns about our products,
you can contact us on
ProductSafety@springernature.com

In case Publisher is established outside the EU,
the EU authorized representative is:
Springer Nature Customer Service Center GmbH
Europaplatz 3, 69115 Heidelberg, Germany

Printed by Libri Plureos GmbH
in Hamburg, Germany